Blackwell's Five-Minute Veterinary Consult

Clinical Companion

Canine and Feline Infectious Diseases and Parasitology

Second Edition

Blackwell's Five-Minute Veterinary Consult

Clinical Companion

Canine and Feline Infectious Diseases and Parasitology

Second Edition

Stephen C. Barr, BVSc, MVS, PhD
Diplomate, American College of Veterinary Internal Medicine (SA)
Professor of Medicine
Department of Clinical Sciences
College of Veterinary Medicine
Cornell University
Ithaca, New York

Dwight D. Bowman, MS, PhD
Professor of Parasitology
Department of Microbiology and Parasitology
College of Veterinary Medicine
Cornell University
Ithaca, New York

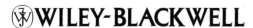

A John Wiley & Sons, Ltd., Publication

This edition first published 2012 © 2012 by John Wiley & Sons, Inc.
First Edition © 2006 Blackwell Publishing Ltd.

Blackwell Publishing was acquired by John Wiley & Sons in February 2007. Blackwell's publishing program has been merged with Wiley's global Scientific, Technical and Medical business to form Wiley-Blackwell.

Registered office: John Wiley & Sons Ltd, The Atrium, Southern Gate, Chichester, West Sussex, PO19 8SQ, UK

Editorial offices: 2121 State Avenue, Ames, Iowa 50014-8300, USA
                      The Atrium, Southern Gate, Chichester, West Sussex, PO19 8SQ, UK
                      9600 Garsington Road, Oxford, OX4 2DQ, UK

For details of our global editorial offices, for customer services and for information about how to apply for permission to reuse the copyright material in this book please see our website at www.wiley.com/wiley-blackwell.

Library of Congress Cataloging-in-Publication Data
Barr, Stephen C.
  Blackwell's five-minute veterinary consult clinical companion : canine and feline infectious diseases and parasitology / Stephen C. Barr, Dwight D. Bowman.—2nd ed.
      p. cm.—(Blackwell's five-minute veterinary consult)
  Rev. ed. of: Blackwell's five-minute veterinary consult clinical companion / Debra F. Horwitz, Jacqueline C. Neilson.
  Includes bibliographical references and index.
  ISBN-13: 978-0-8138-2012-5 (pbk. : alk. paper)
  ISBN-10: 0-8138-2012-X
  I. Bowman, Dwight D.   II. Horwitz, Debra. Blackwell's five-minute veterinary consult clinical companion.   III. Title.
IV. Title: Five-minute veterinary consult clinical companion.   V. Title: Canine and feline infectious diseases and parasitology.
  SF433.H76 2012
  636.7′08969—dc23

                                                                                                2011018220

A catalogue record for this book is available from the British Library.

This book is published in the following electronic formats: ePDF 9780470961414; ePub 9780470961421; Mobi 9780470961438

Set in 10.5/13pt Berkeley by Aptara® Inc., New Delhi, India

Printed and bound in Singapore by Markono Print Media Pte Ltd

1   2012

■ To my friend and mentor, Tom Klei, and to my family, who give reason to all enterprises.

Stephen C. Barr

Contents

Contributors

Portions of chapters in this book have been provided by material contributed to *Blackwell's Five-Minute Veterinary Consult: Canine and Feline* by the following authors:

Edward J. Dubovi
Stephen C. Barr
Sharon Fooshee Grace
Fred W. Scott
Adam J. Birkenheuer
J. Paul Woods
Alfred M. Legendre
Johnny D. Hoskins
Andree D. Quesnel
Leland E. Carmichael
Jo Ann Morrison
Alexander H. Werner
Karen Helton Rhodes
David Twedt
Nita K. Gulbas
Julie Ann Jarvinen
Patrick L. McDonough
Carol S. Foil
W. Dunbar Gram
Karen Kuhl
Jean S. Greek
Margaret C. Barr
Gary D. Norsworthy
Matthew W. Miller
Clay A. Calvert
Clarence A. Rawlings
Jan S. Suchodolski
Jörg M. Steiner

Sharon A. Center
Tania N. Davey
Paul A. Cuddon
Steven A. Levy
Susan E. Little
Scott A. Brown

Preface

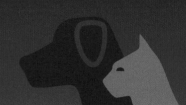

Blackwell's Five-Minute Veterinary Consult Clinical Companion: Canine and Feline Infectious Diseases and Parasitology, Second Edition, is a quick-reference text designed mainly for clinicians, but also for students of veterinary medicine. It assumes a basic knowledge of infectious and parasitic diseases. There are several excellent texts available in infectious diseases of both cats and dogs and also many detailing the parasites of these species. The infectious disease texts offer detailed information regarding the epidemiology and pathophysiology of disease, clinical manifestations, diagnostic techniques, pathology, and therapeutic regimens, and most parasitology texts detail life cycles, parasite morphology, and pathology, with little emphasis on diagnosis and therapy. Although these are excellent reference texts with a place in veterinary libraries and on the shelves of the clinical veterinarian, there are few, if any, texts that include both infectious and parasitic diseases in one volume. This text was written to make clinically relevant information on both infectious and parasitic diseases of cats and dogs available for quick reference in the workplace.

   Blackwell's Five-Minute Veterinary Consult Clinical Companion: Canine and Feline Infectious Diseases and Parasitology, Second Edition, is designed to help the reader recognize various infectious and parasitic diseases common in North America and identify appropriate diagnostic tests to perform. Drug dosages have been presented in table format to allow the busy clinician to access therapeutic information quickly between appointments. Many of the chapters have been adapted from the Infectious Disease section of the third edition of *Blackwell's Five-Minute Veterinary Consult: Canine and Feline,* for which I served as section editor. Chapters from other sections in that text were also used, as were several from *Blackwell's Five-Minute Veterinary Consult Clinical Companion: Small Animal Dermatology, Second Edition,* by Karen Helton Rhodes. Most of the parasitology chapters are unique to this book and include diagnostic images provided by my friend, colleague, and coeditor, Dr. Dwight Bowman.

   New chapters have been added to this edition because of new disease discovery. For example, canine influenza virus first appeared in Florida greyhounds in 2004 and is now more widespread throughout the United States. The appearance of a new isolate of canine parvovirus (CPV-2c) has led to an interesting update of this chapter. Chapters on sarcoptic mange and staphylococcal pyoderma have also been added. Some diseases have purposely been left out (e.g., West Nile virus) because it was felt that their relative impact on canine or feline health did not yet justify a chapter. Other diseases have been addressed within other chapters (e.g., discussion on Wolbachia is in the chapter on Canine Heartworm Disease: Dogs). One chapter (previously Aspergillosis) has been separated into two chapters (Aspergillosis—Nasal and Aspergillosis—Systemic) for ease of reference. All chapters and appendices have been updated with new reference information.

ORGANIZATION AND FORMAT

Like *Blackwell's Five-Minute Veterinary Consult: Canine and Feline*, the organization of this book is based on an alphabetic listing of, in most instances, the etiologic agent. Sometimes the more common version of a disease entity is used as a heading (e.g., Tick Bite Paralysis, Ear Mites) instead of the name of the etiologic agent. Although this might aggravate the purist, we have adhered to this format to aid the fundamental principle of the text—that of a quick reference.

As in the first edition, each chapter in the text is organized into sections of Definition/Overview, Etiology/Pathophysiology, Signalment/History, Clinical Features, Differential Diagnosis, Diagnostics, Therapeutics with Drugs of Choice, Precautions/Interactions, and Comments. This latter section often alludes to the zoonotic potential of the agent in question and occasionally includes comments by the authors based on their experience of the disease. Each section is intentionally kept short, with the information presented in bullet format and usually in incomplete sentences, similar to how one might take notes from a lecture. The purpose of this writing style was to present information as concisely as possible for quick reference. This also allowed us to present the book in a manageable size and at a reasonable cost.

KEY FEATURES

In most cases, color images emphasizing the major diagnostic feature of the disease are presented. The key diagnostic feature itself, where applicable, is highlighted in blue in the text. Where there are a number of drugs involved in treating the disease, the dosage, route of administration, and therapy length are presented in table format for quick reference. A short list of Suggested Readings at the end of each chapter offers the reader the current or most important references for the topic. This reference list is by no means exhaustive.

APPENDICES

Appendices, including core vaccination schedules, antiparasitic products for the treatment of gastrointestinal parasites in dogs, parasiticides for cats, canine heartworm preventives, and canine products with efficacy against arthropods, have been included. A drug formulary extracted from *Blackwell's Five-Minute Veterinary Consult: Canine and*

Feline, Fourth Edition, with emphasis on those agents used against infectious and parasitic diseases, is provided. Several new drugs, particularly in regard to those used in treating parasitic infections, have also been added. In this edition, we have updated and revised Appendices B and C (Cat and Dog Parasitic Therapeutics) and Appendix D (Dog Heartworm Treatments) to make these tables more user-friendly.

Stephen C. Barr

Acknowledgments

To my colleagues who participated in the writing of this book, who provided many color images and expertise along the way, I extend my gratitude. My thanks to Frank Smith and Larry Tilley for their support and guidance for both *Blackwell's Five-Minute Veterinary Consult* and this spin-off project.

Blackwell's Five-Minute Veterinary Consult

Clinical Companion

Canine and Feline Infectious Diseases and Parasitology

Second Edition

Amebiasis

DEFINITION/OVERVIEW

- Facultative parasitic ameba that infects people and nonhuman primates (including dogs and cats)
- Found primarily in tropical areas throughout the world, although still occurs in North America

ETIOLOGY/PATHOPHYSIOLOGY

- *Entamoeba histolytica*—Dogs and cats become infected by ingesting cysts from human feces.
- Encystment of trophozoites seldom occurs in dogs or cats, so they are not a source of infection.
- One of the few organisms transmitted from man to pets but rarely from pets to man
- Trophozoites (the pathogenic stage) inhabit the colonic lumen as commensals or invade the colonic wall, but can disseminate to other organs (rare) including lungs, liver, brain, and skin.
- Trophozoites damage intestinal epithelial cells by secreting enzymes that lyse cells and disrupt intercellular connections.
- Certain bacteria and a diet deficient in protein increase the virulence of the ameba.
- The host's immune response to invasion exacerbates pathology.
- Colonic ulceration results when trophozoites in the submucosa undermine the mucosa.
- *Acanthamoeba castellani* and *Acanthamoeba culbertsoni*—free-living species found in freshwater, saltwater, soil, and sewage; can infect dogs
- Infection with *Acanthamoeba* spp. thought to occur by inhalation of organisms from contaminated water or colonization of the skin or cornea. Hematogenous spread or direct spread from the nasal cavity through the cribriform plate to the central nervous system may occur, resulting in a granulomatous amebic meningoencephalitis.

SIGNALMENT/HISTORY

- Mainly young and/or immunosuppressed animals are infected.

 CLINICAL FEATURES

Dogs

- *E. histolytica* infections are usually asymptomatic.
- Severe infections result in ulcerative colitis to cause dysentery (may be fatal).
- Hematogenous spread results in organ failure (invariably fatal).
- Granulomatous amebic meningoencephalitis (caused by *Acanthamoeba* spp.) causes signs similar to distemper (anorexia, fever, lethargy, oculonasal discharge, respiratory distress, and diffuse neurologic abnormalities).
- Syndrome of inappropriate secretion of antidiuretic hormone has been reported in a young dog with acanthamebiasis causing granulomatous meningoencephalitis with invasion of the hypothalamus.

Cats

- Colitis causes chronic intractable diarrhea (similar to in dogs).
- Systemic amebiasis has not been reported in the cat.
- *Acanthamoeba* has not been reported in the cat.

 DIFFERENTIAL DIAGNOSIS

Dogs

- Causes of bloody diarrhea or tenesmus include the following: constipation; food intolerance/allergy; parasitism (whipworms, leishmaniasis, balantidiasis); HGE; foreign body; irritable bowel syndrome; inflammatory bowel disease; diverticula; infectious (parvovirus, clostridial enteritis, bacterial overgrowth and other bacterial causes, fungal such as histoplasmosis or blastomycosis); neoplasia; ulcerative colitis; endocrinopathy (Addison's disease); toxic (lead, fungal, or plant); and occasionally major organ disease causing colonic ulceration such as renal failure.
- Other causes of diffuse neurologic disease in young animals include the following: infectious (distemper, fungal such as *Cryptococcus, Blastomyces, Histoplasma*, bacterial, protozoal such as *Toxoplasma* and *Neospora*); toxic (lead, organophosphate); trauma; GME; extracranial (hypoglycemia, hepatic encephalopathy); inherited epilepsy; and neoplasia.

Cats

- Other causes of diarrhea include the following: food intolerance/allergy; inflammatory bowel disease; parasitism (giardiasis, parasites such as hookworms, roundworms, tritrichomonas); infectious (panleukopenia, FIV, FeLV producing panleukopenia-like syndrome, bacterial including *Salmonella*, rarely *Campylobacter*); drug (acetaminophen); neoplasia; pancreatitis; and major organ dysfunction.

 DIAGNOSTICS

Diagnostic Feature

- **Microscopic examination—Colonic biopsy (H&E) obtained via endoscopy is the most reliable method.**
- Trophozoites in feces are very difficult to detect, although methylene blue staining improves chances (Fig. 1-1).
- Trichrome and iron-hematoxyline are the ideal fecal stains but must be performed in a reference laboratory.
- Fecal concentration techniques are of little help.
- Brain biopsy may be required to definitively diagnose neurologic forms antemortem.
- A dog reported with granulomatous amebic meningoencephalitis due to *Acanthamoeba* showed elevated WBC counts (70% mononuclear cells), protein, and xanthochromia in CSF.

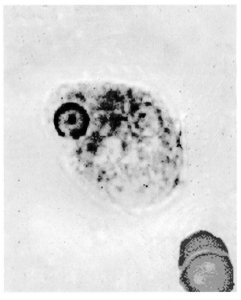

■ **Figure 1-1** Trophozoite of *Entamoeba histolytica* in the feces of a dog. Note the size (about 20 mm) in comparison to the 2 RBCs in the same image (Wright–Giemsa stain, 1500×).

THERAPEUTICS

- Colitis (caused by *E. histolytica*) responds to metronidazole, although dogs continue to shed organisms.
- Systemic forms (particularly neurologic disease) are invariably fatal despite treatment.

Drugs of Choice

- Tinidazole (44 mg/kg, PO, q24h, for 6 days)—found to be more effective than metronidazole in treating amebiasis in people
- Metronidazole (20 mg/kg, PO, q12h, for 7 days)

Precautions/Interactions

- Tinidazole at the above doses has not been associated with any side effects in dogs.
- High doses of metronidazole (usually >30 mg/kg) for extended periods may cause neurologic signs in dogs.

COMMENTS

- Dogs and cats are an unlikely source of infection in people.
- Pets usually acquire infections from the same source as their owners; veterinarians must warn owners of possible risks.
- People and pets are at risk of exposure to free-living amebiasis from the same environmental sources.
- Immunocompetency often determines whether infection will occur.

Abbreviations

CSF, cerebrospinal fluid; FeLV, feline leukemia virus; FIV, feline immunodeficiency virus; GME, granulomatous meningoencephalopathy; HGE, hemorrhagic gastroenteritis; H&E, hematoxylin and eosin; RBC, red blood cell; WBC, white blood cell.

Suggested Reading

Brofman PJ, Knostman KAB, Dibartola SP. Granulomatous amebic meningoenchephalitis causing the syndrome of inappropriate secretion of antidiuretic hormone in a dog. *J Vet Intern Med* 2003;17: 230–234.

Fung HB, Doan TL. Tinidazole: a nitroimidazole antiprotozoal agent. *Clin Ther* 2005;27:1859–1884.

Anaerobic Infections

chapter 2

DEFINITION/OVERVIEW

- Caused by bacteria that require low oxygen tension, are usually normal flora, and elaborate toxins and enzymes leading to extension of the infection into adjacent healthy tissue

ETIOLOGY/PATHOPHYSIOLOGY

- Most common genera—*Bacteroides*, *Fusobacterium*, *Actinomyces*, *Propionibacterium*, *Peptostreptococcus* (enteric *Streptococcus*), *Porphyromonas*, and *Clostridium*.
- Most infections contain at least two different anaerobe species mixed with facultative anaerobes or aerobic bacteria (e.g., *Escherichia coli*).
- Pathogenesis is determined by the body system involved.
- Body areas involved—usually those near a mucosal surface
- Usually caused by normal flora of body—A break in protective barriers allows bacterial invasion.
- Anaerobes—often overlooked as involved in an infectious process

SIGNALMENT/HISTORY

- Predisposing factors—bite wounds, dental disease, open fractures, abdominal surgery, foreign bodies

CLINICAL FEATURES

- Foul odor associated with a wound or exudative discharge
- Gas in the tissue or associated exudates
- Black discoloration of tissue
- Peritonitis

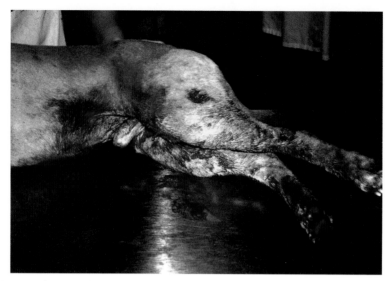

■ **Figure 2-1** Deep bite wounds with considerable tissue damage are likely sources of anaerobic infections.

- Pyothorax
- Pyometra
- Severe dental disease
- Bite wounds with considerable trauma (Fig. 2-1)
- Wounds or deep abscesses that do not heal as anticipated

 DIFFERENTIAL DIAGNOSIS

- Wounds that fail to respond to appropriate medical therapy—Aerobic cultures may be negative; suspect anaerobic organisms.
- Cats with nonhealing wounds—test for FeLV and FIV
- Middle-aged and old animals—Tumor invasion (e.g., in the GIT) may be responsible for establishing infection.

 DIAGNOSTICS

- CBC—neutrophilic leukocytosis and monocytosis common
- Biochemical panel—Abnormalities depend on specific organ involvement.
- Systemic spread of infection may be suggested by signs of septic shock, including leukocytosis with toxic neutrophils, hypoglycemia, increased ALP, and hypoalbuminemia.

Diagnostic Feature

- **Microbiological culture—Collect appropriate samples, such as pus (1–2 ml in stoppered syringe) and tissue (minimum 1 g sample).**
- Minimize exposure to air when collecting and transporting.
- Appropriate transport devices should be on hand before the sample is collected and should include screw-top glass vials with media that accept a Culturette swab and syringes evacuated of all air and capped with a rubber stopper.
- Samples should not be refrigerated prior to submission.
- Often a failure to culture anaerobic bacteria is due to their fastidious nature and errors made in sample collection and submission.

 THERAPEUTICS

- Surgical intervention should not be delayed.
- Surgical removal of devitalized tissue, cleaning of wound, and drainage of pus with the provision for continuous drainage combined with systemic antimicrobial therapy usually gives the best chance of a positive outcome.
- Surgical removal of foreign body is essential if positive outcome is to be achieved.
- Pyothorax—thoracic drainage via chest tube placement
- Removal of swelling to help re-establish local blood flow and increase oxygen tension will help limit spread of tissue damage.

Drugs of Choice

- Amoxicillin with clavulanate—In many cases, this is considered the antibiotic of choice because it is easy, convenient, and has good activity against *Bacteroides.*
- Imipenem—beta lactam with significant activity against serious, resistant infections
- Cefoxitin—the only cephalosporin with reliable activity against anaerobes, but expensive
- Clindamycin—useful for respiratory tract infections
- Metronidazole—effective against all anaerobes, except *Actinomyces* (Table 2-1)
- Aminoglycosides—ineffective
- Trimethoprim-sulfa combinations—ineffective and poor penetration
- Quinolones are routinely ineffective, although newer expanded-spectrum quinolones do have activity against anaerobes (e.g., pradofloxacin).

Precautions/Interactions

- Determine renal and hepatic function to understand how excretion of antibiotics will occur in debilitated patient.
- Support patient appropriately with fluid therapy and nutrition.

TABLE 2-1 Drug Therapy for Anaerobic Infections			
Drug	Dose (mg/kg)	Route	Interval (h)
Penicillin G	20,000–40,000[a]	IM, IV	6–8
Amoxicillin/clavulanic acid	20	PO, IV	8–12
Cefoxitin	10–20	IM, IV	8
Clindamycin	5–10	PO, IV	12
Metronidazole	10	PO, IV	8
Pradofloxacin	5	PO	24

[a]U/kg

COMMENTS

- Antimicrobial therapy alone is unlikely to be successful due to poor drug penetration into exudates and poorly vascularized tissue.
- Antibiotic selection is initially largely empirical (delay in return of culture results)
- Use of antibiotics against both anaerobes and aerobes should be initially selected.

Abbreviations

ALP, alkaline phosphatase; FeLV, feline leukemia virus; FIV, feline immunodeficiency virus; GIT, gastrointestinal tract.

Suggested Reading

Greene CE, Spencer SJ. Anaerobic infections. In: Greene CE, ed. *Infectious Diseases of the Dog and Cat.* Philadelphia: WB Saunders, 2006:381–388.

Meyers B, Schoeman JP, Goddard A, et al. The bacteriology and antimicrobial susceptibility of infected and non-infected dog bite wounds: fifty cases. *Vet Microbiol* 2008;18:360–368.

Silley P, Stephen B, Greife H, et al. Comparative activity of pradofloxacin against anaerobic bacteria isolated from dogs and cats. *J Antimicrob Chemother* 2007;60:999–1003.

Angiostrongylus Infection

chapter 3

DEFINITION/OVERVIEW

- Nematode parasite of the pulmonary arterial tree of dogs in Europe, United Kingdom, Uganda, Australia, and North and South America
- In North America, infections are only reported in the Canadian province Newfoundland-Labrador.
- Important to North American veterinarians as it may be an emerging parasite

ETIOLOGY/PATHOPHYSIOLOGY

- *Angiostrongylus vasorum*—adult worms (1.5–2.5 cm) reside in the pulmonary arteries of dogs
- L1 entering airways—carried up the tracheobronchial tree and swallowed and shed in the feces
- LI in feces—invade molluscan or frog intermediate hosts, where they develop to infective L3
- Molluscan intermediate hosts—eaten by dogs, and L3 migrate to pulmonary artery
- Pulmonary artery obstruction, endarteritis, and pulmonary thrombosis are caused by the adult worms, as well as parenchymal lung damage due to migration of the larvae into the airways.
- Infected dogs develop thrombocytopenia probably as a result of DIC or (as in one dog) immune-mediated thrombocytopenia leading to spontaneous hemorrhage into subcutaneous tissue.
- Natural definitive host—various species of foxes
- PPP 38–57 days (but can be up to 100 days)

SIGNALMENT/HISTORY

- Mainly in rural and stray dogs (due to ingestion of mollusks or frog intermediate hosts)

CLINICAL FEATURES

- Clinical signs vary markedly from asymptomatic to DIC but often involve respiratory signs.
- Chronic cough
- Exercise intolerance
- Weight loss
- Hemoptysis
- Subcutaneous edema consistent with congestive heart failure and parenchymal lung disease
- Respiratory difficulty—increased respiratory rate and tachycardia
- Thrombocytopenia and DIC—spontaneous hemorrhage into subcutaneous tissues
- Aberrant adult worm migration to a number of tissues (eye, left ventricle, urinary bladder, femoral artery, pericardial sac) can occur.

DIFFERENTIAL DIAGNOSIS

A general differential diagnosis for cough includes categories such as the following:

- Cardiovascular and congestive heart failure (pulmonary edema, enlarged heart especially the left atrium, left heart failure, pulmonary emboli, mitral valve insufficiency)
- Allergic (bronchial asthma, eosinophilic pneumonia or granulomatosis, pulmonary infiltrate with eosinophilia)
- Trauma (foreign body, irritating gases, collapsing trachea, hypoplastic trachea)
- Neoplasia (not only of respiratory tree but also associated structures, such as ribs, lymph nodes, and muscles)
- Inflammatory (pharyngitis, tonsillitis, kennel cough from agents such as *Bordetella bronchoseptica*, parainfluenza virus, infectious laryngotracheitis virus, and mycoplasma, systemic fungal pneumonia, bacterial bronchopneumonia, aspiration, chronic pulmonary fibrosis, pulmonary abscess or granuloma, chronic obstructive pulmonary disease)
- Parasites (*Capillaria aerophila, Oslerus [Filaroides] osleri, Filaroides hirthi, Filaroides milksi, Paragonimus kellicotti, Dirofilaria immitis* [heartworm disease])

- Differentiated from canine heartworm disease (caused by *D. immitis*) based on L1 of *A. vasorum* in feces, absence of *D. immitis* antigen, or microfilaria in blood in a dog with radiographic signs consistent with heartworm disease

 # DIAGNOSTICS

- CBC—anemia of chronic disease, thrombocytopenia
- Thoracic radiographs show similar signs as heartworm disease (Fig. 3-1, A and B) and may include increased prominence of the main pulmonary artery, enlarged lobar and peripheral pulmonary arteries, and perivascular parenchymal disease, especially in the caudal lung lobe.
- Right ventricular enlargement may be seen in severe cases.

Diagnostic Feature

- **L1 larvae are identified in transtracheal wash, BAL, and fecal samples using the Baermann technique (Fig. 3-2).**
- False-negative results can occur due to erratic larval shedding, although BAL samples have the fewest false-negative results.
- L1 larvae have a cephalic button, dorsal spine, and kink at the end of the tail that distinguishes it from other L1 larvae found in dog feces.

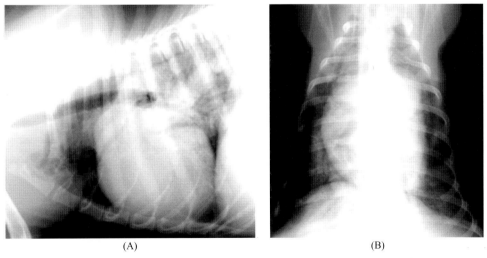

(A)   (B)

■ **Figure 3-1** Lateral (A) and dorsoventral (B) thoracic radiograph showing typical changes of severe *Angiostrongylus* infestation, including increased prominence of the main pulmonary artery, enlarged lobar and peripheral pulmonary arteries, perivascular parenchymal disease, and right ventricular enlargement. These signs must be distinguished from those caused by heartworm disease (*D. immitis*).

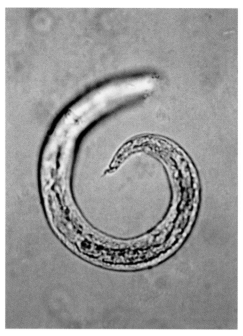

■ **Figure 3-2** L1 larva of *A. vasorum* in the fecal sample of a dog. Note the kink in the tail that makes this larva similar to *Oslerus (Filaroides) osleri*. Clinical cases of *A. vasorum* invariably show abnormalities on thoracic radiographs similar to heartworm disease but not found in *Oslerus* infestations.

- L1 larvae of *A. vasorum* are extremely similar to the lungworm parasite of cats, *Aelurostrongylus abstrusus*; it is possible for larvae of the latter to appear in dog feces after coprophagy.
- An ELISA (detecting E/S antigen) and PCR of blood and fecal samples have recently been reported.

 THERAPEUTICS

- If right-sided heart failure exists, stabilize cardiac function before treating the parasite.

Drugs of Choice

- Milbemycin oxime (0.5 mg/kg, PO, once a week for 4 weeks)
- A single dose of Imidacloprid (10 mg/kg)/Moxidectin (2.5 mg/kg) given as a spot-on (Advocate/Advantage multi; Bayer Animal Health) is effective in eliminating 4th-stage larvae and immature adult worms in experimentally infected dogs, and prevents fecal larval shedding in naturally infected dogs, as does fenbendazole (25 mg/kg, PO, q24h for 20 days).

TABLE 3-1 Drug Therapy for *Angiostrongylus* Infection in Dogs				
Drug	Dose (mg/kg)	Route	Interval (h)	Duration (weeks)
Fenbendazole (Panacur)	25	PO	24	3
Milbemycin oxime	0.5	PO	Once weekly	4
Imidacloprid/Moxidectin	10/2.5	Spot-on	Once	Once
Prednisone[a]	0.5	PO	12	1

[a]Give if signs of pulmonary thromboembolism

COMMENTS

- Naturally infected dogs treated with Imidacloprid/Moxidectin or fenbendazole showed no side effects.
- Clinical and radiographic signs improve rapidly after therapy.
- If pulmonary thromboembolism (presents with signs of cough, fever, mild respiratory distress) occurs after parasiticide therapy, institute strict cage rest and prednisone therapy (0.5 mg/kg, PO, q12h for 3–7 days).

Abbreviations

BAL, bronchoalveolar lavage; CBC, complete blood count; DIC, disseminated intravascular coagulation; ELISA, enzyme-linked immunosorbent assay; E/S, excretory–secretory; FeLV, feline leukemia virus; FIV, feline immunodeficiency virus; GIT, gastrointestinal tract; PPP, prepatent period.

Suggested Reading

Conboy G. Natural infections of *Crenosoma vulpis* and *Angiostrongylus vasorum* in dogs in Atlantic Canada and their treatment with milbemycin oxime. *Vet Rec* 2004;155:16–18.

Schnyder M, Fahrion A, Ossent P, et al. Larvicidal effect of imidacloprid/moxidectin spot-on solution in dogs experimentally inoculated with *Angiostrongylus vasorum*. *Vet Parasitol* 2009;166:326–332.

Willesen JL, Kristensen AT, Jensen AL, et al. Efficacy and safety of imidacloprid/moxidectin spot-on solution and fenbendazole in the treatment of dogs naturally infected with *Angiostrongylus vasorum* (Baillet, 1866). *Vet Parasitol* 2007;147:258–264.

Aspergillosis—Nasal

DEFINITION/OVERVIEW

- An opportunistic fungal infection causing localized (nasal cavity and frontal sinuses) or disseminated disease in both dogs and cats

ETIOLOGY/PATHOPHYSIOLOGY

- *Aspergillus* spp. are common spore-forming molds ubiquitous in the environment, especially in dust, straw, grass clippings, and hay.
- *A. fumigatus* causes nasal aspergillosis, but *A. flavus*, *A. niger*, and *A. nidulans* have also been isolated.
- Infection is thought to occur by direct inoculation of the nasal mucosa.
- Nasal disease does not appear to be related to the systemic form of disease, although one report of a dog developing fungal osteomyelitis 6 months after treatment for nasal aspergillosis raises the possibility.

SIGNALMENT/HISTORY

Dogs

- More commonly affected than cats.
- Dolichocephalic and mesaticephalic breeds
- No sex predilection
- Outdoor dogs and farm dogs—higher prevalence

Cats

- Marginally higher prevalence in Persian cats

Nasal

- Small number of cases reported
- Usually involves frontal (occasionally orbital) sinuses as well

CLINICAL FEATURES

Dogs

- Chronic unilateral or bilateral sanguinopurulent (occasionally serous early or mucopurulent) nasal discharge unresponsive to antibiotics—most common sign
- Sneezing
- Nasal pain
- Epistaxis
- Inappetance
- Lethargy
- Depigmentation or ulceration—common around external nares (but not pathognomonic)
- CNS signs—if cribriform plate involved

Cats

- Mucopurulent nasal discharge
- Sneezing
- Stertor

 # DIFFERENTIAL DIAGNOSIS

- Neoplasia; foreign body; bacterial rhinitis/sinusitis; penicilliosis; *Pneumonyssoides caninum* (nasal mite—dogs); nasopharyngeal polyps (cats); nasal cryptococcosis (cats); dental disease

 # DIAGNOSTICS

- CBC—neutrophilic leukocytosis and monocytosis
- Nasal radiographs—increased radiolucency in affected rostral and maxillary nasal turbinate area (turbinate lysis), especially on open-mouth ventrodorsal and skyline views of frontal sinuses; mixed densities seen due to turbinate destruction and soft tissue dense fungal granulomas or accumulated nasal discharge
- CT and MRI—accurately define extent of disease and allow assessment of the integrity of the cribriform plate; important when considering treatment with local infusion of antifungal agents (Fig. 4-1)
- Rhinoscopy—directly visualize fungal granulomas (Fig. 4-2); appreciate destruction of nasal turbinates (cavernous appearance in severe cases); collect material for culture and cytologic (Fig. 4-3) and histopathologic examination

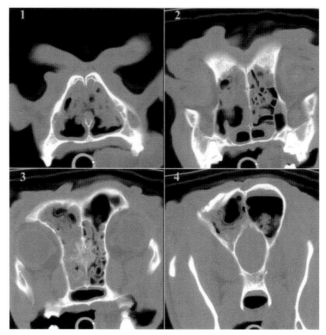

■ **Figure 4-1** A CT scan of a dog with nasal aspergillosis beginning most rostrally (*panel 1*—level of the premolars) and moving caudally (*panel 4*—level of the frontal lobe of the brain). Note the extensive loss of turbinates, especially on the left; involvement of both frontal sinuses; an intact cribriform plate (*panel 3*); and a compressed fracture over the left frontal sinus (*panel 4*), probably the initiating cause of infection in this dog.

- Fungal culture—should be taken from specific lesions or may give false-positive results because the organism is a common contaminant
- Positive culture results—should be confirmed by histopathologic or cytologic examination

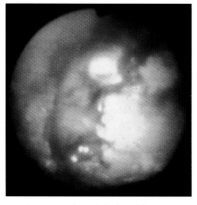

■ **Figure 4-2** *Aspergillus* fungal granulomas as viewed during rhinoscopy.

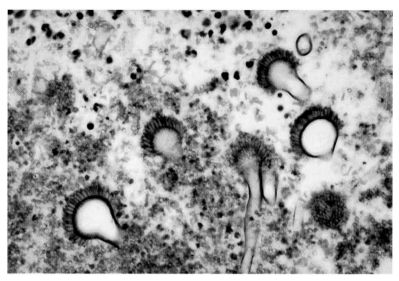

■ **Figure 4-3** Budding heads and microconidia of *Aspergillus* as viewed on cytology.

- Serologic findings (agar gel double diffusion, counterimmunoelectrophoresis, ELISA)—support a diagnosis if made in conjunction with culture and evidence of disease (consistent radiographic changes in nares)
- False-positive results and cross-reactivity with *Penicillium* spp. reported.

Diagnostic Feature

- **Histopathologic findings; positive titer plus culture; positive titer plus appropriate radiographic signs; consistent cytologic findings with fungal plaques identified at rhinoscopic examination**

 THERAPEUTICS

- Systemic antifungal agents (fluconazole, itraconazole)—of limited success unless cribriform plate is breached (as shown on CT or MRI)
- Topical therapy—Clotrimazole infused into the nasal and sinus cavities for 1 hour under general anesthesia is the method of choice (although some still prefer enilconazole).

Method of Nasal Antifungal Therapy

- Prepare patient—general anesthesia with well-fitting cuffed endotracheal tube in place
- Occlude caudal nares by placement of an appropriate-sized Foley catheter (24-French for average-sized dog) in caudal nasopharynx dorsal to soft palate.

- Author prefers using 2 × 2 gauze sponges held in place by monofilament nylon thread placed as follows:
  - Pass the tip of a 1-meter length of nylon suture (no. 3 Supramid Extra II) into the holes of a RRF tube (8-French, 16-inch), which acts as a carrier for the nylon suture material.
  - Pass the RRF tube into the nares on the medioventral floor of the nasal cavity until it can be visualized using a laryngoscope in the oropharynx.
  - Snare the nylon suture with forceps and pull out through the mouth; there is now nylon thread passing from the nares, around the soft palate, and out the mouth.
  - In the center of the nylon thread, tie two 2 × 2 dry gauze sponges and pull them back into the nasophaynx until they are firmly lodged. They are held in place by clamping the nylon thread extending out of the nares in place.
  - The nylon thread exiting the mouth is used to pull the gauze sponges out of the nasopharynx after the procedure is completed.
  - The back of the pharynx may be packed with more gauze sponges (to catch leaks) tied together with nylon thread that protrudes from the mouth for easy retrieval.
- Lavage both nasal cavities (via a 10-French RRF tube)—Use warmed saline (sometimes with 1% Lugol's iodine added) to physically remove mucopurulent material and mildly irritate nasal mucosa.
- Drain well—Air can be gently blown into the nares to dry.
- Place dog in dorsal recumbancy with the nasal opening uppermost (pointing to the ceiling).
- Fill nasal cavities and sinuses with clotrimazole solution and maintain full for 1 hour.
- Large dogs (35 kg) require 50–60 ml clotrimazole for each side.
- When the nasal cavity is full, obstruct the nostril (using Foley catheters—12-French, dental swabs, or tampons) and rotate the head to improve the distribution of the clotrimazole to all nasal and sinus surfaces.
- One hour after treatment is completed, drain clotrimazole by placing the patient in sternal recumbency, open nares to allow solution to drain rostrally, and irrigate with saline to ensure no clotrimazole remains to be swallowed when the dog wakes.
- Remove pharyngeal and nasopharyngeal gauzes through the mouth, and ensure that no clotrimazole is left in the pharynx or nasopharynx.
- Treat pharyngeal or laryngeal irritation postrecovery with one dose of corticosteroids (prednisone 0.5 mg/kg).
- More than one treatment may be required.
- Should extensive sinus involvement be appreciated on CT or radiologic examination, irrigation of the sinuses may be indicated via needles (the author uses Jamshidi bone marrow needles) placed directly into the frontal sinuses (Fig. 4-4) to improve contact of clotrimazole with sinuses should nasal infusions fail.
- Surgical placement of catheters is associated with more complications.
- Enilconazole infusion can be used in place of clotrimazole (as above) or twice daily for 7–14 days via surgically placed frontal sinus catheters (results of single infusion do not appear to be as good as those with clotrimazole).

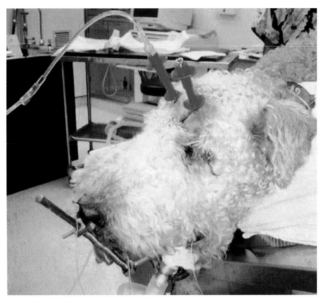

■ **Figure 4-4** Placement of bone marrow needles into frontal sinuses for irrigation with clotrimazole in a dog with intractable nasal aspergillosis.

- Consider enilconazole for treatment failures with clotrimazole—may be associated with greater complication rate (discomfort, aspiration, dislodgement of tubes)

Drugs of Choice

- Clotrimazole (30-ml bottles of 1% solution in PEG).
- Currently, there are three manufacturers of clotrimazole 1% solution in the United States; two (made by Teva and Taro Pharmaceutical) contain the carrier PEG and can be used safely; the third (Vetoquinol; Vet Solutions) contains the carrier PG and should not be used.

Precautions/Interactions

- Clotimazole 1% solutions contain PEG and isopropyl alcohol, which can irritate mucus membranes (larynx and ocular membranes) and has been associated with megaesophagus in some dogs if swallowed.
- Solutions that contain PG can cause severe pharyngitis, laryngitis, and esophagitis and should not be used.
- Ensure that all clotrimazole has been drained out of nares before recovering dog from general anesthesia.
- Protect eyes during the procedure using a generous coating of Paralube or antibiotic ointment in each eye.

- If clotrimazole enters subcutaneous tissues during infusion via needles or catheters placed into the frontal sinuses, facial tissues will swell dramatically and be painful for 24 hours, after which resorption and recovery are uncomplicated.
- Clotrimazole may prolong the recovery from pentobarbital anesthesia, possibly due to hepatic microsomal enzyme inhibitory effects.
- Nasal topical infusion with any drug is contraindicated if the CT shows a damaged cribriform plate; systemic therapy should be attempted.
- Monitor liver enzymes in animals receiving long-term itraconazole and fluconazole.

 COMMENTS

- Local infusion with clotrimazole—approximately 90% success rate
- Success rate can be improved—Perform sinus infusion by trephination during the first treatment if the sinuses are affected, and perform a second clotrimazole infusion 2 weeks after the first irrespective of clinical outcome following the first treatment.
- Persistent cases in which the cribriform plate remains intact should be infused every 2 weeks for four treatments.
- Rhinotomy and turbinectomy should be considered in persistent cases.
- Cats can be treated with clotrimazole infusion in the same manner as dogs.

Abbreviations

BUN, blood urea nitrogen; CBC, complete blood count; CNS, central nervous system; CT, computed tomography; ELISA, enzyme-linked immunosorbent assay; FeLV, feline leukemia virus; FIP, feline infectious peritonitis; FIV, feline immunodeficiency virus; FPV, feline panleukopenia virus; GI, gastrointestinal; MRI, magnetic resonance imaging; PEG, polyethylene glycol; PG, propylene glycol; RRF, red rubber feeding.

Suggested Reading

Davidson A, Mathews KG. Nasal aspergillosis: treatment with clotrimazole. *J Am Anim Hosp Assoc* 1997;33:475–476.
Furrow E, Gorman RP: Intranasal infusion of clotrimazole for the treatment of nasal aspergillosis in two cats. *J Am Vet Med Assoc* 2009;235:1188–1193.
Mathews KG, Davidson AP, Koblik PD, et al. Comparison of topical administration of clotrimazole through surgically placed versus non-surgically placed catheters for treatment of nasal aspergillosis in dogs: 60 cases (1990–1996). *J Am Vet Med Assoc* 1998;213:501–506.

Aspergillosis–Systemic

DEFINITION/OVERVIEW

- An opportunistic fungal infection that causes localized (nasal cavity and frontal sinuses) or disseminated disease in both dogs and cats

ETIOLOGY/PATHOPHYSIOLOGY

- *Aspergillus* spp.—common spore-forming molds ubiquitous in the environment, especially in dust, straw, grass clippings, and hay
- Disseminated disease does not appear to be related to the nasal form of the disease, although one report of a dog developing fungal osteomyelitis 6 months after treatment for nasal aspergillosis raises the possibility.
- *Aspergillus terreus* causes disseminated disease, although *A. deflectus* and *A. fumigatus* have also been isolated.
- Portal of entry unknown—possibly respiratory tract or GI tract followed by hematogenous spread

SIGNALMENT/HISTORY

Dogs

- More commonly affected than cats
- German shepherds—over-represented, but reported sporadically in many other breeds
- Average age—3 years (range 1–9 years); slight bias to females
- Geographic distribution—more commonly reported in California, Louisiana, Michigan, Georgia, Florida, and Virginia, as well as in Western Australia, Barcelona, and Milan

Cats

- Marginally higher prevalence in Persian cats
- Involves mainly the respiratory tract and/or GI tract
- Associated with FIP, FPV, FeLV, FIV, diabetes mellitus, and chronic corticosteroid and antibiotic administration

 # CLINICAL FEATURES

Dogs

- Usually acute onset
- May develop gradually over several months
- Often spinal pain (fungal diskospondylitis)
- Lameness (fungal osteomyelitis)
- Neurologic signs (brain or spinal cord involvement)
- Polyuria/polydipsia
- Hematuria (renal involvement)
- Uveitis (ocular involvement)
- Nonspecific signs of systemic infection—fever, weight loss, vomiting, lymphadenopathy, and anorexia

Cats

- Nonspecific signs of infection—lethargy, depression, vomiting, and diarrhea
- Ocular sign—exophthalmos

 # DIFFERENTIAL DIAGNOSIS

- Bacterial osteomyelitis/diskospondylitis (due mainly to *Staphylococcus* or *Brucella* spp. in dogs); spinal neoplasia; intervertebral disk disease; skeletal neoplasia; bacterial pyelonephritis; bacterial pneumonia; other causes of uveitis (toxoplasmosis, leptospirosis); and other systemic fungal diseases (blastomycosis, histoplasmosis)

 # DIAGNOSTICS

Complete Blood Count

- Nonspecific
- Dogs—often have mature neutrophilic leukocytosis and lymphopenia
- Cats—may have nonregenerative anemia and leukopenia

Biochemical Profile/Urinalysis

- Biochemistry—may see elevations in globulins, creatinine, phosphate, BUN, and calcium
- Urinalysis—may see isosthenuria, hematuria, pyuria, and possible fungal hyphae in the sediment
- Detection of the fungal hyphae can be improved by allowing the sample to incubate at room temperature for 24–48 hours; sediment samples may be examined unstained as wet preparations or may be air dried and stained with Diff-Quick (the hyphae that branch at 45° stain purple).

Other Tests

- Positive fungal serology (agar gel double diffusion, counterimmunoelectrophoresis, and ELISA) support the diagnosis; false-negatives with agar gel immunodiffusion reported; false positives and cross-reactivity with *Penicillium* spp. reported
- Interpret serology in conjunction with other diagnostic tests
- Cats—test for FeLV and FIV because they affect prognosis
- Positive fungal culture from normally sterile body fluids and tissues (e.g., urine, bone, CSF, blood, lymph node, pleural effusions, intervertebral disc aspirates, kidney, spleen)

Radiographic Findings

- Spinal views may show end-plate lysis, attempted bony intervertebral bridging, lysis of vertebral bodies consistent with diskospondylitis, and productive and destructive lesions of the vertebral bodies (Fig. 5-1).
- Bony proliferation and lysis and periosteal reaction are typical of osteomyelitis of the diaphyseal region of long bones.

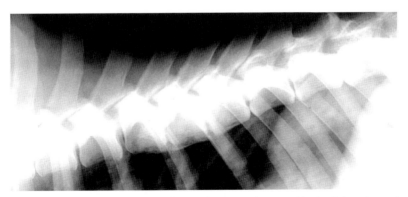

■ **Figure 5-1** Lateral radiographic view of proliferative lesions on the ventral body of thoracic vertebrae in a dog with systemic aspergillosis.

- Pulmonary involvement rare; mixed interstitial/alveolar pattern; enlarged sternal and or tracheobronchial lymph nodes; pleural effusion; productive and destructive lesions of sternebrae

Ultrasonographic Findings

- Kidney—most common site to detect changes; changes seen include renal pelvis dilation ± echogenic debris within pelvis; loss of corticomedullary distinction; renal distortion and mottled appearance of the parenchyma; dilation of proximal ureter; renalomegaly; nodules or masses; hydronephrosis
- Spleen—hypoechoic, lacy, sharply demarcated areas with no Doppler signal suggestive of infarct are most significant ultrasound findings in spleen; other findings include nodules/masses, mottled parenchyma, splenic venous thrombosis
- Other—abdominal lymphadenomegaly; diffuse hepatic hypoechogenicity

MRI Findings

- Useful for further defining brain lesions in animals with CNS signs; changes similar to other infectious and noninfectious inflammatory brain diseases

 # THERAPEUTICS

Dogs

- Treatment rarely curative; may halt progression of clinical signs
- Fluid therapy—indicated by the degree of renal compromise and azotemia

Cats

- Disseminated—likely difficult to treat; data are limited

Drugs of Choice

- Itraconazole, 5–10 mg/kg, PO, q24h (can be divided)—drug of choice for dogs; unlikely to be curative, though the disease may be contained with continued use
- Other drug combinations have been reported, but none have ultimately resulted in reported cure of disease. Some of the combinations reported include the following:
  - Lipid complex amphotericin B (dogs: 2–3 mg/kg, IV, 3 days per week for a total of 9–12 treatments, to cumulative dose of 24–27 mg/kg) + itraconazole 5 mg/kg, PO, q24h
  - Itraconazole (5 mg/kg, PO, q24h) + terbinafine (5–10 mg/kg, PO, q24h)
  - New triazoles: Voriconazole (5 mg/kg, PO, q12h) and Posaconazole (5 mg/kg, PO, q24h) are potential alternatives to cases poorly responsive to itraconazole. They have reportedly been used in combination with lipid complex amphotericin B.

TABLE 5-1 Drug Therapy for Systemic Aspergillosis					
Drug	Formulations (mg)	Dose (mg/kg)	Route	Interval (h)	Duration (weeks)[a]
Fluconazole (Diflucan)	50, 100, 200 tabs powder for oral suspension	1.25–2.5	PO	12	8
Itraconazole (Sporanox)	100 capsules Solution–100 mg/10 ml	5	PO	12	8

[a]Continue at least 2 weeks after clinical recovery

- β-glucan synthase inhibitors Caspofungin, Micafungin, Anidulafungin—may prove useful but very limited clinical information available
- Combination therapy with flucytosine (25–50 mg/kg, PO, q6h, for dogs) and amphotericin B may prove successful, but no published reports are available.

Precautions/Interactions

- Amphotericin B—contraindicated in dogs with pre-existing renal compromise or failure
  - Amphotericin B lipid complex significantly reduced nephrotoxicity.
  - Oral azoles—nausea, intermittent anorexia, liver enzyme elevation
  - Combination of flucytosine and amphotericin B—cutaneous drug eruptions in dogs
  - Avoid midazolam and cisapride with azoles; fatal drug reactions noted in humans
- High-dose (10 mg/kg) itraconazole is associated with ulcerative dermatitis in 5–10% of dogs; recognize early and discontinue, then reinstitute at a reduced dosed, or severe cutaneous and subcutaneous sloughing can occur.

 COMMENTS

- Monitor serial radiographs every 1–2 months, renal function, and urine cultures
- Prognosis of disseminated aspergillosis (especially in German Shepherd dogs) is poor.
- Long-term systemic therapy with itraconazole may alleviate clinical signs in disseminated cases, but seldom results in a cure.

Abbreviations

BUN, blood urea nitrogen; CBC, complete blood count; CNS, central nervous system; CT, computed tomography; ELISA, enzyme-linked immunosorbent assay; FeLV, feline leukemia virus; FIP, feline infectious peritonitis; FIV, feline immunodeficiency virus;

FPV, feline panleukopenia virus; GI, gastrointestinal; MRI, magnetic resonance imaging; PG, propylene glycol; RRF, red rubber feeding

Suggested Reading

Kelly SE, Shaw SE, Clark WT. Long-term survival of four dogs with disseminated *Aspergillus terreus* treated with itraconazole. *Aust Vet J* 1995;72:311–313.

Schultz RM, Johnson EG, Wisner ER, et al. Clinicopathologic and diagnostic imaging characteristics of systemic aspergillosis in 30 dogs. *J Vet Intern Med* 2008;22:851–859.

Astrovirus Infection

DEFINITION/OVERVIEW

- A rare intestinal viral infection of cats, and recently dogs, causing enteritis and diarrhea

ETIOLOGY/PATHOPHYSIOLOGY

- Astrovirus—a small, nonenveloped RNA virus
- More than one serotype may infect cats; only one described in dogs
- Probably causes disease by killing the enterocytes on the villus tips

SIGNALMENT/HISTORY

- No sex, breed, or age predilection, although kittens show more severe disease when infected
- May affect both adults and kittens in a cattery situation
- EM of feces from normal cats (irrespective of age)—suggests that astrovirus may be present in 5–10% of fecal samples of normal cats
- Disease incidence—extremely low

CLINICAL FEATURES

- Small bowel diarrhea often green and watery; may persist 4–14 days
- Diarrhea (with or without vomiting) may be severe and acute enough to produce dehydration and anorexia.

DIFFERENTIAL DIAGNOSIS

- Other causes of acute small bowel diarrhea include the following:
  - Dietary indiscretion
  - Inflammatory bowel disease
  - Food intolerance and allergy
  - Neoplasia (especially GI lymphoma)
  - Drugs (antibiotics)
  - Toxins (lead)
  - Parasites (giardiasis, cryptosporidiosis, tritrichomoniasis)
  - Infectious agents (panleukopenia, FIP, salmonellosis, enteric calici virus, rotavirus)
  - Systemic organ dysfunction (renal, hepatic, pancreatic, cardiac)
  - Metabolic (hyperthyroidism)

 DIAGNOSTICS

- CBC—normal
- Serum biochemical profile—mild acidosis from dehydration
- EM of negatively stained preparations of diarrheic feces—reveals characteristic viral particles (5- to 6-pointed star-shaped surface pattern—30 nm diameter) (Fig. 6-1)

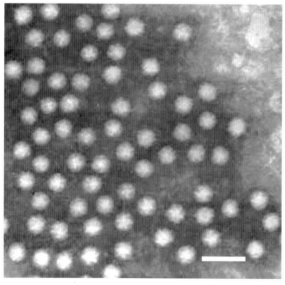

■ **Figure 6-1** EM image of astrovirus in the feces of a cat. Note the distinctive star-shaped surface pattern of each viral particle (bar ×100 nm).

THERAPEUTICS

- Aim of therapy—to control dehydration while seroconversion occurs to eliminate viral infection
- If vomiting present—NPO with parenteral fluids (some cases are mild enough that subcutaneous fluids (0.9% saline with KCl added to 30 U/L) will suffice.
- Antibiotic therapy—not usually indicated unless fever develops, in which case use broad-spectrum coverage and investigate other causes

Drugs of Choice

- N/A

Precautions/Interactions

- No vaccine is available.
- Affected cats should be isolated from others to prevent spread.

 COMMENTS

- Diarrhea is usually not severe enough to warrant treatment, and most healthy cats recover quickly without the need for veterinary care.
- If diarrhea persists, investigate exacerbating conditions or other causes (FIV, FeLV, inflammatory bowel disease, concurrent GI infections such as giardiasis).
- Recent sequence analysis of human and mammalian astroviruses suggests that animal-to-human transmission does not occur.

Abbreviations

CBC, complete blood count; EM, electron microscopy; FeLV, feline leukemia virus; FIP, feline infectious peritonitis; FIV, feline immunodeficiency virus; GI, gastrointestinal; NPO, nothing per os; RNA, ribonucleic acid.

Suggested Reading

Lukashov VV, Goudsmit J. Evolutionary relationships among Astroviridae. *J Gen Virol* 2002; 83:1397–1405.
Toffan A, Jonassen CM, DeBattisti C, et al. Genetic characterization of a new astrovirus detected in dogs suffering from diarrhoea. *Vet Microbiol* 2009;139:147–152.

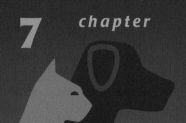

7 *chapter*

Babesiosis

DEFINITION/OVERVIEW

- A protozoal disease (genus *Babesia*) of dogs and cats in which merozoites (piroplasms) infect RBCs
- Degree of illness is usually dependent on the severity and rate of anemia development.
- Anemia is mainly a result of immune-mediated hemolysis but also due to direct piroplasm damage to RBCs.

ETIOLOGY/PATHOPHYSIOLOGY

- Infection (by tick transmission, transplacental, or by blood transfusion) is followed by 2-week incubation period during which piroplasms infect and multiply in RBCs, resulting in RBC damage mainly from immune-mediated processes but also direct RBC lysis.

Dogs

- Large (4–7 mm)
- *Babesia canis* distributed worldwide; three subspecies (some have proposed that these are 3 distinct species) based on biologic, genetic, and geographic distribution
    - *B. canis vogeli*—United States, Africa, Asia, Australia
    - *B. canis rossi*—Africa (most virulent subspecies)
    - *B. canis canis*—Europe, areas of Asia
- Small (2–5 mm); three genetically distinct species
    - *B. gibsoni*—(AKA, *B. gibsoni* [Asia]), worldwide distribution (especially Asia); emerging disease in the United States
    - *B. conradae* (AKA: *B. gibsoni* [California])—infects only dogs and reported only in California
    - *Babesia* (*Theileria*) *annae* (AKA: Spanish dog piroplasm and *B. microti*-like parasite)—reported in Spain and other areas of Europe, and recently in the United States

- Several other single case reports of novel *Babesia* sp. and other piroplasms (i.e., *Theileria equi*) have been published, including *Babesia* sp. (Coco), a large piroplasm identified in splenectomized and immune-suppressed dogs in the United States.

Cats

- Small (2–5 mm)—*B. felis* reported in Africa

 SIGNALMENT/HISTORY

- History of tick attachment
- History of recent dog bite wound may be a risk for *B. gibsoni* (Asia) infection.
- Any age or breed of dog can be infected.
- Severity of disease depends on the strain of the organism and the age and breed of the animal.
- *B. canis* infections are more prevalent in greyhounds (United States).
- *B. gibsoni* (Asia) infections are more prevalent in American pit bull terriers (United States).
- Southern Asia and Africa—Any age or breed dog or cat can be infected.
- United States—cats often infected with a closely related organism (*Cytauxzoon felis*)

 CLINICAL FEATURES

Dogs

- Peracute, acute, chronic, or asymptomatic (in some carrier animals)
- Splenectomy and immunosuppression—severely worsen disease (*B. canis rossi*) or makes it apparent (*B. canis* in the United States)
- Immunosuppression—may result in an increase in parasitemia and manifestation of clinical signs in chronically infected dogs (*B. canis* in the United States)
- Most severe disease—caused by *B. gibsoni* in the United States and *B. canis rossi* in Africa
- *B. canis*—rarely causes clinical disease in the United States
- Signs include the following:
  - Lethargy
  - Anorexia
  - Weight loss
  - Pale mucous membranes (Fig. 7-1)
  - Fever
  - Splenomegaly
  - Lymphadenopathy

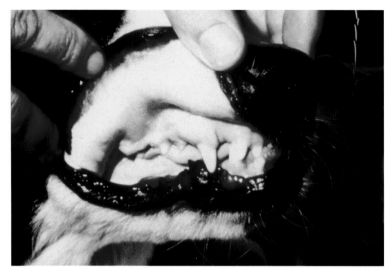

■ **Figure 7-1** Pale mucous membranes typical of anemia are often found in dogs with *B. gibsoni* infections.

- Hemoglobinemia/uria
- Icterus (Fig. 7-2)
- GI signs—Some dogs develop vomiting, diarrhea, and/or dark feces (from increased bilirubin excretion).
- Cerebral babesiosis—weakness, disorientation, collapse (*B. canis rossi* in Africa)
- Renal/urologic disease—results in renal failure (*B. canis rossi* in Africa)

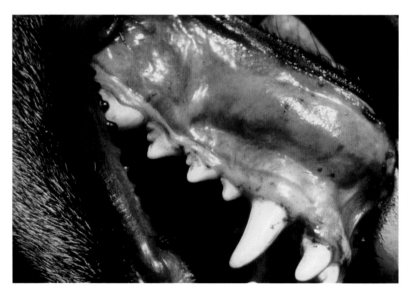

■ **Figure 7-2** Icterus in a dog with *B. gibsoni* usually indicates acute infection with marked intravascular hemolysis.

Cats

- Similar to dogs
- Lethargy
- Anorexia
- Pale mucous membranes
- Icterus

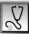 **DIFFERENTIAL DIAGNOSIS**

- Immune-mediated diseases—hemolytic anemia, ITP, ehrlichiosis, RMSF, hemobartonellosis, cytauxzoonosis, SLE
- Non–immune-mediated diseases—hemolytic anemia; heartworm caval syndrome, zinc toxicity, splenic torsion, Heinz body anemia, DIC, PK deficiency, PFK deficiency
- Causes of jaundice—hepatic or posthepatic disease (obstruction or rupture of biliary tract)

 DIAGNOSTICS

Complete Blood Count

- Mild to severe (packed cell volume, 10%) regenerative anemia
- Peracute—Animal may present before a regenerative response has time to occur.
- Anemia—may not be present in all cases (e.g., carriers: greyhounds with *B. canis* in the United States).
- Thrombocytopenia—usually moderate to severe, and can occur without anemia
- Variable leukocytosis or leukopenia

Biochemical Profile/Urinalysis

- Hyperbilirubinemia/uria—if hemolysis acute and severe (African rather than cases in United States)
- Hyperglobulinemia—common in chronic cases (sometimes the only blood chemistry abnormality in these cases)
- Mildly elevated liver enzymes—due to anemia/hypoxia
- Renal failure and metabolic acidosis (*B. canis rossi* in Africa)
- Bilirubinuria—common
- Hemoglobinuria—detected less commonly in the United States than in Africa

Other Tests

- Microscopic examination of stained thin or thick blood smears—can provide definitive diagnosis, but sensitivity depends on experience of microscopist; modified

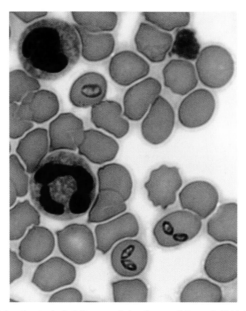

■ **Figure 7-3** RBCs containing the typical piriform and ring forms of *B. canis* (Wright–Giemsa stain).

Wright's stain best for viewing organism; blood from peripheral capillary (ear prick) may improve sensitivity; does not differentiate subspecies using microscopy
- *B. canis*—large piriforms within RBCs but also ring forms (Fig. 7-3)
- *B. gibsoni*—smaller and often single forms are found per RBC (Fig. 7-4)

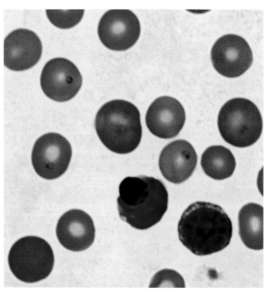

■ **Figure 7-4** RBCs containing the typical piriform and ring forms of *B. gibsoni*. Note the nucleated RBC and polychromasia typical of a regenerating anemia often seen in dogs with *B. gibsoni* (Wright–Giemsa stain, 1500×).

- Serologic examination—IFA; false-negative results in young dogs; does not differentiate species and subspecies; use if microscopic examination negative with high clinical suspicion of disease
- PCR—tests for the presence of *Babesia* DNA in a biologic sample (usually EDTA-anticoagulated whole blood), and can differentiate subspecies and species
  - More sensitive than microscopy
- Coombs' test—usually positive result in dogs with babesiosis, making it necessary to perform other tests to distinguish it from other causes of anemia

 THERAPEUTICS

- Anemic patients—transfusion of whole blood or packed RBCs (for loss of RBC mass)
- Polymerized bovine hemoglobin solution may be used in some anemic animals if fresh blood is not available (not superior to packed RBC).
- Severely affected patients require aggressive fluid therapy for hypovolemic shock from blood loss (usually as a result of thrombocytopenia with bleeding).

Drugs of Choice

- Imidocarb dipropionate (Imizol; Schering-Plough).
  - Preferred therapy
  - May completely clear *B. canis* infections but usually not *B. gibsoni* (Asia)
  - Decreases morbidity and mortality
- Diminazine aceturate
  - Not readily available in the United States and not FDA approved
  - Efficacy similar to that of imidocarb dipropionate
- Metronidazole, clindamycin, and doxycycline
  - Decrease clinical signs, and reduce parasite numbers below the limit of detection of PCR testing, but still may not clear infection
  - Azithromycin—give in combination with atovaquone
  - Effective in treating *Babesia* infections in humans and mice
- Primaquine phosphate—preferred treatment of cats with *B. felis*
- Prednisone—treats immune-mediated component of anemia (Table 7-1)

Precautions/Interactions

- Imidocarb and diminazene
  - May cause pain and swelling at injection site, hypersalivation, nasal drip, shivering, increased lacrimation, diarrhea, vomiting, periorbital edema similar to that with organophosphate toxicity (has inherent anticholinesterase activity)

TABLE 7-1 Drug Therapy for Babesiosis in Dogs

Drug	Dose (mg/kg)	Route	Interval (h)	Duration (days)
Imidocarb dipropionate	5.0–6.6	IM or SC	14 days	2 doses
Diminazine aceturate	3.5–7.0	IM or SC	14 days	2 doses
Metronidazole[a]	25–50	PO	12	7
Clindamycin	12.5–25	PO	12	7–10
Doxycycline	10	PO	12	7–10
Azithromycin	10	PO	24	10
Atovaquone[b]	13.3	PO	8	10
Primaquine phosphate	1	IM	Once	
Prednisone	1	PO	12	5

[a]Give in combination with clindamcyin (25 mg/kg, PO, q12h) and doxycycline (5 mg/kg, PO, q12h) at a dose of 15 mg/kg, PO, q12h. for 4–13 weeks.
[b]Give in combination with azithromycin.

- Do not use these drugs simultaneously with other anticholinesterase agents; side effects can be minimized by administering atropine pretreatment.
- High doses of antibabesial drugs may cause liver and renal damage.
- Metronidazole—Higher doses (>30 mg/kg) can be associated with neurologic toxicity.

COMMENTS

- Imidocarb—current treatment of choice for babesiosis in dogs; few side effects when treated
- It is particularly important to warn owners that the treatment may not completely remove the parasite from the body.
- When a dog from a multi-dog kennel is diagnosed with babesiosis, all dogs in that kennel should be screened for the disease.
- Coinfection with other vector-transmitted pathogens (e.g., *Erhlichia, Hemotropic Mycoplasma, Leishmania*) should be considered.
- Vaccines for *B. canis canis* and *B. canis rossi* are available in Europe, but these vaccines do not confer protection against other *Babesia* spp.
- Tick control is important for disease prevention.
- Acaracides may prevent infection with *Babesia* spp.
- Potential blood donors should test negative for the disease (preferably by 2–3 PCR tests) prior to use.

Abbreviations

AKA, also known as; DIC, disseminated intravascular coagulation; DNA, deoxyribonucleic acid; EDTA, ethylenediamine tetra-acetic acid; GI, gastrointestinal; IFA, immunofluorescent antibody assay; ITP, idiopathic thrombocytopenic purpura; PCR, polymerase chain reaction; PFK, phosphofructokinase; PK, pyruvate kinase, RBCs, red blood cells; RMSF, Rocky Mountain spotted fever; SLE, systemic lupus erythematosus

Suggested Reading

Birkenheuer AJ, Correa MT, Levy MG, et al. Geographic distribution of babesiosis among dogs in the United States and association with dog bites. 150 cases (2000-2003) *J Am Vet Med Assoc* 2005:227942–947.

Birkenheuer AJ, Neel J, Ruslander D, et al. Detection and molecular characterization of a novel large *Babesia* species in a dog. *Vet Parasitol* 2004;124:151–160.

Irwin PJ. Canine babesiosis. *Vet Clin North Am Small Anim Pract* 2010:40;1141–1156.

8

Balantidiasis

DEFINITION/OVERVIEW

- A protozoal infection, usually of pigs, that occasionally infects the colon of dogs (and humans) to produce a hemorrhagic diarrhea

ETIOLOGY/PATHOPHYSIOLOGY

- *Balantidium coli*—large ciliated protozoan found throughout the world, infecting mainly pigs
- *B. coli* trophozoites—inhabit the colon, producing cysts that are passed in the feces to infect other species, including dogs but not cats
- Invasion of the layer between the mucosa and submucosa results in colonic ulceration with hemorrhagic diarrhea.
- Certain colonic bacteria and infection with whipworms (*Trichuris vulpis*) may predispose commensal *B. coli* infection to become pathogenic.
- Extraintestinal invasion of *B. coli* is very rare, unlike that of amebiasis.

SIGNALMENT/HISTORY

- History of contact of dogs with swine (which are usually asymptomatic)

CLINICAL FEATURES

- Clinical signs of hemorrhagic colitis:
    - Mucoid bloody diarrhea
    - Increased frequency of defecation
    - Chronic weight loss

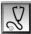 ## DIFFERENTIAL DIAGNOSIS

- Causes of bloody diarrhea or tenesmus, including constipation; food intolerance/allergy; parasitism (whipworms, leishmaniasis, amebiasis); HGE; foreign body; irritable bowel syndrome; inflammatory bowel disease; diverticula; infectious (parvovirus, clostridial enteritis, bacterial overgrowth and other bacterial causes, fungal such as histoplasmosis or blastomycosis); neoplasia; ulcerative colitis; endocrinopathy (Addison's disease); occasionally major organ disease, such as renal failure, causing colonic ulceration

 ## DIAGNOSTICS

- Fecal flotation (using ZSCT) may detect trophozoites (Fig. 8-1) and *B. coli* cysts (Fig. 8-2).
- Staining to reveal the macronucleus of both cysts and trophozoites using acidic methyl green (1 g methyl green mixed with 1 ml glacial acetic acid and 100 ml water) is preferred.

Diagnostic Feature

- **Fresh fecal smear mixed with normal saline often shows trophozoites.**

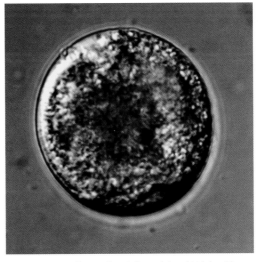

■ **Figure 8-1** Trophozoite of *B. coli* in the feces of an infected dog (Wright–Giemsa stain, 1500×).

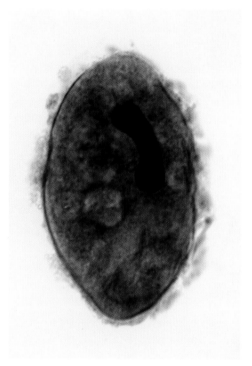

■ **Figure 8-2** Cyst of *B. coli* in a fecal smear from an infected dog (1000×).

 THERAPEUTICS

- Few reports of treatment of *B. coli* in dogs exist in the literature.
- In humans, metronidazole, tetracyclines, and secnidazole have been effective.
- Secnidazole is 80–100% efficacious in people with intestinal amebiasis and giardiasis, and 80% efficacious in cattle with *B. coli*. Secnidazole use in dogs is not reported.

Drugs of Choice

- Metronidazole
- Tetracycline (Table 8-1).
- If secnidazole is available, then this drug would be well worth trying.

Precautions/Interactions

- High doses of metronidazole for extended periods of time may cause neurologic signs in dogs.
- Tetracycline may cause yellow dental staining in young animals.

TABLE 8-1   Drug Therapy for Balantidiasis in Dogs

Drug	Dose (mg/kg)	Route	Interval (h)	Duration (days)
Metronidazole (Flagyl)	15–30	PO	12	7
Tetracycline[a]	22	PO	8	10
Secnidazole[b] (Flagentyl, Sindose)	30	PO	24	5

[a] Many generic formulations.
[b] Use not reported in dogs.

COMMENTS

- Excreted *B. coli* cysts in the feces of infected dogs are a source of infection to humans and other dogs.
- Unlike pigs, dogs do not constitute a significant reservoir of infection for humans.

Abbreviations

HGE, hemorrhagic gastroenteritis; ZSCT, zinc sulfate concentration technique.

Suggested Reading

Barr SC. Balantidiasis. In: Greene CE, ed. *Infectious Diseases of the Dog and Cat.* Philadelphia: WB Saunders; 2006: 744–745.

chapter

9

Bartonellosis

DEFINITION/OVERVIEW

- An intracellular bacterial infection of cats and dogs—Various bacterial species cause different syndromes, from bacteremia in cats to endocarditis in dogs.
- Human syndromes—include CSD (regional lymphadenopathy after a cat scratch), bacillary peliosis, bacillary angiomatosis, relapsing fever with bacteremia, encephalitis, meningitis, neuroretinitis, and endocarditis
- Distribution—worldwide
- Estimated 25,000 human cases per year in the United States, but few fatalities
- Seasonal in human cases—most reported in summer months
- Cat—considered the primary mammalian reservoir and vector for human infections with *Bartonella henselae*

ETIOLOGY/PATHOPHYSIOLOGY

- Fastidious hemotropic gram-negative rod bacterium
- *Bartonella* is thought to invade and multiply within RBCs.
- At least one *Bartonella* species (and probably others) produces a factor that causes vascular endothelial proliferation, a feature of human syndromes—bacillary angiomatosis, bacillary splenic peliosis, and peliosis hepatis.
- *B. henselae*—two primary genetically different types with at least two subgroups per type; even genomic variation during course of infection (making vaccine development very difficult)

Cats

- Infected with five *Bartonella* spp.—*B. henselae, B. clarridgeiae, B. koehlerae, B. quintana,* and *B. bovis* (most of which are zoonotic); infections with species other than *B. henselae* and *B. clarridgeiae* are rare.
- *B. henselae* bacteremia occurs in about 5–40% of cats in the United States (highest in warmer, humid climates, where it can be as high as 90%).
  B. clarridgeiae—10% of cats with bacteremia

44

- Mixed infections of *B. henselae* (which contains at least two subgroups) and *B. clarridgeiae* occur.
- Transmission—does not occur without the presence of infected cat fleas (*Ctenocephalides felis felis*); infected flea dirt injected intradermally is infectious; *B. henselae* can survive for 3 days in flea dirt.
- Transmission can occur via blood transfusion (even if given subcutaneously or intradermally).
- Transmission between cats does not occur if fleas are not present.
- Bacteremia with *B. henselae* and *B. clarridgeiae*—chronic and recurrent, probably for years
- *Bartonella* organisms have been seen within RBCs, in blood and other tissues (vascular endothelial cells), but may occur in other locations within the body.

Dogs

- Infected with four *Bartonella* species—*B. vinsonii* subsp. *berkhoffii*, *B. henselae*, *B. clarridgeiae*, and *B. elizabethae*
- Ticks and fleas may be vectors for transmission of *B. vinsonii* subsp. *berkhoffii* to dogs.
- *B. vinsonii* subsp. *berkhoffii*—experimentally, causes no clinical signs but mild immunosuppression and persistent bacteremias (up to 247 days)
- Natural cases—rare disease caused by *B. henselae* (peliosis hepatis) and *B. vinsonii* subsp. *berkhoffii* (endocarditis, granulomatous rhinitis, and granulomatous lymphadenitis)

 SIGNALMENT/HISTORY

Cats

- Seroprevalence highest for *B. henselae*—worldwide occurrence
- Highest seroprevalence—in warm humid climates, older cats, and those most exposed to fleas
- Prevalence of bacteremia in cats in the United States is 5–40% (highest in warm humid climates).
- Flea infestation appears to be necessary for the transmission of *B. henselae* from cats to humans, but direct transmission to humans via a flea bite is speculative.
- Until recently—was not thought to cause disease in the cat

Dogs

- Seroprevalence of *B. henselae*—approximately 3–9% in the United States
- High seroprevalence in coyotes for *B. vinsonii* subsp. *berkhoffii*—approximately 25–75%, suggesting they may be the reservoir host for this species

- Endocarditis cases—variable, but often include weight loss, syncope, collapse, and sudden death
- Hepatic disease—depression, weight loss, and vomiting

 ## CLINICAL FEATURES

Cats

- In natural cases, clinical signs are rare.
- Uveitis is thought by some to be caused by *Bartonella*, but in one study, healthy cats were more likely to be seropositive for *Bartonella* than were cats with uveitis.
- After intradermal inoculation of *B. henselae*—develop abscess at inoculation site, lymphadenomegaly, periodic fever, and mild neurologic signs (nystagmus, whole-body tremors, focal motor seizures, and behavior changes)
- Histologic lesions—include peripheral lymph node hyperplasia, splenic follicular hyperplasia, lymphocytic cholangitis/pericholangitis, lymphocytic hepatitis, lymphoplasmacytic myocarditis, and interstitial lymphocytic nephritis
- Reproductive failure has occurred in some cats infected experimentally with *B. henselae*.
- Experimental infections with *B. koehlerae*—no clinical signs
- Endocarditis—associated with two cats infected with *B. henselae*
- To date—no proven association between *Bartonella* infection and anemia, gingivostomatitis, neurologic conditions, or uveitis in cats
- To date—*Bartonella* infections have not been verified to cause chronic illness in cats.
- Cats with rhinosinusitis—no support for any pathogenic role by *Bartonella*.
- Cats with plasmacytic pododermatitis or peliosis hepatis—*Bartonella* DNA could not be found in tissues from these cats.

Dogs

- *B. vinsonii* subsp. *berkhoffii*—associated with endocarditis, cardiac arrhythmias, granulomatous rhinitis, and granulomatous lymphadenopathy
- Dogs experimentally infected with *B. vinsonii* subsp. *berkhoffii* show no clinical signs (transient fever in some).
- Ocular signs— uveitis, chorioretinitis
- *B. henselae*—identified by PCR in the liver of a dog with peliosis hepatis; another with granulomatous hepatitis

Humans

- Erythematous papule at inoculation site (scratch, bite)—then unilateral regional lymphadenopathy (painful, often suppurative) in 3–10 days (>90% of cases)
- Symptoms—mild fever, chills (infrequent), anorexia, myalgia, and nausea

- Atypical manifestations (usually in immunosuppressed patients, in up to 25% of cases)—encephalopathy (1–7%), palpebral conjunctivitis (3–5%), meningitis, osteolytic lesions, granulomatous hepatitis, and pneumonia

DIFFERENTIAL DIAGNOSIS

- Other causes of endocarditis—bacterial
- Other causes of hepatic dysfunction—Differentiate from other causes by ruling out other causes of dysfunction and demonstrating *Bartonella* organisms associated with pathology.

DIAGNOSTICS

- Diagnosis of a disease caused by *Bartonella* is not easy because so many healthy animals are seropositive and PCR-positive.
- CBC, serum biochemistry, and urinalysis are noncontributory, although they may show elevations of hepatic enzymes in dogs with liver syndromes; some cats have persistent eosinophilia.
- Serologic assays—IFA test and ELISA are available, but value is questionable given that 12% of cats with *B. henselae* bacteremia are seronegative, and many animals that have cleared the bacteremia are seropositive.
- The positive predictive value of a positive serologic test for bacteremia is low in cats (40–45%); the positive predictive value of a negative serologic test is high (90–97%).
- Predictive value for serology tests in dogs is not assessed, but in coyotes, negative (29%) and positive (73%) predictive values are lower than in cats.
- Blood or tissue culture—use 1–2 ml EDTA blood (freeze to release organisms from RBCs) in enriched blood containing media—positive in 1–3 weeks.

Diagnostic Feature

- **Blood culture is the most reliable definitive test for detecting active infection in cats; it may be necessary to perform several due to the relapsing nature of bacteremia.**
- Blood culture in dogs—considered insensitive because endocarditis cases are usually negative; need to culture heart valve
- PCR assay of blood—no more sensitive than cultures
- PCR assays—available through some laboratories (e.g., North Carolina State University and UC Davis)
- PCR results—Advantages over blood culture are that it is usually quicker and can detect species of *Bartonella* involved.

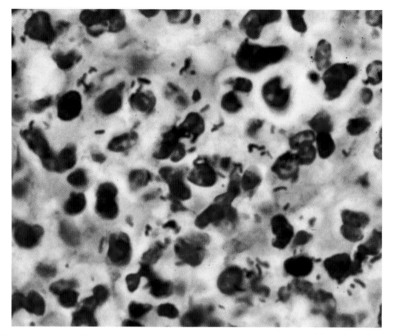

■ **Figure 9-1** Aspirate from the lymph node of a human with cat scratch fever and local lymphadenophathy showing *Bacillus* bacteria (Warthin–Starry silver stain, 1000×).

- In humans—may see bacillus in lymph node aspirates using Warthin–Starry silver stain (Fig. 9-1)

 THERAPEUTICS

Humans

- Supportive treatment, including bed rest and heat on swollen lymph nodes
- Doxycycline, erythromycin, and rifampin are recommended.
- Treat for 2 weeks in immunocompetent, 6 weeks in immunocompromised, individuals.

Cats

- Efficacy of antibiotics—much worse in cats than in humans
- Indication for treating infected cats with no clinical signs is questionable; no regimen of antibiotic treatment has been proven effective for definitively eliminating infections in cats.
- Treat only those cats showing clinical signs of disease.
- If treated, follow-up blood cultures (taken 3 weeks after antimicrobial therapy had been discontinued) are needed to confirm treatment success.

TABLE 9-1 Drug Therapy for Bartonellosis in Dogs and Cats				
Drug	**Dose (mg/kg)**	**Route**	**Interval (h)**	**Duration (weeks)**
Enrofloxacin (Baytril)	5	PO	12	4–6
Doxycycline (Vibramycin)	5–10	PO	12	4–6
Azithromycin (Zithromax)	5–15	PO	12	4–6

- Control fleas.

Dogs

- Dogs with clinical signs and that are seropositive—treat with antibiotics

Drugs of Choice

- Doxycycline and azithromycin (Zithromax; Pfizer)—probably the drugs of choice, although there is little controlled data; treat for a minimum of 4–6 weeks
- Enrofloxacin (Baytril; Bayer); doxycycline (Vibramycin; Pfizer) is also effective but resistance has been documented (Table 9-1)

Precautions/Interactions

- In humans, thoroughly cleanse all cat scratches or bites.
- Prevent cats from contacting open wounds.
- Immunocompromised persons should avoid young cats.
- Enrofloxacin causes retinal degeneration and blindness in some cats when doses over 5 mg/kg are used.
- Resistance to fluoroquinolones—documented in naturally occurring infections in man so is no longer recommended
- Doxycycline may cause esophagitis and stricture; higher doses seem to be more effective in clearing infection (in cats).
- Azithromycin—reduce dosage with hepatic or biliary dysfunction
- Treat cats vigorously for fleas.

COMMENTS

- The involvement of *Bartonella* spp. as a cause of significant disease in the cat is yet to be fully elucidated.
- Occasional case reports implicate some *Bartonella* spp. as causes of certain rare diseases in dogs.
- The zoonotic potential of *Bartonella* infection in dogs and cats is still uncertain, although dogs have been suggested to serve as chronically infected blood reservoirs of *Bartonella* spp. that may spread by arthropod vectors to people.

Abbreviations

CBC, complete blood count; CSD, cat scratch disease; EDTA, ethylenediamine tetra-acetic acid; ELISA, enzyme-linked immunosorbent assay; FIV, feline immunodeficiency virus; IFA, immunofluorescent antibody test; PCR, polymerase chain reaction; RBCs, red blood cells; UTIs, urinary tract infections.

Suggested Reading

Breitschwerdt EB. Feline bartonellosis and cat scratch disease. *Vet Immunol Immunopathol* 2008;123:167–171.

Guptill-Yoran L. Feline bartonellosis. *Vet Clin North Am Small Anim Pract* 2010;40:1073–1090.

Guptill-Yoran L, Breitschwerdt EB, Chom BB. Bartonellosis In: Greene CE, ed. *Infectious Diseases of the Dog and Cat*. Philadelphia: WB Saunders, 2006: 510–524.

Blastomycosis

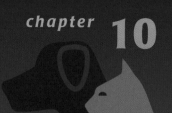

chapter 10

DEFINITION/OVERVIEW

- A systemic mycotic infection affecting dogs, and rarely cats, most commonly in the Mississippi, Ohio, and Tennessee River basins

ETIOLOGY/PATHOPHYSIOLOGY

- *Blastomyces dermatitidis*—small soil fungus
- Small spores (conidia)—shed from the mycelial phase of the organism growing in soil
- Conidia—inhaled and enters the terminal airway
- At body temperature, spores become yeast, which initiates lung infection.
- From this focus of mycotic pneumonia—yeast disseminates hematogenously throughout the body
- The immune response to the invading organism—Pyogranulomatous infiltrate to control the organism, resulting in organ dysfunction.
- Of affected dogs, 85% have lung disease.
- Eyes, skin, lymphatic system, and bones are commonly affected.
- CNS, testes, prostate, mammary gland, nasal cavity, gums, and vulva are less commonly affected.

SIGNALMENT/HISTORY

- Historically, most commonly reported complaints:
  - Weight loss
  - Depressed appetite
  - Cough or dyspnea
  - Lameness
  - Draining skin lesions
- History of exposure to wet soil by rivers, streams, or lakes
- Often history of construction or soil disturbance

Dogs

- Breed predilection—large-breed dogs (>25 kg) most often affected, especially sporting breeds (probably reflects exposure rather than susceptibility)
- Age predilection—2–4 years (uncommon >7 years)
- Sex predilection—males

Cats

- Age predilection—young to middle age; can occur in indoor cats

 CLINICAL FEATURES

Dogs

- Fever up to 104°F (40°C)—approximately 50% of patients
- Harsh, dry lung sounds associated with increased respiratory effort are common.
- Generalized or regional lymphadenopathy—with or without skin lesions
- Uveitis—with or without secondary glaucoma and conjunctivitis, ocular exudates, corneal edema, retinal granulomas
- Lameness—common because of fungal osteomyelitis
- Testicular enlargement and prostatomegaly are seen occasionally.

Cats

- Increased respiratory effort
- Granulomatous skin lesions

 DIFFERENTIAL DIAGNOSIS

- Respiratory signs—a general differential diagnosis for respiratory signs and cough includes such categories as:
  - Cardiovascular (pulmonary edema; enlarged heart, especially the left atrium; pleural effusion; pulmonary emboli)
  - Allergic (bronchial asthma, chronic bronchitis, eosinophilic pneumonia, or granulomatosis, pulmonary infiltrate with eosinophilia)
  - Trauma (foreign body, irritating gases, collapsing trachea)
  - Neoplasia (not only of the respiratory tree but also associated structures such as ribs, lymph nodes, muscles)
  - Inflammatory (pharyngitis; tonsillitis; kennel cough from such agents as *Bordetella bronchiseptica*, parainfluenza virus, infectious laryngotracheitis virus, and mycoplasma; bacterial bronchopneumonia; chronic pulmonary fibrosis; pulmonary abscess or granuloma; chronic obstructive pulmonary disease)

- Parasites [*Oslerus (Filaroides) osleri, Crenosoma vulpis, Capillaria aerophila, Filaroides milksi, Paragonimus kellicotti, Dirofilaria immitis*—heartworm disease)
- Lymph node enlargement—similar to lymphosarcoma; differentiated by cytologic examination of lymph node aspirate
- Combination of fever and respiratory disease with eye, bone, or skin involvement in a young dog—suggests the diagnosis

 DIAGNOSTICS

- CBC—changes reflect mild to moderate inflammation (neutrophilic leukocytosis ± left shift, monocytosis)
- High-serum globulins with borderline low-albumin concentrations—dogs with chronic infections
- Hypercalcemia—in some dogs, secondary to the granulomatous changes
- *Blastomyces* yeasts can be found in the urine of dogs with prostatic involvement.
- Urine antigen test—useful for making a diagnosis if organisms cannot be found on cytologic or histopathologic examination; sensitivity of >90%; some cross-reaction with other fungal agents (histoplasma)
- Positive AGID—strongly supports diagnosis, with a specificity of 90%; in endemic areas, dogs can be positive but not have disease
- Negative AGID—common in dogs with early infection
- Radiographic findings—lungs usually show generalized interstitial-to-nodular infiltrates (Fig. 10-1) with tracheobronchial lymphadenopathy (common) but can see nonuniform distribution of lesions
- Chest radiographic findings—inconsistent with bacterial pneumonia but must be differentiated from metastatic neoplasia (especially hemangiosarcoma)
- Chylothorax secondary to blastomycosis—can occur in dogs
- Focal lytic and proliferative radiographic bone lesions—must be differentiated from osteosarcoma
- Cytologic findings—organisms usually (but not always) plentiful in lesions

Diagnostic Feature

- **Cytology—most definitive method of diagnosis; aspirates from lymph nodes and lungs, impression smears of draining skin lesions, or tracheal wash fluid are often best sources of infective material (Fig. 10-2)**
- Histopathologic findings—bone biopsies, enucleated eyes, or single firm skin pyogranulomas sometimes needed to confirm diagnosis if cytologic examination unsuccessful
- Do not attempt culture of lesions in-hospital, because cultures can be a source of infection to humans; instead send culture material out to diagnostic laboratory if culture is needed.

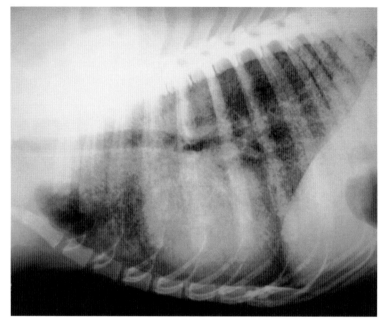

■ **Figure 10-1** Lateral thoracic radiograph of a dog with blastomycosis showing diffuse fine interstitial-to-nodular infiltrates.

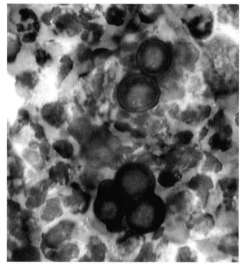

■ **Figure 10-2** Cytologic findings of exudate from a skin lesion showing broad-based, thick-walled budding *Blastomyces* yeast cells on a background of degenerate neutrophils and red blood cells (Diff-Quick stain, 400×).

THERAPEUTICS

- Usually outpatient—oral itraconazole treatment if patient is stable
- Severely dyspneic dogs require an oxygen cage for a minimum of 1 week before lung improvement is sufficient for comfort in room air.
- About 25% have worsening of lung disease during the first few days of treatment, owing to an increase in the inflammatory response after the *Blastomyces* organisms die and release their contents (inflammatory response may be dampened by judicious use of anti-inflammatory glucocorticoids with antifungals).
- Removal of an abscessed lung lobe may be required when medical treatment cannot resolve infection.

Drugs of Choice

Itraconazole

Dogs
- Give with a fat-rich meal, such as canned dog food, for the first 3 days to achieve a therapeutic blood concentration as soon as possible.
- Dogs with neurologic signs should be treated with amphotericin B or fluconazole.
- Treat for a minimum of 60 days or for 1 month after all signs of disease have disappeared.
- Avoid corticosteroid use unless life-threatening dyspnea is present (dexamethasone—0.2 mg/kg, q24h, for 2–3 days in conjunction with itraconazole treatment).

Cats
- Have drug compounded by an appropriate pharmacy or open the 100-mg capsules containing pellets and mix with palatable food.

Alternative Drugs

- Amphotericin B—use in dogs that cannot take oral medication or that do not respond to itraconazole (see *Histoplasmosis*)
- Lipid complex form of amphotericin B—less nephrotoxic than other forms; use in dogs with renal dysfunction that cannot take itraconazole
- Ketoconazole (cheaper alternative to itraconazole)—lower response rate; higher rates of anorexia, malaise, and hepatopathy; higher recurrence rate; not recommended
- Fluconazole—more expensive but fewer side effects than other conazoles and better penetration into ocular and CNS tissues; IV preparation available
- See Table 10-1

TABLE 10-1 Drug Therapy for Blastomycosis in Small Animals

Drug	Species	Dose (mg/kg)	Route	Interval (h)	Duration (days)[a]
Itraconazole	B	5	PO	12[b]	60
Fluconazole	B	5[c]	PO, IV	12	60
AMB deoxycholate	D	0.5	IV	3 times weekly	[d]
	C	0.25	IV	3 times weekly	[e]
AMB-lipid complex (Abelcet)	D	1–2.5	IV[f]	3 times weekly	[g]

[a] Continue treatment at least 30 days beyond resolution of clinical signs.
[b] Dogs—after 3 days, reduce dosing interval to q24h.
[c] Cats—up to a maximum total daily dose of 200 mg.
[d] To a total dose of 12 mg/kg.
[e] To a total dose of 4–10 mg/kg, or until renal toxicity occurs.
[f] IV infusion rate—2.5 mg/kg/hr.
[g] Use for 1 month or until renal toxicity occurs.
B, both cats and dogs; C, cats; D, dogs.

Precautions/Interactions

Itraconazole Toxicity

- Anorexia—most common sign; attributed to liver toxicity; monitor serum ALT monthly (itraconazole induces ALT) for duration of treatment or when anorexia occurs; temporarily discontinue drug for patients with anorexia and ALT activities >200; after appetite improves, restart at half the previously used dose; avoid antacids as they reduce itraconazole absorption
- Ulcerative dermatitis—seen in some dogs; the result of vasculitis; dose-related condition; temporarily discontinue drug; when ulcers have resolved, restart at half the previously used dose
- Teratogenic effects of itraconazole—none reported at therapeutic doses in rats and mice; embryotoxicity found at high doses; no dog or cat studies; one dog started on itraconazole halfway through her pregnancy delivered a normal litter

 COMMENTS

- Inform owner when treatment is costly and requires a minimum of 60–90 days.
- Determine duration of treatment based on resolution of clinical signs and follow-up chest radiographs.
- Considerable permanent lung changes may occur after the infection has resolved, making determination of persistent active disease difficult.
- At 60 days of treatment, if active lung disease is seen, continue treatment for an additional 30 days.
- If lungs are normal, stop treatment and obtain repeat radiographs in 30 days.

- At 90 days of treatment, if condition is the same as at day 60, changes are residual.
- Fibrosis on radiographs indicates inactive disease. If condition is better than at day 60, continue treatment for 30 more days. If lesions are significantly worse than at 60 days, change treatment to amphotericin B and then obtain another radiograph.
- At 120 days of treatment, obtain another radiograph; continue treatment as long as there is improvement in the lungs. If there is no further improvement and no indication of active disease, the lesions are probably scarring.
- Prognosis is death; 25% of dogs die during the first week of treatment. Early diagnosis improves chance of survival.
- Severity of lung involvement and invasion into the CNS affect prognosis.
- Recurrence in about 20% of dogs usually within 3–6 months after completion of treatment, even with 60–90 days of treatment; it may occur up to 15 months after treatment. A second course of itraconazole treatment will cure most patients. Drug resistance to itraconazole has not been observed.
- Inform owners that there is no spread from animals to humans, except through bite wounds; also inform them when inoculation of organisms from dog bites has occurred.
- Caution—avoid cuts during necropsy of infected dogs; avoid needle sticks when aspirating lesions
- Warn clients of the following: Blastomycosis is acquired from an environmental source and that they may have been exposed at the same time as the patient. A common source of exposure has been documented in duck and raccoon hunters. The incidence in dogs is 10 times more than that in humans. Encourage clients with respiratory and skin lesions to inform their physicians that they may have been exposed to blastomycosis.

Abbreviations

AGID, agar gel immunodiffusion; ALT, alanine aminotransferase; CBC, complete blood count; CNS, central nervous system

Suggested Reading

Crews LJ, Feeney DA, Jessen CR, et al. Radiographic findings in dogs with pulmonary blastomycosis: 125 cases (1989-2006) . *J Am Vet Med Assoc* 2008;232:215–221.

Krawiec DR, McKiernan BC, Twardock AR, et al. Use of amphotericin B lipid complex for treatment of blastomycosis in dogs. *J Am Vet Med Assoc* 1996;209:2073–2075.

Legendre AM. Blastomycosis. In: Greene CE, ed. *Infectious Diseases of the Dog and Cat.* Philadelphia: WB Saunders, 2006:569.

Legendre AM, Rohrbach BW, Toal RL, et al. Treatment of blastomycosis with itraconazole in 112 dogs. *J Vet Intern Med* 1996;10:365–371.

Spector D, Legendre AM, Wheat J, et al. Antigen and antibody testing for the diagnosis of blastomycosis in dogs. *J Vet Intern Med* 2008;22:839–843.

Bordetellosis: Cats

DEFINITION/OVERVIEW

- A contagious bacterial disease of cats (and dogs—see *Infectious Canine Tracheobronchitis*) primarily causing respiratory abnormalities and establishing chronic infections

ETIOLOGY/PATHOPHYSIOLOGY

- *Bordetella bronchiseptica*—a small, aerobic gram-negative coccobacillus (Fig. 11-1)
- Infections spread rapidly—usually by direct contact from seemingly healthy cats to others in the same environment
- Infected queens may not shed organisms prepartum but serve as a source of infection to newborn kittens when shedding begins postpartum.
- Stress may serve as a cause of shedding.

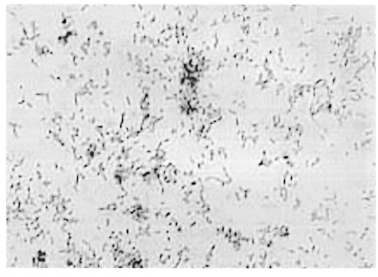

■ **Figure 11-1** Gram stain of *B. bronchiseptica*.

SIGNALMENT/HISTORY

- Most severe in kittens <6 weeks old and kittens living in less than ideal hygienic conditions
- Occurs at all ages and often with pre-existing, subclinical airway disease (e.g., feline herpesvirus and calicivirus infections)
- Predisposition is seen in cats with coexisting subclinical airway disease, such as congenital anomalies, chronic bronchitis, allergic bronchitis, and viral URI.
- No breed or gender predilection recognized

 CLINICAL FEATURES

- May be nonexistent, mild, or severe—for example, kittens with life-threatening pneumonia
- Signs—usually begin ~5 days after exposure to infecting agent
- Bacterial agent—spreads rapidly from apparently healthy cats to others in the same environment
- Fever
- Sneezing
- Nasal discharge
- Mandibular lymphadenopathy
- Spontaneous or induced cough—characteristic of uncomplicated disease

Severe Disease

- Fever—may note constant, low-grade, or fluctuating fever (39.4–40°C [103–104°F])
- Cough—usually moist and productive
- Nasal discharge
- Lethargy
- Anorexia
- Dyspnea as a result of severe pneumonia that can lead to death
- Lung sounds—often normal, but may detect increased intensity of normal sounds, crackles, or (less frequently) wheezes

 DIFFERENTIAL DIAGNOSIS

- Specific diagnosis is difficult.
- Clinical signs mimic those seen with other respiratory disease agents.
- Several agents may be involved concurrently.

- Consider viral URI with secondary bacterial infections other than *Bordetella* (*Pasturella* spp.).
- In severe disease in the individual cat, historic exposure to point source of infection 5 days previously can help differentiate from other severe URIs.

 ## DIAGNOSTICS

- CBC—neutrophilic leukocytosis with a left shift in cases of severe pneumonia
- Serum chemistry profile and urinalysis—usually normal
- Bacterial isolation from oropharyngeal swab specimens—relatively easy during active clinical disease
- PCR—of oropharyngeal swabs or transtracheal wash/bronchoalveolar lavage
- Both bacterial culture and PCR lack sensitivity.
- Bacterial isolation during chronic carrier state—difficult because few organisms are shed
- Thoracic radiographs—unremarkable with uncomplicated disease
- Radiologic examination—useful for ruling out noninfectious causes; may demonstrate an interstitial and alveolar lung pattern with a cranioventral distribution typical of bacterial pneumonia; a diffuse interstitial lung pattern typical of viral pneumonia; a mixed lung pattern (combination of alveolar, interstitial, and peribronchial lung patterns)
- Bacterial cultures by endotracheal wash or tracheobronchial lavage via bronchoscopy—helpful in ruling out other bacterial agents but is rarely indicated except in the case of chronic cough

 ## THERAPEUTICS

- Outpatient—strongly recommended for uncomplicated disease.
- Inpatient—strongly recommended for complicated disease or pneumonia
- Isolation—essential to keep inpatients isolated from the rest of hospital population
- Fluid therapy—with complicated disease or pneumonia
- Cage rest—for at least 14–21 days with uncomplicated disease or for at least the duration of radiographic evidence of pneumonia

Drugs of Choice

- Antibiotic therapy—Ideally, antibiotic should be selected based on culture and sensitivity results.
- Amoxicillin/clavulanic acid—good for kittens
- Doxycycline—very effective, and is the drug of choice
- Tetracyclines—organism usually very susceptible (Table 11-1)

TABLE 11-1 Drug Therapy for Bordetellosis in Cats				
Drug	Dose (mg/kg)	Route	Interval (h)	Duration (days)
Amoxicillin/clavulanic acid	10–20	PO	12	10–14
Doxycycline	3–5	PO, IV	12	10–14
Tetracycline	10	PO	8	10–14

Azithromycin and pradofloxacin—similar efficacy as amoxicillin
- Antimicrobial therapy should continue for at least 10 days beyond resolution of radiographic abnormalities.

Precautions/Interactions

- Tetracycline and related drugs may cause drug-induced fever.
- Doxycycline at high doses has been associated with esophageal stricture in cats; give with food or water.
- Amoxicillin may cause anorexia in cats.

COMMENTS

- Uncomplicated disease should respond to treatment in 10–14 days.
- Diagnosis of uncomplicated disease—question if respiratory signs persist 14 days or more after initiating treatment
- Severe disease—typical course of 2–6 weeks
- Repeat thoracic radiography in severe cases, at least 14 days beyond resolution of all clinical signs.
- Affected cats may shed organisms for at least 19 weeks postinfection.
- Shedding of *B. bronchiseptica* in respiratory secretions of asymptomatic carriers accounts for the persistence of disease in catteries, animal shelters, boarding facilities, and veterinary hospitals.
- *B. bronchiseptica*–infected dogs can be a source of infection for cats.
- Cats can presumably be a source of infection for dogs.
- Kittens in infected environment—seroconvert at 7–10 weeks of age
- Mortality—mainly occurs in kittens <7 weeks of age
- Modified live vaccine available (Protex-Bb; Intervet)—not recommended for routine use
- Vaccination—consider for cats entering or residing in multiple-cat environments in which *B. bronchiseptica* infections associated with clinical disease have been documented
- Zoonosis—Spread of *B. bronchiseptica* from cats to immunocompromised people has been implicated in human infections.

Abbreviations

CBC, complete blood count; PCR, polymerase chain reaction; URI, upper respiratory tract infection.

Suggested Reading

Egberink H, Addie D, Belak S, et al. *Bordetella bronchiseptica* infection in cats. ABCD guidelines on prevention and management. *J Feline Med Surg* 2009;11:610–614.

Helps CR, Lait P, Damhuis A, et al. Factors associated with upper respiratory tract disease caused by feline herpesvirus, feline calicivirus, *Chlamydophila felis* and *Bordetella bronchiseptica* in cats: experience from 218 European catteries. *Vet Rec* 2005;156:669–673.

Botulism

chapter 12

DEFINITION/OVERVIEW

- Disease caused by ingestion of a preformed neurotoxin from a bacterium found in carrion and spoiled foodstuff (raw meat)
- Diagnosis is virtually always based on clinical disease.

ETIOLOGY/PATHOPHYSIOLOGY

- *Clostridium botulinum* type C—obligate anaerobic spore-forming gram-positive rod
- Found worldwide
- Very resistant to disinfectants and environmental exposure
- Botulinal neurotoxin—inhibits acetylcholine release at the neuromuscular junctions and autonomic cholinergic synapses
- Results in diffuse neuromuscular blockade and autonomic dysfunction

SIGNALMENT/HISTORY

- Natural cases—only described in dogs
- Cats—natual infection in 8 cats (4 of which died) after eating pelican carrion recently reported
- Risk factor—ingestion of toxin (usually associated with eating dead decomposing birds, especially ducks)
- Clinical signs occur within hours to 6 days of toxin ingestion.
- Several dogs within a kennel, household, or neighborhood may be affected at once.
- Historically—may initially show vomiting/diarrhea, gastroenteritis from eating carrion
- Acute hind limb weakness ascending to trunk—then front limb, neck, and muscles innervated by cranial nerves become involved
- Gait—initially stiff or short-strided progressing to recumbency within 12–24 hours

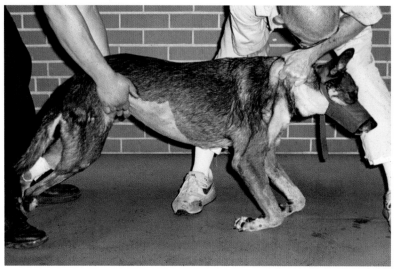

■ **Figure 12-1** Dog with botulism showing tetraparesis with profound lower motor neuron dysfunction, hypotonia, and hyporeflexia, but with normal pain perception (courtesy of Dr. A. deLahunta, Cornell University).

 ## CLINICAL FEATURES

- Severity of signs depends on how much toxin was ingested.
- Signs vary from mild paraparesis to tetraplegia and respiratory muscle paralysis leading to death.
- Patient usually presents with generalized lower motor neuron weakness to tetraplegia with hypotonia, and hyporeflexia (Fig. 12-1).
- Tail tone and movements are preserved.
- Patient remains alert with normal pain perception.
- Cranial nerve dysfunction is present as dysphagia, voice change (weakness), droopy face with poor eyelid closure, poor jaw and tongue tone, megaesophagus.
- Autonomic abnormalities are mydriasis with decreased PLR, ileus or constipation, urine retention or frequent voiding of small volumes, and decreased lacrimation (dry eye).
- Muscle atrophy is marked after 7 days.

 ## DIFFERENTIAL DIAGNOSIS

Three main conditions from which botulism must be differentiated include:
- Idiopathic polyradiculoneuritis—may follow raccoon bite, systemic illness or vaccination; cranial nerve involvement usually limited to facial and pharyngeal/laryngeal paresis; no autonomic signs; hyperesthesia may be present; diffuse denervation potentials on EMG examination because of demyelination of peripheral nerves

- Tick bite paralysis
  - North America—cranial nerve involvement unusual or mild; no autonomic signs; rapid recovery after tick removal
  - Australia—cranial nerve and autonomic signs present; more severe signs may develop after tick removal; EMG: few, if any fibrillation potentials and marked reduction in amplitude of evoked motor potentials
- Myasthenia gravis—exercise-induced weakness; rapid improvement after short period of rest; megaesophagus common, but cranial nerve involvement often limited to moderate facial and pharyngeal/laryngeal paralysis; normal spinal reflexes if patient ambulatory

 DIAGNOSTICS

- CBC and serum biochemical panel—usually normal
- Identify toxin (in ingested material, serum, vomit, and feces) by neutralization test in mice or in vitro tests measuring toxin antigenicity. However, toxin testing is rarely successful and a diagnosis is often made on clinical grounds only.
- Serology to identify a rise in titer of antibodies to *C. botulinum* type C has been used to confirm infection in a dog; titers showed a 4-fold elevation 3 weeks (but not by 10 days) postinfection.
- Radiographic examination may reveal megaesophagus with or without aspiration pneumonia.
- EMG examination—no or few denervation potentials (come back during recovery phase)
- Reduced amplitude of evoked motor potentials

 THERAPEUTICS

- Those in respiratory distress—respiratory support in intensive care facility
- Swallowing difficulties—Placement of a PEG tube will alleviate complications of megaesophagus.
- Care of recumbent patient—frequent turning; good padding; attend to urine scald or place urinary catheter
- Laxatives or enemas—if recent ingestion
- Perform physical therapy (both passive and active)—to prevent tendon contraction and limit muscle atrophy
- Antibiotics—unhelpful because intestinal colonization of organism does not occur
- Antibiotics—indicated if secondary aspiration pneumonia or UTI present
- Medicate dry eye if present.

Drugs of Choice

- Type C or polyvalent containing type C antitoxin—only effective before toxin has bound nerve endings (dosage: 10,000–15,000 U, IV or IM, twice at 4-hour interval)

Precautions/Interactions

- Aminogycosides, procaine penicillin, tetracyclines, phenothiazines, and magnesium may potentiate neuromuscular blockade.
- Antitoxin has the potential to cause anaphylaxis.
- Test for anaphylaxis before use—0.1 ml, ID, 20 minutes before systemic administration

 COMMENTS

- Maximum severity of signs—usually reached within 12–24 hours after signs first start to develop
- Signs disappear in reverse order from the order in which they appeared, but more slowly.
- Complete recovery usually occurs within 1–3 weeks.

Abbreviations

CBC, complete blood count; EMG, electromyography; PEG, percutaneous endoscopic gastrostomy; PLR, pupillary light reflex; UTI, urinary tract infection.

Suggested Reading

Bruchim Y, Steinman A, Markovitz M, et al. Toxicological, bacteriological and serological diagnosis of botulism in a dog. *Vet Rec* 2006;158:768–769.

Elad D, Yas-Natan E, Aroch I, et al. Natural *Clostridium botulinum* type C toxicosis in a group of cats. *J Clin Microbiol* 2004;42:5406–5408.

chapter 13

Brucellosis

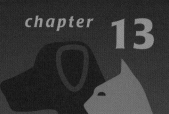

DEFINITION/OVERVIEW

- A contagious disease of dogs characterized by abortion and infertility in females, epididymitis and testicular atrophy in males, and occasionally diskospondylitis

ETIOLOGY/PATHOPHYSIOLOGY

- *Brucella canis*—an intracellular gram-negative coccobacillus
- Target tissues—include those high in gonadal steroids (gravid uterus, fetus, epididymis, and prostate gland) and lymphoid tissues (lymph nodes, spleen, and bone marrow)
- Occasionally grows in other tissues (intervertebral disks, anterior uvea, meninges).

SIGNALMENT/HISTORY

- Most common in beagle dogs, but no known genetic predisposition
- Overall prevalence unknown
- Highest prevalence in dogs from rural areas (particularly of the southern states) and certain kennels (Labrador retrievers over-represented)
- Also high in stray dogs (strays in Mexico have a 25–30% seroprevalence)
- Pets are occasionally affected.
- No age preference, but it is more common in sexually mature dogs.
- Females are more commonly affected than males.

CLINICAL FEATURES

- Suspect disease whenever a female dog aborts or has reproductive failures or males have genital disease.
- Affected dogs (especially females) usually appear healthy or have vague signs of illness.

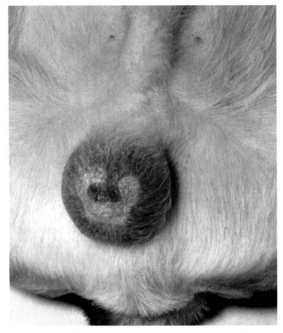

■ **Figure 13-1** Scrotal dermatitis may develop in dogs with *B. canis* due to self-trauma (rubbing scrotum on ground, licking) as a result of pain from epidydimitis.

- Lethargy
- Loss of libido
- Lymphadenopathy
- Back pain
- Abortion—a consistent sign
- Abortion—commonly occurs 6–8 weeks after conception (although pregnancy may terminate at any stage)
- Males may have swollen scrotal sacs, scrotal dermatitis (Fig. 13-1), enlarged and firm epididymis (Fig. 13-2), unilateral or bilateral testicular atrophy.
- Chronic and recurrent unilateral anterior uveitis without other systemic signs of disease; also includes iris hyperpigmentation, vitreal infiltrates, and multifocal chorioretinitis
- Diskospondylitis—spinal pain with ataxia
- Glomerulonephritis—weight loss, elevated blood pressure; rare

 DIFFERENTIAL DIAGNOSIS

- Abortions or chronic infertility—maternal, fetal, or placental abnormalities; systemic infections (canine distemper, herpesvirus, *Brucella abortus*, *Escherichia coli*, leptospirosis, toxoplasmosis, neosporosis); chronic endometritis; hypothyroidism

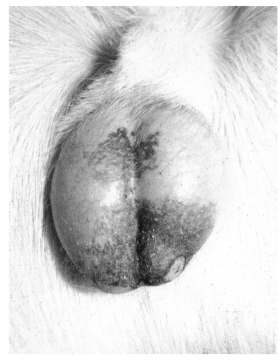

■ **Figure 13-2** Epidydimitis is a common finding in dogs with *B. canis*.

- Epididymitis and scrotal edema—inguinal hernias, blastomycosis, RMSF
- Diskospondylitis—most often caused by *Staphylococcus* but also fungal infections, actinomycosis, *Streptococcus* spp., nocardiosis, and others

 DIAGNOSTICS

- CBC and biochemical profile—usually normal
- Chronically infected dogs–hyperglobulinemia with hypoalbuminemia
- Urinalysis and biochemistry—may reflect protein-losing nephropathy if glomerulonephritis exists (hypoalbuminemia, proteinuria)
- Urinalysis—usually normal even if bacteria can be cultured from urine
- CSF—pleocytosis (mainly neutrophils) with elevated protein in meningioencephalitis; normal in diskospondylitis
- Serology—three main tests (all susceptible to error):
  - RSAT—commercially available; becomes positive 3–4 weeks postinfection; rapid and very good at identifying true-negative status; high rate of false-positive results (50%), so positive results must be confirmed by other tests
  - Mercaptoethanol tube agglutination test—semiquantitative test; similar to RSAT in its lack of specificity

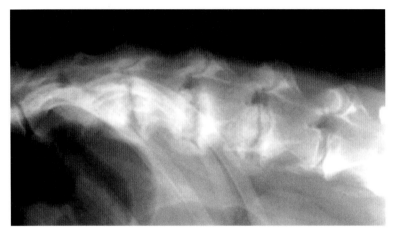

■ **Figure 13-3** Lateral radiograph of lumbar vertebrae of a dog with diskospondylitis caused by *B. canis*.

- AGID—highly sensitive (if uses cell wall lipopolysaccharide antigen of *B. canis*), but can give false-positive results in negative dogs; if soluble antigens (extracted from bacterial cytoplasm) are used, test is highly specific for antibodies against other *Brucella* spp. (*B. suis*, *B. abortus*) that infect dogs; may give false-negative results if performed soon after infection.
- Procedure for serologically testing dogs—First use RSAT; if positive, confirm using an AGID.
- Organism—can be isolated from the blood (if no antibiotics have been used) 2–4 weeks postinfection, and persist for 8 months to 5 years.
- Best results for blood culture—most likely to be positive 1–28 months postinfection.
- Cultures of vaginal discharges after abortion—usually positive
- Culture of semen—usually positive if collected in a sterile manner
- Semen examination—commonly reveals sperm abnormalities 5–8 weeks postinfection, aspermia in dogs with bilateral testicular atrophy
- Lymph node biopsies—shows lymphoid hyperplasia with plasma cell hyperplasia, intracellular bacteria (special stain: Brown–Brenn).
- Imaging—may reveal diskospondylitis lesions (Fig. 13-3), as well as splenomegaly and osteomyelitis in some dogs; radiographic changes often slow in developing and may not be present even when pain is present
- PCR—shown to be more sensitive than blood culture and serology in detecting infection in human patients

THERAPEUTICS

- Antibiotic treatment—recommended only for nonbreeding dogs or those that have been spayed or castrated
- Antibiotic therapy outcome—uncertain at best

- If attempting antibiotic treatment in intact dogs, be aware that the risk of transmission to other dogs still remains.
- Aim of antibiotic treatment—to have dogs seroconvert to negative and be abacteremic for at least 3 months
- Best treatment efficacy—achieved by high-dose doxycycline in combination with injectable streptomycin
- If streptomycin is not available, substitute gentamicin for streptomycin.
- Using gentamicin in combination with doxycycline improves the overall efficacy of treatment (over doxycycline alone) but is not as efficacious as using doxycycline and streptomycin in combination.
- Dogs with diskospondylitis often experience recurrence of hyperesthetic episodes, requiring repeated treatments with doxycycline; surgical intervention is rarely if ever needed.
- Enrofloxacin—recently shown to be effective, and may have added antibacterial effects when combined with doxycycline or gentamicin
- Multiple drug combination therapy—Gentamicin or streptomycin, doxycycline, enrofloxacin, and rifampin have been successful in treating ocular disease in dogs.

Drugs of Choice

- Doxycycline
- Gentamicin
- Enrofloxacin (Table 13-1)

Precautions/Interactions

- Use of doxycycline is contraindicated in pregnant or lactating bitches.
- Use doxycycline with caution in pups <6 months of age—risk of tooth discoloration
- Avoid the development of esophagitis—Give doxycycline with food or liquids.
- Gentamicin—nephrotoxic; monitor for casts in urine; avoid giving drug to animals with dehydration, renal disease, or cardiac failure or with other drugs that may exacerbate renal disease, including tetracyclines (but not including doxycycline)
- Enrofloxacin—avoid in young (<12 months), growing animals as can cause cartilaginous injury; avoid in dogs with marked renal insufficiency

TABLE 13-1 Drug Therapy for Brucellosis in Dogs				
Drug	Dose (mg/kg)	Route	Interval (h)	Duration (weeks)
Doxycycline	12–15	PO	12	4
Gentamicin	5	SC	24	1[a]
Enrofloxacin[b]	5	PO	24	4

[a] Repeat after 1 week.
[b] Combine with doxycycline or gentamicin for added bacterial effects.

COMMENTS

- Control of brucellosis in a kennel—problematic
- First confirm—by isolation of the organism before antibiotic treatments are initiated
- Quarantine infected kennels—All confirmed infected animals should be eliminated.
- Animals should not be admitted or released from the kennel until the disease has been eradicated.
- All dogs in the infected kennels—serotest for at least 3 months after seronegative status has been achieved, especially before each breeding
- If infected dogs are to be treated with antibiotics, they should be neutered and moved to separate housing.
- Clean kennels—use quaternary ammonium compounds or iodophors
- Identify carrier dogs—essential, because these are usually responsible for transmission to other kennels
- New acquisitions into a kennel—only admit if serologically negative on testing on two occasions 1 month apart
- Warn clients—*B. canis* is infectious to humans.
- Contact with aborting bitches—main source of infection to humans
- Clinical signs in humans—relatively mild (fevers, fatigue, malaise, lymphadenopathy) and easily treated with tetracyclines

Abbreviations

AGID, Agar gel immunodiffusion; CBC, complete blood count; CSF, cerebral spinal fluid; RMSF, Rocky Mountain spotted fever; RSAT, rapid 2-ME slide agglutination test.

Suggested Reading

Carmichael LE, Greene CE. Canine brucellosis. In: Greene CE, ed. *Infectious Diseases of the Dog and Cat*. Philadelphia: WB Saunders, 2006:369–381.

Keid LB, Soares RM, Vasconcellos SA, et al. Comparison of agar gel immunodiffusion test, rapid slide agglutination test, microbiological culture, and PCR for the diagnosis of canine brucellosis. *Res Vet Sci* 2009;86:22–26.

Ledbetter EC, Landry MP, Stokol T, et al. *Brucella canis* endophthalmitis in 3 dogs: clincial features, diagnosis, and treatment. *Vet Ophthalmol* 2009;12:183–191.

Lucero NE, Corazza R, Almuzara MN, et al. Human *Brucella canis* outbreak linked to infection in dogs. *Epidemiol Infect* 2009;5:1–6.

Wanke MM, Delpino MV, Baldi PC. Use of enrofloxacin in the treatment of canine brucellosis in a dog kennel (clinical trial). *Theriogenology* 2006;66:1573–1578.

Campylobacteriosis

chapter 14

DEFINITION/OVERVIEW

- A gastrointestinal bacterial infection of dogs and cats (and other mammals)—causes a superficial erosive enterocolitis resulting in diarrhea

ETIOLOGY/PATHOPHYSIOLOGY

- *Campylobacter jejuni*—fastidious microaerophilic gram-negative curved bacteria often isolated from the feces of normal cats and dogs
- Infection occurs by the fecal–oral route from contaminated food, water, fresh meat, and environment.
- Localizes in mucus-filled crypts of small intestine—bacteria produce enterotoxin, cytotoxin, cytolethal-distending toxin, and invasin
- May invade intestinal mucosa—leads to ulceration, edema, congestion of the intestine, resulting in hematochezia, leukocytes in the feces (occasionally septicemia) with bacteria shed in feces for weeks to months afterward
- Young dogs (but not cats) with diarrhea—more animals shed organisms than nondiarrheic animals

Campylobacter spp often found in raw meat diets (especially chicken) fed to dogs and cats.

SIGNALMENT/HISTORY

- Found in dogs; less commonly cats
- Higher prevalence in puppies and kittens (birth to 6 months of age)
- Organism often found in dogs and cats with chronic diarrhea
- Risk factors are kennels with poor hygiene, immunosuppression or GI parasitism, or other concurrent causes of diarrhea.

CLINICAL FEATURES

- Diarrhea—ranges from mucus-like and watery to blood-streaked; sometimes chronic
- Tenesmus common
- Fever (rare and usually mild)
- Anorexia
- Intermittent vomiting may accompany diarrhea.
- Young animals (<6 months)—signs more severe
- Adults—usually asymptomatic carriers

 ## DIFFERENTIAL DIAGNOSIS

- Other causes of acute enterocolitis—dietary indiscretion; IBD; neoplasia (especially GI lymphoma); drugs (antibiotics); toxins (lead); parasites (cryptosporidiosis, trichomoniasis, giardiasis, whipworms); infectious agents (parvovirus, FIP, salmonellosis, rickettsia, GI bacterial overgrowth, clostridia, histoplasmosis, leishmaniasis, pythiosis, other rare infections); systemic organ dysfunction (renal, hepatic, pancreatic, cardiac); metabolic (hypoadrenocorticism, feline hyperthyroidism)

 ## DIAGNOSTICS

- CBC—leukocytosis only with septicemia
- Biochemical panel—reflects effects of diarrhea and dehydration
- Fecal smear—high leukocyte count
- Gram stain of feces (leaving counterstain [safranin] on for longer than usual)—will demonstrate curved gram-negative "seagull" bacteria (Fig. 14-1)
- Wet mount of feces (1 drop mixed with 1 drop of saline, coverslip) viewed on phase (condenser down) at 403× magnification will show large numbers of curved, highly motile bacteria with characteristic darting motility.
- Transportation to laboratory—organisms remain viable in feces at room temperature for 3 days, 7 days if refrigerated
- Fecal culture—grown for 48 hours on special *Campylobacter* blood agar plates
- Species-specific quantitative PCR—targets the 60-kDa chaperonin gene of different *Campylobacter* spp.

 ## THERAPEUTICS

- Mild diarrhea—treated with antibiotics as outpatients
- Self-limiting—usually

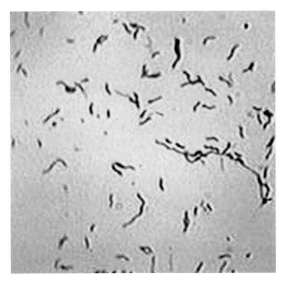

■ **Figure 14-1** *Campylobacter* organisms in the feces of a dog. Note the large number of curved bacteria often referred to as "seagull" shaped (1500×).

- Severe neonatal diarrhea—may require oral fluid therapy if not vomiting
- If dehydrated—IV fluid support, or plasma (if albumin <2.0 mg/dl)
- Antibiotics—recommended if signs of systemic illness or diarrhea persists beyond 5 days, also in immunosuppressed patients

Drugs of Choice

- Erythromycin
- Tylosin—Tylan soluble powder (Elanco; 100-g containers; <3 g/tsp)
- Neomycin
- Enrofoxacin (Table 14-1)

Precautions/Interactions

- Erythromycin may cause GI irritability, resulting in vomiting, anorexia, and diarrhea.
- Enrofloxacin can produce adverse effects of arthropathy in dogs 4–28 weeks of age.

TABLE 14-1 Drug Therapy for Campylobacteriosis in Dogs and Cats				
Drug	Dose (mg/kg)	Route	Interval (h)	Duration (days)
Enrofloxacin	5–20[a]	PO	24	7
Erythromycin	10–20	PO	8	5
Tylosin	11	PO	8	7
Neomycin	10–20	PO	8	5

[a]5 mg/kg for cats

- If GI irritability occurs—stop until signs abate, then restart at half the dose; slowly, over 48 hours, work back up to full dose

 COMMENTS

- Erythromycin is the drug of choice.
- Repeat fecal culture after completion of treatment.
- Zoonosis—Good hand-cleaning hygiene is usually sufficient to prevent infection of humans.
- Reduce fecal contamination in kennel situations—remove solid waste, disinfect runs and food and water bowls
- Avoid feeding raw-meat diets to dogs and cats.

Abbreviations

FIP, feline infectious peritonitis; GI, gastrointestinal; IBD, inflammatory bowel disease; PCR, polymerase chain reaction.

Suggested Reading

Altekruse SF, Tollefson LK. Human campylobacteriosis: a challenge for the veterinary profession. *J Am Vet Med Assoc* 2003;223:445–452.

Chaban B, Ngeleka M, Hill JE. Detection and quantification of 14 *Campylobacter* species in pet dogs reveals an increase in species richness in feces of diarrheic animals. *BMC Microbiol* 2010;10:73.

Elwood C, Devauchelle P, Elliott J, et al. Emesis in dogs: a review. *J Small Anim Pract* 2010;51:4–22.

Fox JG. Enteric bacterial infections. In: Greene CE, ed. *Infectious Diseases of the Dog and Cat*. Philadelphia: WB Saunders, 2006:339–343.

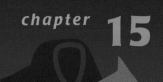

Candidiasis

DEFINITION/OVERVIEW

- Opportunistic yeast (part of the normal flora of the mouth, nose, ears, and GI and genital tracts) that causes disease by colonizing damaged tissues of dogs and cats

ETIOLOGY/PATHOPHYSIOLOGY

- *Candida albicans*—normal flora on mucous membranes of cats and dogs
- Recovery of organisms from mucous membranes—does not imply disease
- Opportunistic—colonizing damaged tissues or invading normal tissues of immuno-suppressed animals
- Pathogenic role—determined by identifying a fungemia, infiltration of organisms into the tissues, or signs of organisms in presumed sterile sites (e.g., urinary bladder)
- Conditions that suppress the immune system—increase the likelihood of isolation in asymptomatic animal
- FIV—*C. albicans* has been isolated from throat cultures five times more often in FIV-infected cats than in asymptomatic, non–FIV-infected cats of a similar age and sex.
- Infection—rare
- Infection—usually associated with neutropenia (secondary to parvovirus, retrovirus infection, bone marrow suppression), diabetes mellitus, retrovirus-induced immuno-suppression, chronic glucocorticoid treatment, prolonged antibiotic treatment, and gastrotomy tubes, indwelling urinary catheters, urethrostomy, IV catheters, and incomplete emptying of the bladder

SIGNALMENT/HISTORY

- Cats—occurs less commonly than in dogs
- Historically—skin damaged by burns, trauma, or necrotizing dermatitis predisposes to infection
- Urinary tract—preferred site in diabetic cats, secondary to indwelling catheters, and cats that have urinary retention due to strictures secondary to urethrostomy

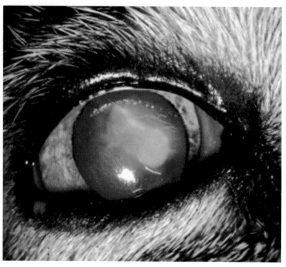

■ **Figure 15-1** Chronic keratitis in a cat caused by *C. albicans* (courtesy of Dr. R. Riis, Cornell University).

CLINICAL FEATURES

- Urinary bladder involvement—cystitis (pollakiuria, hematuria, proteinuria, WBCs in urine)
- Ear infection—head shaking and scratching
- Oral cavity involvement—drooling
- Keratitis—rare, occasionally seen after extensive use of intraocular antibiotic-steroid treatment (Fig. 15-1)
- Inflammation around IV catheters or gastrotomy tubes
- Ulcerative, red skin lesions
- Systemic disease with pericarditis, spondylitis, and neurologic signs

DIFFERENTIAL DIAGNOSIS

- Suspect candidiasis—when a primary infection (otitis, cystitis) does not respond to treatment, especially with antibiotics, but becomes worse

DIAGNOSTICS

- Urinalysis—may show yeast form or clumps of mycelial elements (pseudohyphae) accompanied by an increase in inflammatory cells (Fig. 15-2); normal fat globules in cat urine may adhere, giving the appearance of budding yeast.

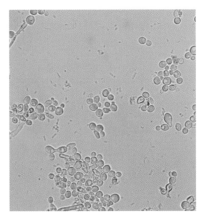

■ **Figure 15-2** Urinalysis from a dog with *C. albicans* infection of the urinary bladder showing the yeast form with some mycelial elements and increased numbers of inflammatory cells (courtesy of Dr. T. Stokol, Cornell University).

- Pyuria without bacterial growth—culture for fungi and *Mycoplasma* organisms
- Collect urine sample by cystocentesis—A culture of a large number of yeast colonies strongly supports a diagnosis.
- Neutropenic patients—inflammatory response may be absent
- Biopsy sometimes needed to determine whether *Candida* is truly a pathogen—requires demonstration of organisms penetrating the tissues
- Otitis (dogs)—Culture of *Candida* organisms or identification of yeast or mycelial elements on ear cytologic examination suggests the diagnosis.
- Blood cultures may identify fungal organisms.

 THERAPEUTICS

- Try to remove inciting factor:
  - Regulate diabetes mellitus.
  - Remove indwelling catheters.
  - Treat underlying cause of neutropenia.
  - Improve immune suppression, if possible (remove or modify chemotherapeutic drugs).

Drugs of Choice

Topical

- Treatment of infected mucous membranes
- Nystatin (e.g., Nilstat cream)
- Clotrimazole (e.g., Lotrimin cream)
- Miconazole (e.g., Conofite cream)

TABLE 15-1 Drug Therapy for Candidiasis in Dogs and Cats

Drug	Dose (mg/kg)	Route	Interval (h)	Duration (weeks)
Nystatin cream (100,000 U/g)	—	Topical	8–12	2
Clotrimazole cream (1%)	—	Topical	6–8	1
Miconazole cream (2%)	—	Topical	12–24	3
Fluconazole	5	PO	12	4
Itraconazole	5–10	PO	12–24	4
Clotrimazole solution (1%)[a]	10–30 ml	Bladder infusion	48	—

[a]Infuse into the bladder every other day for 3 treatments.

Systemic

- Fluconazole (Diflucan; Pfizer)—very effective; excreted unchanged in the urine, achieving a high concentration in commonly infected sites
- Itraconazole (Sporanox; Janssen)—effective but not as effective as fluconazole; use if the organism becomes resistant to fluconazole; not recommended for UTI because it is not excreted in the urine
- Clotrimazole (Lotrimin solution; Schering-Plough Animal Health)—infused into the bladder if urinary tract *Candida* infection resistant to fluconazole (Table 15-1)

Precautions/Interactions

- Fluconazole and itraconazole—hepatic toxicity; monitor serum ALT monthly and check if patient becomes anorexic; withdraw drug if ALT >200 U or with anorexia
- After signs have resolved—obtain repeat culture of sites of infection; continue treatment for 2 weeks more; repeat culture examination 2 weeks after completion of treatment and again if signs recur

 COMMENTS

- Prognosis—should resolve within 2–4 weeks of treatment
- Genetic similarities between human and animal isolates suggest a potential for transfer of *C. albicans* between species.

Abbreviations

ALT, alanine aminotransferase; FIV, feline immunodeficiency virus; GI, gastrointestinal; IV, intravenous; UTI, urinary tract infection; WBC, white blood cell.

Suggested Reading

Forward ZA, Legendre AM, Khalsa HDS. Use of intermittent bladder infusion with clotrimazole for treatment of candiduria in a dog. *J Am Vet Med Assoc* 2002;220:1496–1498.

Greene CE, Chandler FW. Candidiasis, torulopsosis, rhodotorulosis. In: Greene CE, ed. *Infectious Diseases of the Dog and Cat*. Philadelphia: WB Saunders,2006:627–633.

Jin Y, Lin D. Fungal urinary tract infections in the dog and cat: a retrospective study (2001-2004). *J Am Anim Hosp Assoc* 2005;41:373–381.

Pressler BM, Vaden SL, Lane IF, et al. *Candida* spp. urinary tract infections in 13 dogs and 7 cats: predisposing factors, treatment, and outcome. *J Am Anim Hosp Assoc* 2003;39:263–270.

Canine Coronavirus Infection

DEFINITION/OVERVIEW

- A viral infection causing sporadic outbreaks of vomiting and diarrhea (CECoV) or respiratory infection (CRCoV) in dogs

ETIOLOGY/PATHOPHYSIOLOGY

- Coronaviruses undergo rapid evolution, are highly variable, and differences in virulence between individual isolates are likely.
- Distribution—worldwide, including wild canids
- CECoV-feces—primary source of infection; infection—inapparent usually
- Virus—restricted to upper two-thirds of the small intestine and associated lymph nodes
- Crypt cells spared—unlike in CPV
- Mild to severe enteritis may occur—most dogs recover uneventfully
- Death—reported in young pups
- Virus shedding—in feces for about 2 weeks
- Simultaneous infection with CPV—results in severe diarrhea; often fatal
- CRCoV-respiratory secretions and fomites primary source of infection
- Associated with the kennel cough complex
- Can have assymptomatic carriers

SIGNALMENT/HISTORY

- Only wild and domestic dogs are known to be susceptible to disease.
- Cats can have inapparent infections.
- No age or breed predilection
- Stress (e.g., intensive training, crowding) is greatest risk factor.
- Sporadic outbreaks occur in dogs attending shows and in kennels, where the introduction of new dogs is frequent.

- Crowding and unsanitary conditions promote clinical illness.
- CRCoV may be seasonal, with infections more common in winter.

 CLINICAL FEATURES

- CECoV adults—most infections inapparent
- Puppies—may develop severe, fatal enteritis
- Incubation period—short (1–3 days)
- Sudden onset of vomiting—usually only once
- Vomiting—followed by diarrhea
- Diarrhea—may be explosive; yellow–green or orange; loose or liquid; typically malodorous
- Diarrhea—may persist for a few days up to 3 weeks; may recur later
- Young pups may suffer severe, protracted diarrhea and dehydration with anorexia and depression common.
- CRCoV—mild respiratory effects, mainly coughing

 DIFFERENTIAL DIAGNOSIS

- Consider all causes of diarrhea, including systemic or metabolic disease as well as specific intestinal disorders.
- Other causes of acute enterocolitis in very young puppies—dietary indiscretion or intolerance; drugs (antibiotics); toxins (lead); parasites (cryptosporidiosis, giardiasis, hookworms, roundworms); infectious agents (parvovirus, salmonellosis, GI tract bacterial overgrowth, campylobacteriosis, clostridial enterotoxicosis); systemic organ dysfunction (renal, hepatic, pancreatic, cardiac); metabolic (hypoadrenocorticism, hypoglycemia); GI tract foreign body
- Other causes of acute respiratory disease in young animals—other infectious causes of kennel cough, including viral (adenovirus-2, parainfluenza, herpes, canine influenza, distemper), bacterial (*Bordetella bronchiseptica, Streptococcus equi zooepidemicus*) and *Mycoplasma cynos*, fungal (blastomycosis, histoplasmosis), and some parasitic (*Crenosoma vulpis*), *Oslerus osleri, Filaroides*, migatory parasites, heartworm), aspiration pneumonia

 DIAGNOSTICS

- CBC and serum biochemical profile—usually normal unless severe dehydration
- Serologic tests—available but not standardized

- Antibody titers—generally low; may not indicate recent infection because of high rate of asymptomatic infection
- Viral isolation for CECoV—from feces in feline cell cultures at onset of diarrhea will identify virus; prolonged and often impractical. Isolation for CRCoV is difficult and not recommended.
- PCR—using type/strain-specific probes
- Immunofluorescent staining of frozen sections of the small intestine in fatal cases—may reveal viral antigen in cells lining the villous epithelium
- Electron microscopy of feces—typical CCV particles (interpretation requires expertise)
- Because other enteric infections augment the disease, check feces for CPV and parasites.

 # THERAPEUTICS

- Most affected dogs recover without treatment.
- CECoV—Hospitalization for supportive fluid and electrolyte treatment is indicated in severe infections with dehydration in very young puppies.
- CRCoV—treatment as for kennel cough complex

Drugs of Choice

- Antibiotics—administer if enteritis is severe, or sepsis or respiratory illness are present
- Use GI tract antibiotics—ampicillin, ceftiofur, cefazolin, gentamicin (Table 16-1)

Precautions/Interactions

- CCV—highly contagious and will spread rapidly
- Strict isolation and sanitation—essential in the kennel
- Infections by other enteric pathogens—believed to augment the disease

TABLE 16-1 Antibiotic Therapy to Consider for Use in Canine Coronaviral Enteritis

Drug	Dose (mg/kg)	Route	Interval (h)	Duration (days)
Ampicillin	10–20	IV, IM, SC	6–8	5
Ceftiofur (Naxcel)	2–5	SC	12	5
Cefazolin (Ancef, Kefzol)	22	IV, IM	8	5
Gentamicin[a]	2–4	IM, SC	8	5

[a] Ensure animal is well hydrated before administration; check for nephrotoxicity by examining urine sediment. Can be given in combination with ampicillin.

COMMENTS

- Vaccines (for CECoV only)—controversial
- Inactivated and live viral vaccines available—appear to be safe but efficacy unknown, except for brief periods (2–4 weeks) after vaccination
- Vaccination—not recommended
- Vaccines for CECoV do not cross-protect against CRCoV.
- Diarrhea—may persist 10–12 days and may recur
- Prognosis—normally good, except severe infections in young pups
- Prognosis—majority recover after a few days of illness
- Fluid or soft stools—may persist for several weeks
- Virus—readily inactivated by disinfectants, drying, or steam cleaning

Abbreviations

CBC, complete blood count; CCV, canine coronavirus; CECoV, canine enteric coronavirus; CPV, canine parvovirus; CRCoV, canine respiratory coronavirus; GI, gastrointestinal; PCR, polymerase chain reaction.

Suggested Reading

Decaro N, Buonavoglia C. An update on canine coronaviruses: viral evolution and pathobiology. *Vet Microbiol* 2008;132:221–234.

Erles K, Brownlie J. Canine respiratory coronavirus: an emerging pathogen in the canine infectious respiratory disease complex. *Vet Clin North Am Small Anim Pract* 2008;38:815–825.

McCaw DL, Hoskins JD. Canine viral enteritis. In: Greene CE. *Infectious Diseases of the Dog and Cat.* Philadelphia: WB Saunders, 2006;63–73.

17 *chapter*

Canine Distemper

DEFINITION/OVERVIEW

- A viral infection of dogs causing acute to subacute febrile and often fatal disease with respiratory, GI, and CNS manifestations

ETIOLOGY/PATHOPHYSIOLOGY

- Morbillivirus (in the Paramyxoviridae family)—affects many different species of the order Carnivora
- Mortality rate—varies greatly among species
- Natural route of infection—airborne and droplet exposure
- Nasal cavity, pharynx, and lungs—Macrophages carry the virus from these structures to local lymph nodes, where virus replication occurs.
- Within 1 week postinfection, virtually all lymphatic tissues become infected.
- Spreads via viremia to surface epithelium of respiratory, GI, and urogenital tracts and to the CNS.
- Fever (for 1–2 days) and lymphopenia—may be the only findings during initial period
- Further development of disease depends on the virus strain and the immune response.
- Strong cellular and humoral immune response may remain subclinical.
- Weak immune response—subacute infection; may survive longer
- Failure of immune response—death within 2–4 weeks postinfection
- Seizures and other CNS disturbances—frequent causes of death
- Affects—all lymphatic tissues; surface epithelium in the respiratory, alimentary, and urogenital tracts; endocrine and exocrine glands; and nervous tissues
- Domestic dogs—restricted to sporadic outbreaks
- Wildlife (raccoons, skunks, fox)—fairly common

SIGNALMENT/HISTORY

- Most carnivores are affected—Canidae, Hyaenidae, Mustelidae, Procyonidae, Viverridae; also felidae (large cats in zoos and wild)
- Young animals—more susceptible than are adults

CLINICAL FEATURES

- Fever, first peak—occurs 3–6 days postinfection; may pass unnoticed
- Fever, second peak—several days later (and intermittent thereafter); usually associated with nasal and ocular discharge, depression, and anorexia
- Fever followed by GI and/or respiratory signs—often enhanced by secondary bacterial infection
- CNS—many infected dogs; often, but not always, after systemic disease; depends on the virus strain
- CNS presentation—either acute gray matter disease (seizures and myoclonus with depression) or subacute white matter disease (incoordination ataxia, paresis, paralysis, and muscle tremors). Some dogs die 4–5 weeks postinfection from noninflammatory demyelinating disease; others recover with minimal CNS injury.
- Meningeal signs of hyperesthesia and cervical rigidity—may be seen in both
- Optic neuritis and retinal lesions—not uncommon; sometimes injected scleral blood vessels from anterior uveitis
- Hardening of the footpads (hyperkeratosis) and nose—some virus strains; now much less common
- Enamel hypoplasia of the teeth after neonatal infection—common
- In utero infection of fetuses in antibody-negative bitches—rare
- May lead to abortion or persistent infection—Infected neonates may develop fatal disease by 4–6 weeks of age.

 ## DIFFERENTIAL DIAGNOSIS

- Consider—in any young, unvaccinated dog with multifocal CNS disease and other organ involvement
- Kennel cough—Distemper can mimic the respiratory disease in young pups.
- Enteric signs—differentiate from CPV and CCV infections, parasitism (giardiasis, hookworms, roundworms), bacterial infections, gastroenteritis from toxin ingestion, or IBD
- CNS form—differentiate from granulomatous meningoencephalomyelitis, protozoal encephalitis (toxoplasmosis, neosporosis), cryptococcosis or other infections (meningitis, ehrlichiosis, RMSF), pug dog encephalitis, and lead poisoning

 ## DIAGNOSTICS

- CBC—lymphopenia during early infection

Diagnostic Feature

- **Blood cell inclusions—occasionally seen in circulating lymphocytes and, rarely, in monocytes, neutrophils, and RBCs (Fig. 17-1)**
- Radiology—MRI-sensitive for visualization of demylination
- Serology—limited value; positive antibody results do not differentiate between vaccination and exposure to virulent virus

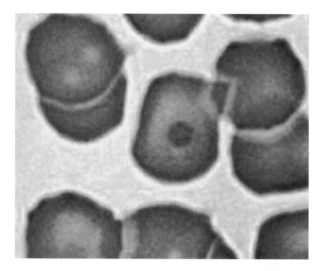

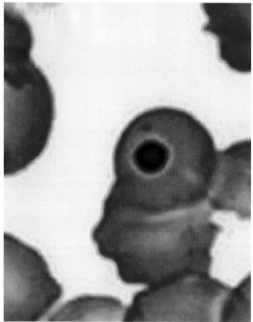

■ **Figure 17-1** Inclusion bodies within the red blood cells of a dog infected with CDV. Distinguishable from Howell–Jolly bodies because CDV inclusions tend to be darker staining and larger (A, Wright's stain; B, Giemsa stain, 1400×.)

- Acute disease—Patient may die from acute disease before neutralizing antibody can be produced.
- IgM responses—may be seen for up to 3 months after exposure to virulent virus and for up to 3 weeks after vaccination
- CDV antibody in CSF—offers definitive evidence of distemper encephalitis because antibody is locally produced and not elevated even in vaccinated animals; may see false-positive titers if CSF is contaminated by blood during collection process or if a bleed into the CNS has occurred
- To avoid false-positive CSF antibody results—compare ratio of CDV antibody titer in CSF to serum; if >1 in association with consistent clinical signs, strongly indicative of distemper encephalitis
- To increase predictive value of this ratio comparison even further—compare ratio to corresponding CSF/serum antibody ratio for another infectious agent against which the dog has been vaccinated (e.g., CPV or CAV); if CDV is greater, the only way elevation can occur is by the presence of distemper encephalitis.
- Vaccination or CDV infection without CNS involvement—will not increase CDV antibody titers in CSF
- Viral antigen or viral inclusions—in buffy coat cells and conjunctival or vaginal imprints; negative results do not rule out the diagnosis.
- PCR on buffy coat and urine sediment cells—more sensitive
- CSF—test for cell and protein content, CDV-specific antibody, interferon, and viral antigen early in disease course
- Tissue immunofluorescence and/or immunocytochemistry, virus isolation, and/or PCR—preferred tissues from lungs, stomach, urinary bladder, lymph nodes, and brain
- Virus may persist in skin for up to 60 days postinfection—PCR and immunocyto-chemistry may help in identifying CDV in skin biopsies; high false-negative rate

 THERAPEUTICS

- Inpatients and in isolation—to prevent infection of other dogs
- Symptomatic nursing care—including intravenous fluids (with anorexia and diarrhea) or parenteral nutrition
- Once fever and secondary bacterial infections are controlled, patients usually begin to eat again.

Drugs of Choice

- Antiviral drugs—none known to be effective
- Antibiotics—to reduce secondary bacterial infection, because CDV is highly immuno-suppressive

- Anticonvulsant therapy—phenobarbital, potassium bromide; to control myoclonus and seizures
- Vaccination—MLV-CD—prevents infection and disease
- Two types of MLV-CD available:
  - Canine tissue culture–adapted vaccines (e.g., Rockborn strain)—induce complete immunity in virtually 100% of susceptible dogs; rarely, a postvaccinal fatal encephalitis develops 7–14 days after vaccination, especially in immunosuppressed animals.
  - Chick embryo–adapted vaccines (e.g., Onderstepoort, Lederle strain)—safer; postvaccinal encephalitis does not occur; only about 80% of susceptible dogs seroconvert.
- Other species—Chick embryo can safely be used in a variety of zoo and wildlife species (e.g., gray fox); Rockborn type is fatal in these animals.
- Killed vaccines—useful for species for which either type of MLV-CD is fatal (e.g., red panda, black-footed ferret)
- Canarypox recombinant CDV vaccine
- Because most pups lose protection from maternal antibody at 6–12 weeks of age, give 2–3 vaccinations during this period.
- Heterotypic (measles virus) vaccination—recommended for pups that have maternal antibody; induces protection from disease but not from infection

Precautions/Interactions

- Corticosteroids—not to be used because they augment the immunosuppression and may enhance viral dissemination; anti-inflammatory levels may provide short-term control of signs.
- Tetracyclines—may produce renal tubular necrosis at high doses; produce yellow discoloration of teeth in young animals
- Fluoroquinolones—may produce arthropathy in dogs up to 6 months of age; potentiate seizures in epileptic animal.

    COMMENTS

- Inform client—mortality rate is about 50% once the dog has contracted CDV
- Death—typically occurs 2 weeks to 3 months postinfection
- Dogs that appear to recover from early catarrhal signs may later develop fatal CNS signs, such as myoclonus (which may continue for several months).
- Owners can avoid infection of pups by isolation to prevent infection from wildlife (e.g., raccoons, fox, skunks) or from CDV-infected dogs.
- Recovered dogs are not carriers.
- Zoonotic risk—possible that humans may become subclinically infected with CDV
- Immunization against measles virus also protects humans against CDV infection.

Abbreviations

CAV, canine adenovirus; CBC, complete blood count; CCV, canine coronavirus; CDV, canine distemper virus; CNS, central nervous system; CSF, cerebrospinal fluid; CPV, canine parvovirus; GI, gastrointestinal; IBD, inflammatory bowel disease; MLV-CD, modified live virus of canine distemper; PCR, polymerase chain reaction; RBCs, red blood cells; RMSF, Rocky Mountain spotted fever.

Suggested Reading

Bathen-Noethen A, Stein VM, Puff C, et al. Magnetic resonance imaging findings in acute canine distemper virus infection. *J Small Anim Pract* 2008;49:460–467.

Greene CE, Appel MJ. Canine distemper. In: Greene CE, ed. *Infectious Diseases of the Dog and Cat.* Philadelphia: WB Saunders, 2006:25–41.

Haines DM, Martin KM, Chelack BJ, et al. Immunohistochemical detection of canine distemper virus in haired skin, nasal mucosa, and footpad epithelium: a method for antemortem diagnosis of infection. *J Vet Diagn Invest* 1999;11:396–399.

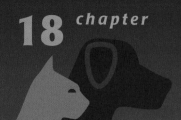

Canine Herpesvirus Infection

DEFINITION/OVERVIEW

- A rare systemic viral disease (although the virus is common in nature)—affects puppies <3 weeks of age, resulting in high mortality; is a cause of conjunctivitis/keratitis in adult dogs
- Other canine species susceptible—wolves and coyotes

ETIOLOGY/PATHOPHYSIOLOGY

- Canine herpesvirus—often found latent in several tissues, including the trigeminal nerve ganglia
- Virus—may be excreted in nasal secretions in response to stress or corticosteroid use
- Poor regulation of body temperature and immature immune response mechanisms—probably result in susceptibility of young puppies
- Clinical disease very rare in pups <3 weeks of age—all organ systems involved
- Pups—acquire infection as they pass through vagina during birth in an infected bitch
- Mature nonpregnant dogs—often have subclinical infections (nasopharynx and external genitalia)
- Transplacental infections during last 3–4 weeks of gestation—can result in fetal deaths, often with mummification; abortions; birth of dead or dying pups
- Localized genital infection—occurs in both sexes

SIGNALMENT/HISTORY

- Puppy infections—sudden death usually occurs 9–14 days after birth
- Sudden death—can occur as early as first day of life and as late as day 30 after birth
- No breed predilection—most often reported in purebred dogs, however

CLINICAL FEATURES

- Neonatal pups—4- to 6-day incubation period; sudden onset with death 12–36 hours later
- Some die with no signs; some develop mild signs—survive, but later develop ataxia, persistent vestibular signs, and blindness
- Signs include:
  - Dyspnea
  - Serous to mucopurulent nasal discharge
  - Anorexia
  - Yellow to green soft stool
  - Crying
  - CNS signs
  - Petechial hemorrhages on mucous membranes
  - Gasping before death
- Surviving pups—may suffer deafness, blindness, encephalopathy, or renal damage
- Mature females—lymphofollicular or hemorrhagic lesions on vaginal mucosa (Fig. 18-1)
- Mature dogs—may be a more common cause of conjunctivitis than once thought; keratitis reported but incidence is unknown. Immunosuppressive drugs may provoke reactivation of latent CHV with associated transient ocular disease.

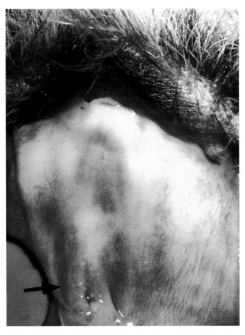

■ **Figure 18-1** Vulval mucous membrane of a bitch. Note the lymphofollicular lesions and superficial excoriation on the vulva (*arrow*) (courtesy of Dr. L. Carmichael, Cornell University).

- Infection of dams during last 3 weeks of gestation—fetal infection with death and mummification or ill pups that die shortly after birth; increased seroprevalence in kennels with reproductive problems

 DIFFERENTIAL DIAGNOSIS

- Other causes of sudden death in newborn pups—bacterial (brucellosis, coliform bacteria, streptococci, umbilical infections); toxoplasmosis; neosporosis; toxins; all fail to display the typical pathologic lesions of CHV
- CPV type 1 (canine minute virus)—causes enteric and respiratory disease; distinguished from CHV by characteristic gross pathologic changes of CHV
- Distemper and canine hepatitis (CAV type 1)—very rare and no characteristic renal gross pathologic changes

 DIAGNOSTICS

- CBC—thrombocytopenia occurs occasionally
- Serology—of little value

Diagnostic Feature

- **Diagnostic method of choice—gross and histopathology**
- Gross lesions—disseminated focal necrosis and hemorrhage in:
  - Kidneys—diffuse hemorrhagic areas, necrotic foci, hemorrhagic infarcts (pathognomonic in young pups; Fig. 18-2)
  - Lungs, liver, adrenal glands—diffuse foci of hemorrhage and necrosis

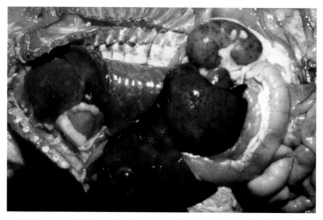

■ **Figure 18-2** Opened thorax and abdomen of a puppy that died of canine herpesvirus infection. Note the pathognomonic hemorrhagic infarcts over the kidney and liver surfaces (courtesy of Dr. L. Carmichael, Cornell University).

- ▪ Small intestine—variably affected
- ▪ Lymph nodes, spleen—generalized enlargement (consistent finding).
- ▪ Histopathologic examination—focal perivascular necrosis in kidneys, lung, liver, spleen, intestine, brain; necrotizing lesions in fetal placentas
- ▪ Immunohistochemistry—viral antigens in most organs, especially in lesion areas
- ▪ Viral isolation (on refrigerated samples, not frozen)—easily from lung or kidney
- ▪ Real-time PCR from DNA isolated from samples of suspected tissues (e.g., conjunctival swabs)

 # THERAPEUTICS

- ▪ Treatment—not recommended
- ▪ Antiviral drug therapy—unsuccessful
- ▪ Immune sera from a recovered bitch—may be beneficial in reducing pup deaths when given before onset of illness

Drugs of Choice

- ▪ No vaccine available

 # COMMENTS

- ▪ Normal litters can be expected from bitches that have previously suffered pup losses or abortion.
- ▪ Isolate pregnant dams (especially young bitches) when introduced into a kennel— Adults commonly shed latent CHV in nasal secretions for 1–2 weeks after encountering newly introduced dogs.
- ▪ Use of immunosuppressive drugs in adult animals may induce recrudescence of latent CHV, possibly leading to ocular disease (conjunctivitis and/or keratitis).

Abbreviations

CAV, canine adenovirus; CBC, complete blood count; CHV, canine herpesvirus; CNS, central nervous system; CPV, canine parvovirus.PCR; polymerase chain reaction.

Suggested Reading

Green CE, Carmichael LE,. Canine herpesvirus infection. In: Greene CE, ed. *Infectious Diseases of the Dog and Cat.* Philadelphia: WB Saunders, 2006:47–53.
Ledbetter EC, Hornbuckle WE, Dubovi EJ. Virologic survey of dogs with naturally acquired idiopathic conjunctivitis. *J Am Vet Med Assoc* 2009;235:954–959.

Canine Influenzavirus Infection

DEFINITION/OVERVIEW

- An acute to subacute contagious viral disease of dogs causing respiratory disease, easily confused with other causes of kennel cough

ETIOLOGY/PATHOPHYSIOLOGY

- H3N8 virus—an orthomyxovirus with a direct genetic link to equine influenza virus H3N8 (United States) or to an avian H3N2 virus (South Korea)
- Acquisition—Natural route of infection is airborne particles or oral contact with contaminated surfaces.
- Replication—restricted to upper and lower respiratory tract epithelial cells with possible involvement of alveolar macrophages
- Incubation period—2 to 4 days
- Antibody response—detectable by 8 days PI; titers remain detectable for >1 year
- H3N8 CIV infections in dogs—first detected in greyhound racetracks in the United States in 2004; currently enzootic in nonracing dogs in at least three regions, including Florida, Colorado, and the eastern seaboard from Connecticut to Virginia
- H3N2 CIV—first detected in South Korea in 2007; genetic lineage and extent of the epizootic of this virus has not been reported, but the virus seems to be restricted to South Korea.

SIGNALMENT/HISTORY

- All breeds and age groups of dogs are susceptible to infection, mainly because CIV is a new virus and there is little population immunity.
- Greyhounds—develop more severe signs with H3N8 CIV, but other factors (such as virus strain) contribute to disease pattern
- H3N2 CIV infections—seem to be more severe than H3N8 CIV
- Most cases have a history of group housing—day care centers, rescue shelters, or contact with dogs that have recently been in group housing

CLINICAL FEATURES

- 60–80% of infected dogs develop clinical signs.
- Fever (rarely >104°F)—3 to 6 days PI
- Clear nasal discharge progressing to thick mucoid discharge (due to secondary bacterial infection)
- More severe form—higher temperatures with development of pneumonia 6–10 days PI.
- Cough—developed by many dogs; can last for several weeks

 DIFFERENTIAL DIAGNOSIS

- A general differential diagnosis for cough includes categories such as:
  - Cardiovascular (pulmonary edema; pleural effusions; enlarged heart, especially the left atrium; pulmonary emboli)
  - Allergic (bronchitis, eosinophilic pneumonia or granulomatosis, pulmonary infiltrate with eosinophilis)
  - Trauma (foreign body, irritating gases, collapsing trachea)
  - Neoplasia (not only of the respiratory tree but also associated structures, such as ribs, lymph nodes, muscles)
  - Inflammatory (pharyngitis, tonsillitis, bacterial bronchopneumonia, chronic pulmonary fibrosis, pulmonary abscess or granuloma, chronic obstructive pulmonary disease)
  - Parasites (*Capillaria aerophila, Oslerus [Filaroides] osleri, Filaroides hirthi, F. milksi, Paragonimus kellicotti, Dirofilaria immitis*—heartworm disease)
- Kennel cough—often a clinical diagnosis based on a history of sudden onset, recent exposure to likely pathogens (boarding), lack of recent vaccinations for the respiratory pathogens, lack of other clinical signs other than cough, and cough easily induced upon even slight tracheal palpation

 DIAGNOSTICS

- CBC and serum biochemistry profile—usually unremarkable, although a CBC may show a stress leukogram or leukocytosis with a left shift (in response to bacterial pneumonia)
- Thoracic radiology—bronchopneumonia, cranioventral pattern if have bacterial pneumonia; if bacteria are not present, lung lesions are more severe in the right crania, right middle, accessory, and left cranial areas of the lung.
- HI serum test—measures serum antibodies to virus to assess exposure

- Antigen capture ELISA tests—currently give an unacceptable level of false-negative results
- PCR or viral isolation of nasal swab—most effective during the first 1–3 days after the onset of clinical signs and is undetectable 7 days PI, although in rare cases, virus can be detected using RT-PCR out to 10 days PI
- Nasal swabs—keep moist by applying a few drops of saline prior to sending to the lab; can use other transport medium except bacterial transport medium
- More than 7 days after the onset of clinical signs—HI serum test best for detecting exposure to virus

 THERAPEUTICS

- Contagious period for CIV—extends for 6 days after the onset of clinical signs; continued coughing of affected animals beyond 6 days is not a sign of virus shedding.
- Isolate infected dogs to prevent spread; treat uncomplicated cases as outpatients.
- Hospitalize pneumonia cases that require IV fluid support.
- Enforced rest—for at least 3 weeks (uncomplicated) and 8 weeks (pneumonia)

Drugs of Choice

- Antiviral drugs – efficacy not reported
- Broad-spectrum antibiotics in uncomplicated cases—amoxicillin/clavulanic acid, doxycycline, or TMS
- Severe cases that are resistant to first-choice antibiotic therapies above—combination therapy of an aminoglycoside (gentamicin or amikacin) with a cephalosporin (cefazolin). May use enrofloxacin as alternative to gentamicin.
- In severe cases (bronchopneumonia)—continue at least 2 weeks past radiographic resolution of signs
- Resistant bacteria (*B. bronchiseptica* and others)—important to culture and establish the bacterial sensitivity; may need to deliver antibiotics by nebulization (kanamycin 250 mg; gentamicin 50 mg; polymyxin B 333,000 IU) for 3–5 days
- Cough suppressants—butorphanol (Torbutrol [Fort Dodge] or hydrocodone bitartrate [Hycodan; [DuPont Pharma]) often effective in suppressing a dry, nonproductive cough
- Bronchodilators (theophylline or aminophylline)—offer little help but may relieve clinically apparent wheezing

Precautions/Interactions

- Do not use cough suppressants in patients with pneumonia or productive coughs.
- TMS—multiple adverse reactions, including:
  - KCS—monitor tear production weekly throughout treatment

- Hepatotoxicity—anorexia, depression, icterus; monitor ALT—if prolonged therapy
- Megaloblastic-folate acid deficiency anemia—especially in cats after several weeks; supplement with folinic acid (2.5 mg/kg/day)
- Immune-mediated polyarthritis, retinitis, glomerulonephritis, vasculitis, anemia, thrombocytopenia, urticaria, toxic epidermal necrolysis, erythema multiforme, and conjunctivitis—remove from drug
- Renal failure and interference with renal excretion of potassium—leading to hyperkalemia
- Salivation, diarrhea, and vomiting (cats)
- May interfere with thyroid hormone synthesis (dogs)—check T_3 and T_4 after 6 weeks.
- TMS—Use with caution in neonates and pregnant patients.
- Fluoroquinolones—avoid use in pregnant, neonatal, or growing animals (medium-sized dogs <8 months of age; large or giant breeds <12–18 months of age) because of cartilage lesions
- Fluoroquinolones and theophylline derivatives—used together may increase the plasma theophylline concentrations to toxic levels

 COMMENTS

- If infection becomes established in a kennel facility—evacuate the kennel for 1–2 weeks; disinfect with sodium hypochlorite (1:30 dilution), chlorhexidine, or benzalkonium
- Uncomplicated cases—should resolve within 10–14 days; if coughing continues beyond 14 days, question the diagnosis or look for secondary bacterial pneumonia.
- Mortality rate—highly variable; linked mainly to degree of secondary bacterial infections, strain of virus, and intensity of veterinary care
- Vaccination—one currently USDA licensed (Nobivac Canine Flu H3N8; Intervet Schering Plough Animal Health)
- Zoonotic risk—no evidence that CIV can infect humans; the virus in horses directly linked to CIV has not been linked to human disease.
- Horses—Experimentally, CIV is not able to establish a productive infection in challenged horses.
- Cats—H3N8 can infect cats, but no natural disease has been detected.
- Birds—Avian origin CIV (South Korea) can be transmitted to birds.

Abbreviations

CBC, complete blood count; CIV, canine influenza virus; ELISA, enzyme-linked immunosorbent assay; HI, hemagglutination inhibition; PCR, polymerase chain reaction; PI, postinfection.

Suggested Reading

Dubovi EJ. Canine influenza. *Vet Clin North Am Small Anim Pract* 2010;40:1063–1071.

Gibbs EPJ, Anderson TC. Equine and canine influenza: a review of current events. *Anim Health Res Rev* 2010;29:1–9.

Harder TC, Vahlenkamp TW. Influenza virus infections in dogs and cats. *Vet Immunol Immunopathol* 2010;134:54–60.

chapter 20

Canine Lungworm (*Crenosoma*)

DEFINITION/OVERVIEW

- A helminth parasite usually of foxes, wolves, and raccoons, but can invade the bronchial tree of domestic dogs to produce a productive chronic cough and a bronchointerstitial pattern on thoracic radiographs

ETIOLOGY/PATHOPHYSIOLOGY

- *Crenosoma vulpis*—a metastrongyloidae parasite
- Eggs and L1 larvae—laid in the respiratory tree of infected dogs, ascend the trachea, and are swallowed back into the GI tract and passed in the feces
- L1 larvae—infect snails and slugs, where they develop to L3 larvae
- Dogs—become infected by eating infected mollusks or small amphibians and reptiles, which may serve as paratenic hosts
- PPP = 19–21 days

SIGNALMENT/HISTORY

- Affects dogs of all ages
- Usually a history of unusual exposure to outdoors, such as might occur with a suburban dog visiting a rural region for a period of time
- Infected dogs usually present during mid to late summer.
- Occurs mainly in northeastern parts of North America, with higher incidence in the Atlantic Canadian provinces, especially New Brunswick, Newfoundland-Labrador, Nova Scotia, and Prince Edward Island.

CLINICAL FEATURES

- Productive cough that is unresponsive to antibiotics
- Cough develops approximately 2–3 weeks after likely exposure to parasite and remains for several months if untreated.

- Cough easily elicited on tracheal palpation (unlike cough caused by *Oslerus* [*Filaroides*] *osleri*)
- Dogs rarely debilitated by disease

 ## DIFFERENTIAL DIAGNOSIS

- A general differential diagnosis for cough includes categories such as:
  - Cardiovascular (pulmonary edema; enlarged heart, especially the left atrium; left-sided heart failure; pulmonary emboli)
  - Allergic (bronchial asthma, eosinophilic pneumonia or granulomatosis, pulmonary infiltrate with eosinophilia)
  - Trauma (foreign body, irritating gases, collapsing trachea, hypoplastic trachea)
  - Neoplasia (not only of the respiratory tree but also associated structures such as ribs, lymph nodes)
  - Inflammatory (pharyngitis, tonsillitis, kennel cough from such agents as *Bordetella bronchoseptica*, parainfluenza virus, infectious laryngotracheitis virus, and mycoplasma; bacterial bronchopneumonia; fungal pneumonia; aspiration pneumonia; chronic pulmonary fibrosis; pulmonary abscess or granuloma; chronic obstructive pulmonary disease)
  - Parasites (*Capillaria aerophila*, *Oslerus* [*Filaroides*] *osleri*, *Filaroides hirthi*, *Filaroides milksi*, *Paragonimus kellicotti*, *Dirofilaria immitis*—heartworm disease)
- The L1 of all the canine lungworms (*F. hirthi*, *Oslerus* [*Filaroides*] *osleri*, *Crenosoma vulpis*, and *F. milksi*) are very similar. *Oslerus* (*Filaroides*) *osleri* is best differentiated from the others by demonstrating nodules at the bifurcation of the trachea; the tail has a small kink making it similar to *F. milksi*. Thoracic radiographic changes for *F. hirthi*, *C. vulpis*, and *F. milksi* can be similar, but the L1 of *F. milksi* has a kinked tail; the other two do not. Differentiating *F. hirthi* and *C. vulpis* is difficult and requires comparing L1 larval differences: *F. hirthi* organisms have blunt, rounded oral ends, whereas *C. vulpis* organisms have bluntly conical oral ends and a straight-sided, more gradually tapering cone than that of *F. hirthi*. From a therapeutic perspective, differentiation of these latter two is unimportant because they are treated similarly.

 ## DIAGNOSTICS

Diagnostic Feature

- L1 larvae can be identified in the feces using either ZSCT (specific gravity, 1.18), or Baermann's technique, which is usually more sensitive than finding parasites in a transtracheal wash (Fig. 20-1). Because of intermittent fecal shedding, several consecutive fecal samples may need to be examined.

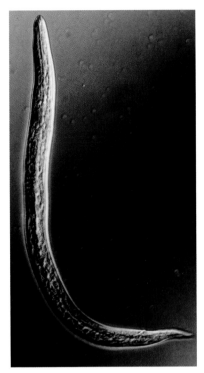

■ **Figure 20-1** L1 larvae of *C. vulpis* in an infected dog's feces. Note the nonkinked tail, which distinguishes this larva from *Oslerus* (*Filaroides*) *osleri*, and the relatively long esophagus that distinguishes this larva from those of Strongyloides and Ancylostoma.

- Transtracheal wash usually contains L1 larvae (some L1 larvae are in eggs), eosinophils, and some neutrophils.
- CBC occasionally demonstrates mild eosinophilia.
- Thoracic radiographs often show a diffuse bronchointerstitial pattern throughout the pulmonary parenchyma (Fig. 20-2).

 THERAPEUTICS

- Response to drug therapy—usually rapid and complete with cessation of cough 3 days after beginning treatment with anthelmintic and prednisone
- Radiographic changes—should be completely resolved by 6 weeks post-treatment

Drugs of Choice

- Fenbendazole—not approved for use in dogs for this parasite
- Febantel—not approved for use in dogs for this parasite
- Milbemycin oxime—not approved for use in dogs for this parasite

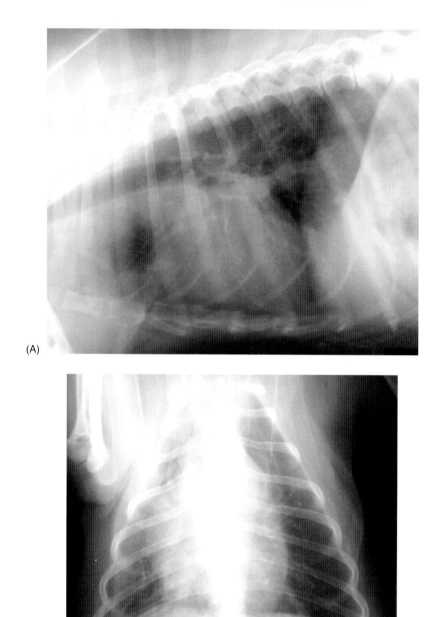

(A)

(B)

■ **Figure 20-2** Lateral (A) and dorsoventral (B) thoracic radiographs of a dog with *C. vulpis* infestation. Note the diffuse bronchointerstitial lung pattern.

TABLE 20-1	Drug Therapy for *Crenosoma vulpis* Infection in Dogs			
Drug	Dose (mg/kg)	Route	Interval (h)	Duration (days)
Fenbendazole (Panacur)	50	PO	24	3
Febantel	14	PO	24	7
Milbemycin oxime	0.5	PO	once	
Prednisone	0.5	PO	12	5

- Prednisone—improves inflammation caused by the products of parasites killed off by anthelmintic therapy (Table 20-1)

 # COMMENTS

- The severity of the cough can be similar to that caused by kennel cough.
- Foxes do not acquire infections if raised on wire but do if raised on dirt; control of a dog's access to dirt and intermediate hosts should prevent infection.

Abbreviations

CBC, complete blood count; GI, gastrointestinal; PPP, prepatent period; ZSCT, zinc sulfate concentration technique.

Suggested Reading

Conboy G. Helminth parasites of the canine and feline respiratory tract. *Vet Clin North Am Small Anim Pract* 2009;39:1109–1126.

Canine Lungworm
(*Filaroides*)

DEFINITION/OVERVIEW

- Adults of this helminth parasite live in the lung parenchyma of dogs, producing few clinical signs in most cases.
- May cause severe pneumonia (especially after treatment) in some cases

ETIOLOGY/PATHOPHYSIOLOGY

- *Filaroides hirthi*—Metastrongyloidea nematode parasite
- Adults—curl up in lung parenchyma; release thin-shelled eggs or L1 larvae into airways
- L1 larvae—coughed up and swallowed, appear in feces
- L1 larvae—infective; horizontal transmission is common
- PPP = 5 weeks
- A second helminth, *Filaroides milksi*, has been very rarely demonstrated to cause verminous pneumonia in dogs in North America, Japan, and Belgium; details of life cycle, pathogenicity, and chemotherapy are unknown.

SIGNALMENT/HISTORY

- Although any dog can become infected (client-owned dogs from Alabama, Georgia, New York, Pennsylvania, Texas, and Washington have been reported infected), most infections are seen in dogs housed closely together (breeding facilities of research colony dogs), where horizontal transmission and autoinfection are common.
- Transmission by the fecal–oral route from a brood bitch to offspring is common.
- Young (<3 years), small breeds—once treated specifically for infection or if immuno-suppressed, can show severe signs of pneumonia

CLINICAL FEATURES

- Most are asymptomatic
- Those with clinical signs present with a mild cough on exercise.
- Dogs immunosuppressed with corticosteroids for long periods (weeks), suffering from Cushing's disease, or that have undergone prolonged nutritional stress may show severe and fatal signs of pneumonia.
- In dogs with severe pneumonia, a cycle of autoinfection causing massive worm numbers to develop in the lungs usually precedes the fatal pneumonia.

DIFFERENTIAL DIAGNOSIS

- A general differential diagnosis for cough includes categories including the following:
  - Cardiovascular (pulmonary edema; enlarged heart, especially the left atrium; left-sided heart failure; pulmonary emboli)
  - Allergic (bronchial asthma, eosinophilic pneumonia or granulomatosis, pulmonary infiltrate with eosinophilia)
  - Trauma (foreign body, irritating gases, collapsing trachea, hypoplastic trachea)
  - Neoplasia (not only of the respiratory tree but also associated structures, such as ribs, lymph nodes)
  - Inflammatory (pharyngitis; tonsillitis; kennel cough from such agents as *Bordetella bronchoseptica*, parainfluenza virus, infectious laryngotracheitis virus, and mycoplasma; bacterial bronchopneumonia; fugal pneumonia; aspiration pneumonia; chronic pulmonary fibrosis; pulmonary abscess or granuloma; chronic obstructive pulmonary disease)
  - Parasites (*Capillaria aerophila, Oslerus* [Filaroides] *osleri, Crenosoma vulpis, Paragonimus kellicotti, Dirofilaria immitis*—heartworm disease).
- The L1 of all the canine lungworms (*F. hirthi, Oslerus* [Filaroides] *osleri, Crenosoma vulpis,* and *F. milksi*) are very similar. *Oslerus (Filaroides) osleri* is best differentiated from the others by demonstrating nodules at the bifurcation of the trachea; the tail has a small kink making it similar to *F. milksi*. Thoracic radiographic changes for *F. hirthi, C. vulpis,* and *F. milksi* can be similar, but the L1 of *F. milksi* has a kinked tail, whereas the other two do not. Differentiating *F. hirthi* and *C. vulpis* is difficult, requiring comparing L1 larval differences: *F. hirthi* organisms have blunt, rounded oral ends, whereas *C. vulpis* organisms have bluntly conical oral ends and a straight-sided, more gradually tapering cone than *F. hirthi*. From a therapeutic perspective, differentiation of these latter two is unimportant because they are treated similarly.

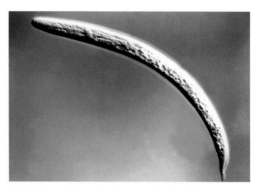

■ **Figure 21-1** L1 larva of *F. hirthi* in the feces of a dog. L1 of *F. hirthi* are very similar to, although thicker than, those of *C. vulpis* (no kinked tail and long esophagus), and thoracic radiographic changes can be similar. A careful history is required for the clinician to differentiate between the two. The L1 larvae of *F. hirthi* are best concentrated in the feces using ZSCT instead of Baermann's technique.

 # DIAGNOSTICS

Diagnostic Feature

- **L1 larvae—best identified in feces using ZSCT (specific gravity, 1.18) instead of Baermann's technique; L1 larvae do not escape from the feces easily (Fig. 21-1).**
- Transtracheal wash—probably the most effective method of identifying L1 larvae; mild increase in eosinophil count also
- Thoracic radiographs—Lesions include linear and nodular interstitial infiltrates and occasional alveolar and peribronchial patterns.
- After anthelmintic treatment, pulmonary infiltrates often become more nodular and consolidated.

 # THERAPEUTICS

- Patients can experience severe clinical signs 2–5 days after the onset of anthelmintic therapy.
- The author has found that treating for 5 days with anti-inflammatory levels of corticosteroids during the early stages of anthelmintic therapy decreases the severity and longevity of signs resulting from dying of parasites.

Drugs of Choice

- Fenbendazole
- Prednisone (Table 21-1)

TABLE 21-1 Drug Therapy for *F. hirthi* in Dogs

Drug	Dose (mg/kg)	Route	Interval (h)	Duration (days)
Fenbendazole (Panacur)	50	PO	24	10–14
Albendazole (Valbazen)	25	PO	12	5[a]
Ivermectin[b]	1	SC	Once[c]	
Prednisone	0.5	PO	12	5

[a]Repeat in 2 weeks after end of first course.
[b]Use ivermectin with albendazole to control infections in research colonies.
[c]Repeat in 1 week.

Precautions/Interactions

- Albendazole—effective therapy but possible side effects; can cause teratogenesis and myelosuppression in dogs and cats
- Fenbendazole—can be used safely in pregnant and nursing bitches, stud male dogs, and puppies

 # COMMENTS

- If infected dogs are in contact with others, all dogs should be treated to attempt to break the horizontal transmission cycle.
- Feces from all dogs should be screened using ZSCT; all dogs with positive test results should be isolated and treated.
- In a colony of experimental dogs, rigorous attempts must be made to clear the infection because lungworm lesions can lead to spurious results in drug toxicologic and carcinogenicity studies.

Abbreviations

PPP, prepatent period; ZSCT, zinc sulfate concentration technique.

Suggested Reading

Conboy G. Helminth parasites of the canine and feline respiratory tract. *Vet Clin North Am Small Anim Pract* 2009;39:1109–1126.

22 *chapter*

Canine Parvovirus Infection

DEFINITION/OVERVIEW

- Viral infection causing systemic illness with primarily GI and immunologic effects in young dogs (6–16 weeks of age) and occasionally cats
- Clinically characterized by anorexia; vomiting; bloody, watery diarrhea; and sepsis as a result of absolute neutropenia

ETIOLOGY/PATHOPHYSIOLOGY

- CPVs are small, nonenveloped, single-stranded DNA viruses; two are pathogenic to dogs—CPV-1 (minute virus of canines) and CPV-2 (causing GI tract disease).
- CPV-1—uncertain pathogenicity; has been associated with "fading puppy syndrome"; causes lethargy, loose stools, respiratory distress, and sudden death in 1- to 3-day-old pups
- CPV-2—first appeared in 1977; known simply as canine parvovirus and is closely related to feline panleukopenia virus and mink enteritis virus
- CPV-2a appeared in 1980, and CPV-2b in 1984—different antigenic structures, increased pathogenicity, and shorter incubation period (4–5 days vs. 5–8 days) compared with CPV-2
- CPV-2c—reported in Italy in 2000; spread throughout the world and the United States by 2007
- CPV-2a, -2b, and -2c—also replicate in cats
- MLV vaccines made against the original CPV-2 and -2b—protect against all 2a, 2b, and 2c
- Route of infection—fecal/oral followed by viral replication in tonsilar lymphoid tissue initially, with subsequent spread to other lymphoid tissue (bone marrow, mesenteric nodes, thymus)
- Viremia occurs by day 3–5 postinfection and precedes clinical signs—Virus can be detected in intestinal epithelial cells by day 4 postinfection.
- Fecal shedding occurs soon after viremia, with large amounts of virus excreted in feces in clinically affected dogs.
- Fecal shedding usually lasts no longer than day 12 postinfection.

- CPV targets rapidly dividing cells in the intestine (crypt cells of distal duodenum and jejunum), bone marrow, and, under exceptional circumstances, myocardial tissue.

Enteritis

- Commonly seen in pups 6–16 weeks of age
- Dividing crypt cells are killed; enteric cells moving up the villus to be lost into the intestinal lumen are not replaced by new cells; leads to denuded villus
- Takes about 2 weeks for complete villus repair to occur
- Virtually all clinical signs are a consequence of crypt cell and lymphoid/bone marrow destruction.
- Severe cases develop sepsis and endotoxemia from gram-negative enteric bacteria (CPV infection alone in gnotobiotic dogs produces minimal signs).
- Sepsis causes circulatory collapse, multiple organ failure, and death.

Bone Marrow

- CPV causes necrolysis of both myeloid and erythroid stem cells in marrow—Because RBCs have long half-lives (approximately 120 days), few effects are seen on the RBC indices, although anemia may occur as a result of blood loss from the bowel.
- Leukocyte counts reflect both peripheral consumption and myeloid destruction, with marked reduction beginning from day 3 to 5 postinfection.
- Myeloid destruction with profound reductions in WBC counts—occurs with, or just after, the onset of clinical signs (day 6 postinfection)
- In recovery—WBC count > 4.5, lymphocyte count > 1, monocyte count > 0.15, eosinophil count > 0.1 with a left shift are accurate predictors of a good outcome
- A marked rise in lymphocytes in the first 24 h postadmission in survivors (more significant that total WBC count)
- An increase in monocytes usually precedes a rise in PMNs in survivors.
- The appearance of eosinophils 48 h after admission—good prognostic indicator

Myocardial Disease

- Cardiac myocytes can only support CPV growth in first 2 weeks of puppy's life, so must be infected in utero or within first weeks of life—Puppies with any degree of passive immunity from dam (today virtually 100%) are immune and will not become infected (syndrome rarely seen today, but was common in late 1970s).
- Although viral damage occurs in first 2 weeks—myocarditis not seen until pups are 6–8 weeks of age; causes acute death

 SIGNALMENT/HISTORY

- Young dogs—usually between 6 and 16 weeks of age
- Certain dog breeds—rottweilers, Doberman pinschers, pit bull terriers, German shepherds, English springer spaniels, Alaskan sled dogs, and perhaps Labrador

retrievers—seem more predisposed (more severe infection and can be infected as adults).
- Cats can be infected with CPV-2a and -2b and show clinical signs similar to those seen in dogs, but this is rare.

CLINICAL FEATURES

- Can be extremely variable depending on age, immunity, copathogens (parasites or enteric bacteria), and infective dose
- Crowding and poor sanitation reduce the chances of successful response to immunization in kennels.
- However, crowding and poor sanitation do not enhance severity of disease in individuals—not unusual to have some pups in a litter unaffected while others die acutely.
- Depression
- Anorexia
- Vomiting—with or without pyrexia
- Pups vomit repeatedly—sometimes with roundworms in vomitus
- Profuse mucoid then bloody diarrhea—with rapid severe weight loss (Fig. 22-1)

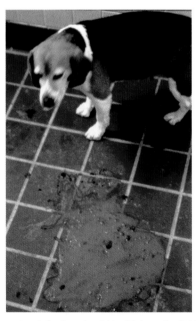

■ **Figure 22-1** A diagnosis of parvovirus infection should be high on the list in a puppy between 6 and 16 weeks of age displaying clinical signs of depression, anorexia, vomiting, and bloody diarrhea (courtesy of Dr. Leland Carmichael, Cornell University).

- Tachycardia—pale, tacky (5–8% dehydration) mucous membranes, abdominal pain or discomfort
- Signs of cerebella hypoplasia—although occurs in dogs very rarely, more often found in feline panleukopenia infection

 ## DIFFERENTIAL DIAGNOSIS

- All causes of diarrhea, including systemic or metabolic disease, as well as specific intestinal disorders, should be considered, although those affecting puppies should receive a higher priority.
- Other causes of acute enteritis: dietary indiscretion, foreign body, IBD, HGE, intussusception, drugs (antibiotics); toxins (lead), parasites (roundworms, cryptosporidiosis, giardiasis, coccidiosis, whipworms), infectious agents (salmonellosis, *Campylobacter* spp., GI tract bacterial overgrowth, clostridiosis, coronavirus), systemic organ dysfunction (renal, hepatic, pancreatic), metabolic (hypoadrenocorticism), and neoplasia (GI tract lymphoma or adenocarcinoma) in older dogs
- Parvovirus may be distinguished from other causes of acute diarrhea by the presence of a profound neutropenia apparent even on a stained direct blood smear without cell counts (Fig. 22-2).

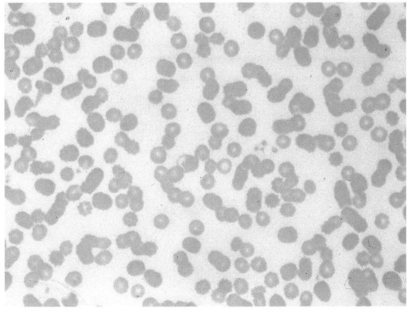

■ **Figure 22-2** A blood smear showing a profound neutropenia in a puppy with depression, anorexia, vomiting, and bloody diarrhea is virtually diagnostic of parvovirus infection.

DIAGNOSTICS

- CBC—profound neutropenia and lymphopenia
- Neutrophils—often show toxic changes
- Rebound leukocytosis with left shift—in recovery
- Biochemical profile—reflects dehydration; electrolyte abnormalities (metabolic acidosis, hypokalemia) and hypoglycemia are common.
- Panhypoproteinemia initially as the signs progress—Hypoalbuminemia may become progressively more severe with persistent diarrhea.
- Chemistry profile—may reflect multiorgan failure with sepsis
- Imaging (radiology or abdominal ultrasonography)—perform to rule out foreign body, intussusception; radiographs shows fluid-filled bowel without gas; ultrasound shows fluid filled atonic tract, small intestinal mucosal layer thinning, hyperechoic mucosal speckling, corrugations, and sometimes indistinct wall layering and irregular luminal–mucosal surfaces
- Fecal ELISA (Snap Parvo Antigen Test Kit; IDEXX Laboratories)—for parvovirus antigen; false-negative results may be seen due to relatively short time of viral shedding; false-positive results may be seen with recent vaccination (prior 5–15 days); test is effective in detecting CPV in cat feces also.
- Less commonly used tests—viral isolation, fecal PCR, electron microscopy, fecal hemagglutionation assay, serum for hemagglutination inhibition

THERAPEUTICS

- Intensive therapy with hospitalization—significantly improves survival
- Isolate from other patients—affected patients excrete large amounts of virus
- Puppies that are not vomiting and not significantly dehydrated—treat on an outpatient basis
- Intravenous crystalloid fluid therapy is mainstay of therapy—account for dehydration and ongoing losses from vomiting and diarrhea
- Avoid subcutaneous fluid administration in neutropenic patients to avoid abscess formation.
- Extreme care in catheter maintenance should be taken—A high proportion (up to 22%) of CPV patients develop bacterial colonization of IV catheters.
- Colloid therapy may be useful in patients with hypoalbuminemia—Whole blood and plasma may also be used if blood loss in diarrhea is severe.
- Enteral nutrition via a nasogastric feeding tube soon after admission—improves morbidity, time to recovery, and survivability of CPV-affected dogs; vomiting my make this challenging but all efforts should be made to control vomiting and institute early feeding.
- Glutamine supplementation—improves enterocyte health

- When ready to initiate food—use a bland diet (Hill's i/d, Purina EN), with gradual transition to normal diet

Drugs of Choice

- Antiemetics—use if vomiting protracted; Metoclopramide or the serotonin receptor antagonist ondansetron are preferred. Phenothiazines (promethazine, chlorpromazine) may worsen lethargy and hypotension.
- H$_2$ blockers (famotidine)—may reduce nausea
- Antibiotics—to prevent and treat sepsis; use broad-spectrum agents to include gram-negative organisms; ampicillin, cefazolin, ceftiofur, sometimes in combination with gentamicin (unless patient is very young or dehydrated), metronidazole
- Anthelmintic therapy (fenbendazole)—for concurrent parasitism should be considered once vomiting has ceased.rFeIFNS—may improve survivability of CPV-affected dogs (not available in the United States) (Table 22-1)
- Equine endotoxin antiserum, granulocyte colony-stimulating factor, TNF, corticosteroids, and NSAIDs—do not seem to improve survivability or recovery time
- Vaccination—MLV given at 6, 9, and 12 weeks (a third dose at 16–22 weeks may be given in susceptible breeds, e.g., rottweiler, Doberman); all current MLV vaccines protect against all known CPV subtypes.
- Intranasal modified live CPV-2b vaccine—also provides good protection
- Main reason for vaccine failure—interference from maternal antibody

TABLE 22-1 Drug Therapy for Canine Parvovirus Infections

Drug	Dose (mg/kg)	Route	Interval (h)	Duration (days)
Metoclopramide	0.2–0.4	SC	6–8	5[a]
	1–2	IV–CRI	—	5[a]
Ondansetron	0.5–1	IV	12–24	5[a]
Famotidine	0.5–1	SC, IM	12–24	5
Ampicillin	10–20	SC, IM, IV	6–8	10[b]
Cefazolin	22	IM, IV	8	10[b]
Ceftiofur	2.2–4.4	SC	12	10[b]
Gentamicin	2–4	SC, IM	8	5[c]
Fenbendazole	50	PO	24	3[d]
rIFNS	2,500,000 U/kg	IV	24	3

[a]Or as long as needed
[b]Or until oral medications can be taken
[c]Not for use in dehydrated patient; monitor for nephrotoxicity
[d]Use once vomiting has stopped.
CRI, constant rate infusion; rIFNS, recombinant feline interferon omega.

- Yearly booster vaccination—advised by most vaccine manufacturers, but dogs probably only require booster vaccination every 3 years
- Dogs acquire natural boostering throughout their lives from exposure to wild-type CPV isolates in the environment—negates the need for regular booster vaccination
- Dogs recovering from infection—develop life-long immunity negating the need for future vaccination

Precautions/Interactions

- Avoid fluoroquinolones in puppies because of risk of cartilage defects.
- Avoid use of gentamicin in dehydrated patients—Monitor use of gentamicin by examining urine for appearance of casts to avoid nephrotoxicity.
- Avoid any surgical intervention while severe neutropenia is present.
- Extended antibiotic therapy may result in development of oral and intestinal candidiasis.

 COMMENTS

- Recovery—usually complete within 7–10 days, even in those severely affected
- Complications of infection—can include intussusception, DIC, endotoxic shock, or sepsis
- CPV—ubiquitous in the environment and extremely resistant
- CPV—can be killed using a 1 : 32 dilution of bleach

Abbreviations

CBC, complete blood count; CPVs, canine parvoviruses; DIC, disseminated intravascular coagulation; DNA, deoxyribonucleic acid; ELISA, enzyme-linked immunosorbent assay; GI, gastrointestinal tract; HGE, hemorrhagic gastroenteritis; IBD, inflammatory bowel disease; MLV, modified live vaccine; NSAIDs, nonsteroidal anti-inflammatory drugs; PCR, polymerase chain reaction; RBCs, red blood cells; rFeIFNS, recombinant feline interferon omega; TNF, tumor necrosis factor; WBC, white blood cell.

Suggested Reading

Goddard A, Leisewitz AL, Christopher MM, et al. Prognostic usefulness of blood leukocyte changes in canine parvovirus enteritis. *J Vet Intern Med* 2008;22:309–316.

Goddard A, Leisewitz AL. Canine parvovirus. *Vet Clin North Am Small Anim Pract* 2010;40:1041–1053.

Larson LJ, Schultz RD. Do two current canine parvovirus type 2 and 2b vaccines provide protection against the new type 2c variant? *Vet Ther* 2008;9:94–101.

Mari K, Maynard L, Eun HM, et al. Treatment of canine parvoviral enteritis with interferon-omega in a placebo-controlled field trial. *Vet Rec* 2003;152:105–108.

chapter 23

Canine Tracheal Worm (*Oslerus*)

DEFINITION/OVERVIEW

- A helminth parasite that forms nodules within the mucosa at the bifurcation of the trachea of dogs
- Causes cough, respiratory distress, and eventually tracheal obstruction

ETIOLOGY/PATHOPHYSIOLOGY

- *Oslerus (Filaroides) osleri*—Metastrongyloidea parasite
- Adult parasites—live in fibrous nodules within the tracheal bifurcation submucosa/mucosa; release eggs containing L1 larvae directly into the tracheal lumen.
- L1 larvae—directly infective to other dogs (a unique feature of these parasites; other infective larvae require further development before becoming infective)
- Dogs acquire infection directly from L1 in feces from infected dogs or when an infected dam regurgitates food that is eaten by pups, or exposes pups to infected saliva while grooming.
- Regurgitated food becomes contaminated with L1 larvae as the food passes over the oropharynx.
- Pups eating regurgitated food become infected—a feature more common of wild canids (particularly coyotes, but also wolves, foxes, dingoes); may explain why infection is more common in wild canids than in domestic dogs

SIGNALMENT/HISTORY

- Usually found in young dogs (4–6 months of age)—usually become infected months earlier because the nodules take about 70 days to develop after infection
- Infected dogs—often have a history of contact with wild canids or at least frequent terrain where wild canids live; become infected by eating infected regurgitated food or feces
- PPP = 10–14 weeks

CLINICAL FEATURES

- First signs—harsh cough (often exercise induced or in cold weather)
- Tracheal pressure—usually does not elicit the cough, unlike other causes of tracheo-bronchitis in the dog
- After coughing several times, dog often retches a brown phlegm, which is usually swallowed.
- Advanced and severe stages of disease—the trachea becomes so obstructed with nodules that harsh wheezes can be auscultated over the hilar region, especially on expiration (Fig. 23-1).
- Tachypnea
- Increased inspiratory effort
- Prolonged expiration

 # DIFFERENTIAL DIAGNOSIS

- A general differential diagnosis for cough includes categories such as:
  - Cardiovascular (pulmonary edema; enlarged heart, especially the left atrium; left-sided heart failure; pulmonary emboli)
  - Allergic (bronchial asthma, eosinophilic pneumonia or granulomatosis, pulmonary infiltrate with eosinophilia)
  - Trauma (foreign body, irritating gases, collapsing trachea, hypoplastic trachea)
  - Neoplasia (not only of the respiratory tree but also associated structures such as ribs, lymph nodes)
  - Inflammatory (pharyngitis; tonsillitis; kennel cough from such agents as *Bordetella bronchoseptica*, parainfluenza virus, infectious laryngotracheitis virus, and mycoplasma; bacterial bronchopneumonia; fungal pneumonia; aspiration pneumonia; chronic pulmonary fibrosis; pulmonary abscess or granuloma; chronic obstructive pulmonary disease)
  - Parasites (*Capillaria aerophila, Filaroides hirthi, Crenosoma vulpis, Paragonimus kellicotti, Dirofilaria immitis*—heartworm disease)
- The L1 of all the canine lungworms (*Filaroides hirthi, Oslerus [Filaroides] osleri, Crenosoma vulpis,* and *Filaroides milksi*) are very similar. *Oslerus (Filaroides) osleri* is best differentiated from the others by demonstrating nodules at the bifurcation of the trachea; the tail has a small kink making it similar to *F. milksi*. Thoracic radiographic changes for *F. hirthi, C. vulpis,* and *F. milksi* can be similar, but the L1 of *F. milksi* has a kinked tail and the other two do not. Differentiating *F. hirthi* and *C. vulpis* is difficult, requiring comparing L1 larval differences: *F. hirthi* have blunt, rounded oral ends, whereas *C. vulpis* have bluntly conical oral ends and a straight-sided, more gradually tapering cone than *F. hirthi*. From a therapeutic perspective, differentiation of these latter two is unimportant because they are treated similarly.

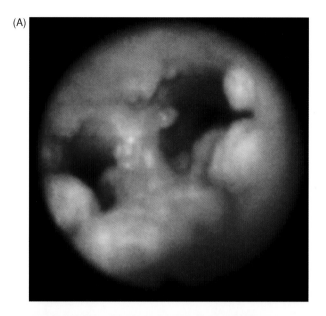

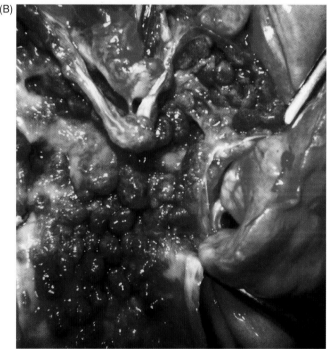

■ **Figure 23-1** Endoscopic view (A) and gross pathology specimen (B) of the tracheal bifurcation of a dog with *Oslerus (Filaroides) osleri* infestation. Note the nodes protruding into the tracheal lumen and, in the gross specimen, totally obliterating the lumen even down into bronchioles.

DIAGNOSTICS

Diagnostic Feature

- **In large-breed dogs, bronchoscopy will reveal the nodules at the tracheal bifurcation and down into the mainstem bronchus.**
- Biopsies of nodules through the bronchoscope—reveal sections of adult parasites, eggs, and many L1 larvae (Fig. 23-2).
- In small-breed dogs (where bronchoscopy cannot be used), transtracheal wash reveals L1 larvae (Fig. 23-3) and L1 larvae within eggs (Fig 23-4).
- Transtracheal wash is superior to fecal examination in demonstrating L1 larvae.

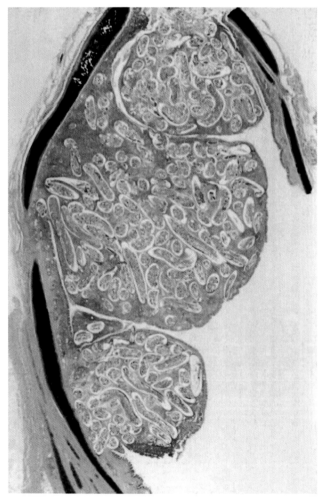

■ **Figure 23-2** Histologic section of the trachea at the level of the bifurcation. Note the adult worm coiled within the nodule protruding from the mucosa.

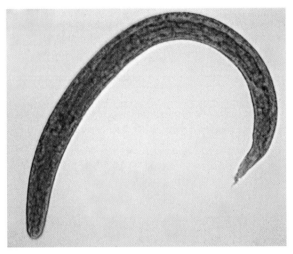

■ **Figure 23-3** L1 larva of *Oslerus* (*Filaroides*) *osleri* from a fecal. The kinked tail and relatively long esophagus distinguishes this L1 from those of *Strongyloides* and *Ancylostoma* spp.

- Fecal examinations for L1 larvae—often produce false-negative results; may need multiple fecal examinations to find L1 larvae (Fig. 23-5)
- ZSCT (specific gravity, 1.18)—superior to Baermann's technique because of the lethargy of these larvae
- The larvae of *O. (Filaroides) osleri* are indistinguishable from those of *F. hirthi*—Identifying the location of the lesion will help differentiate infestations by these parasites.
- Thoracic radiographs: trachea—may show soft tissue densities within the tracheal lumen at the bifurcation on severe infestations
- Thoracic radiographs: diaphragm—may be flattened and lung volume increased on expiratory films in dogs with severe tracheal obstruction

 THERAPEUTICS

- The author finds that physical removal of the nodules visualized during bronchoscopy using the biopsy forceps attachment of the endoscope (in medium and large-breed dogs) greatly improves respiratory signs such as cough and inspiratory difficulty.
- In severe cases, nodules may need to be removed during several procedures over days.
- During this procedure, the dog may require continuous ventilatory support with a high-frequency jet ventilator (using a rate of 100 breaths/min, a drive pressure of 20 psi, and an inspiratory fraction of 0.30).
- After nodule removal, tracheal mucosal inflammation and respiratory discomfort can be markedly reduced by administering prednisone.

TABLE 23-1 **Drug Therapy for** *Oslerus (Filaroides) osleri* **in Dogs**

Drug	Dose (mg/kg)	Route	Interval (h)	Duration (days)
Oxfendazole (Synanthic)	10	PO	24	28
Fenbendazole (Panacur)	50	PO	24	10–14
Ivermectin	0.4	PO or SC	Once[a]	
Prednisone	0.5	PO	12	5

[a]Repeat every 3 weeks for 4 treatments.

Drugs of Choice

- Oxfendazole (Synanthic Bovine Dewormer Suspension 9.06%; Fort Dodge Animal Health)—not registered for use in the dog (Table 23-1)
- Other anthelmintics (ivermectin, fenbendazole) have shown efficacy, whereas others (milbemycin, levamisole, albendazole, and pyrantal pamoate) are ineffective.

Precautions/Interactions

- Although not reported in dogs treated with oxfendazole, albendazole (a related benzimidazole) can cause myelosuppression in dogs. Given the few dogs ever treated with oxfendazole, it is advisable to perform a CBC at 2 and 4 weeks after starting oxfendazole treatment in dogs.

 COMMENTS

- Prevent dogs from frequenting terrain used by wild canids or from eating regurgitated food or feces of infected dogs (wild canids particularly).
- The feces of infected dogs, although of relatively low infectivity compared with regurgitated material, should be disposed of to prevent other in-contact dogs from becoming infected.

Abbreviations

CBC, complete blood count; PPP, prepatent period; ZSCT, zinc sulfate concentration technique.

Suggested Reading

Conboy G. Helminth parasites of the canine and feline respiratory tract. *Vet Clin North Am Small Anim Pract* 2009;39:109–1126.

Kelly PJ, Mason PR. Successful treatment of *Filaroides osleri* infection with oxfendazole. *Vet Rec* 1985;116:445–446.

Outerbridge CA, Taylor SM. *Oslerus osteri* tracheobronchitis: treatment with ivermectin in 4 dogs. *Can Vet J* 1998;39:238–240.

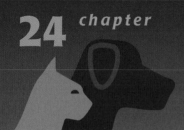

24 *chapter*

Chagas Disease (American Trypanosomiasis)

DEFINITION/OVERVIEW

- A systemic protozoal infection of dogs, initially causing acute myocarditis, that may progress to chronic dilated cardiomyopathy
- Diffuse neurologic signs are occasionally seen

ETIOLOGY/PATHOPHYSIOLOGY

- *Trypanosoma cruzi*—zoonotic hemoflagellated protozoan transmitted in the feces of vectors (*Triatomina protracta* and *Triatomina sanguisuga* or "kissing bug")
- Infection in dogs—can occur by eating infected vectors or by organisms in the feces of the vector entering a bite wound or mucous membrane, by blood transfusion, or by the transmammary or transplacental route of transmission
- After intracellular multiplication at site of entry, parasitemia develops (trypomastigotes)—followed by invasion of cardiac myocytes, where more cycles of multiplication/cell rupture/add to parasitemia occurs (coincides with acute myocarditis)
- Peak parasitemia—occurs 14–21 days postinfection
- Parasitemia levels drop as antibody titer to protozoa rises.
- Subpatent infection—occurs 30 days postinfection
- Dogs that survive acute myocarditis—enter protracted asymptomatic stage with insidious progression in some patients to end-stage dilated cardiomyopathy 1–5 years later
- United States—occurs in dogs (and reservoir hosts and vectors) mostly in Texas, but also in other southern and southeastern coastal states (as far north as Virginia); reservoir hosts and vectors also reported in the west (California, New Mexico) and as far north as Maryland

SIGNALMENT/HISTORY

- Acute myocarditis—dogs <2 years of age; chronic disease in older dogs
- Dogs diagnosed at an older age (>5 years) tend to survive longer (2–5 years) than younger (<5 years) dogs (survive up to 5 months).

- Hunting breeds and male dogs are overrepresented.
- Cats—infected in South America; not reported in North America

 CLINICAL FEATURES

Acute Myocarditis (Occasionally Encephalitis)

- Sudden death
- Lethargy
- Depression
- Weakness
- Exercise intolerance
- Syncope
- Generalized lymphadenopathy
- Pale mucous membranes
- Poor capillary refill
- Both left- and right-sided heart failure—tachycardia with reduced QRS complexes and prolonged P-R interval (heart block)
- Neurologic weakness, ataxia, chorea, seizures

Chronic Dilated Cardiomyopathy

- Weakness
- Exercise intolerance
- Syncope
- Occasionally sudden death
- Ventricular tachycardias

 DIFFERENTIAL DIAGNOSIS

- Cardiomyopathy, congenital cardiac disease, traumatic myocarditis
- Distemper, *Neospora* spp., toxoplasma

 DIAGNOSTICS

Acute Stage

Diagnostic Feature

- **Trypomastigotes on blood smear (Fig. 24-1) or on a buffy coat**
- Visualized organisms (403 objective) above the buffy coat in a microhematocrit tube spun down for PCV
- Antibody titer (ELISA or IFA)—may be negative in acute cases; repeat in 3 weeks

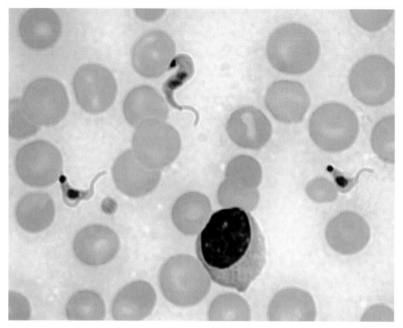

■ **Figure 24-1** Trypomastigotes of *T. cruzi* in the blood smear of a dog (Wright–Giemsa stain, 1000×).

- Blood culture—LIT medium (special laboratory—CDC)
- Thoracic radiologic examination—cardiomegaly and pulmonary edema, slight pleural effusion
- ECG—AV block, depression of R wave and QRS amplitude, right bundle branch block (Fig. 24-2)
- Echocardiography—usually normal

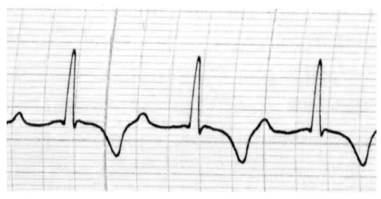

■ **Figure 24-2** Electrocardiogram showing second-degree heart block and depressed QRS complexes typical of those found in acute Chagas disease.

Chronic Stage

Diagnostic Feature

- Antibody titers are very sensitive and specific if they rule out *Leishmania* spp.; cross-reaction with *Leishmania* spp.
- On-site immunochromatographic antibody tests (developed for human diagnostic use in South America) have high sensitivity and specificity when used in dogs; excellent tool for survey work not only in dogs but also wildlife.
- PCR—very useful during indeterminate and chronic stages when blood trypomastigotes are very difficult to demonstrate; high specificity but low sensitivity unless samples from multiple tissues (including blood) are examined
- Trypomastigotes—sometimes found in lymph nodes or effusions, but virtually impossible to find in blood; may culture in LIT if use a large blood volume (50 ml)
- Thoracic radiologic examination—enlarged cardiac silhouette, ascites, pleural effusion
- ECG—low QRS amplitude, right bundle branch block, ventricular arrhythmias (initially VPC, then multiform, then degenerates into all types) (Fig. 24-3)
- Echocardiography—reduced ejection fraction, fractional shortening, thinning of the right and left ventricular free wall; initially right, then bilateral, chamber dilation

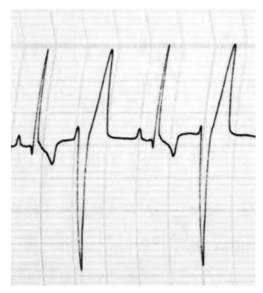

■ **Figure 24-3** Electrocardiogram showing ventricular arrhythmias typical of those found in chronic Chagas disease.

TABLE 24-1 Drug Therapy for Chagas Disease (American Trypanosomiasis)

Drug[a]	Table Size (mg)	Dose (mg/kg)	Route	Interval (h)	Duration (months)
Benznidazole (Ragonil)	100	5–10	PO	24	2
Nifurtimox (Lampit)	120	2–7	PO	6	3–5
Cythioate (Proban)		3.3	PO	48[b]	

[a]Both benznidazole and nifurtimox are available from the CDC.
[b]Give until vector numbers greatly reduced, then reduce to twice a week.

 # THERAPEUTICS

- Medical treatment rarely produces a clinical cure.
- In severe cases of acute myocarditis coupled with high parasitemia, prognosis is poor and zoonotic risk higher (to those handling blood products), so consider euthanasia.
- If dogs survive acute disease, progression to chronic stage tends to occur more quickly (in about 1–2 years) in dogs diagnosed at a younger age (<2 years) than dogs diagnosed at an older age (>4 years), which survive longer (3–5 years).
- Treat cardiac failure and arrhythmias specifically.

Drugs of Choice

Acute Stage

- Benznidazole (Ragonil; Roche SA)—preferred drug; produces cures in humans and dogs
- Nifurtimox (Bayer 2502 or Lampit; Bayer AG)—combined with corticosteroids may remove parasitemia and improve mortality (Table 24-1)
- Both drugs—available in the United States only from the CDC

Chronic Stage

- Neither nifurtimox nor benznidazole show efficacy during the chronic stage of disease.
- Cythioate (Proban)—effective in reducing vector populations; Fipronil Spot-on (Frontline Top Spot; Merial) has been shown to be ineffective in preventing reduviidae from feeding on dogs.

Precautions/Interactions

- Neither drug is registered for use in dogs.
- Nifurtimox side effects are common and usually limit treatment to 3–4 weeks; side effects include anorexia, vomiting, weight loss, CNS signs, polyneuritis, pulmonary infiltrates, and skin eruptions.

- Benznidazole side effects are less common than those with nifurtimox; include vomiting

COMMENTS

- Zoonosis—Transmission to humans can occur by accidental injection of infected blood into a person.
- Warning—Warn laboratory staff of potential infectivity of samples from a suspected patient.
- Risk of infection from dog to human by vector is very low because of the absence of specific species of vectors (that do not occur in North America but do in South America).
- Kennel of dogs are infected—investigate mode of transmission so source of infection can be recognized and blocked
- Chronic disease—Organisms may be difficult to identify on histopathologic examination of the cardiac tissue (pseudocysts containing amastigotes; Fig. 24-4), necessitating the use of immunohistochemistry (Fig. 24-5) or tissue PCR.
- Serum antibody titer—usually still present in spite of drug treatment, although reported to drop in humans treated with benznidazole

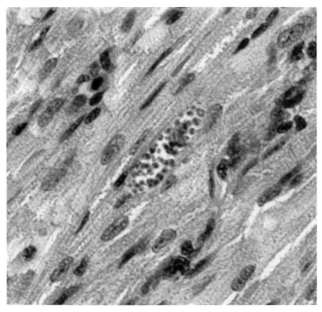

■ **Figure 24-4** Pseudocyst of *T. cruzi* within the myocardium of an infected dog (hematoxylin and eosin stain, 1000×).

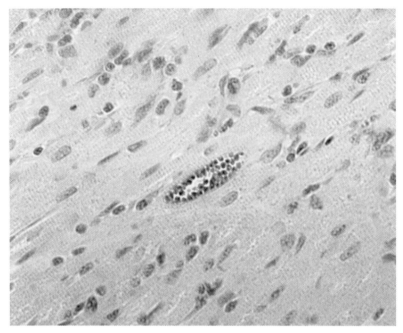

■ **Figure 24-5** Pseudocyst of *T. cruzi* within the myocardium of an infected dog (immunohistochemistry stain, 1000×).

Abbreviations

AV, atrioventricular; CDC, Centers for Disease Control and Prevention; CNS, central nervous system; ECG, electrocardiogram; ELISA, enzyme-linked immunosorbent assay; IFA, immunofluorescence assay; LIT, liver infusion tryptose; PCR, polymerase chain reaction; PCV, packed cell volume; VPC, ventricular premature contraction.

Suggested Reading

Araujo FM, Bahia MT, Magalhaes NM, et al. Follow-up of experimental chronic Chagas' disease in dogs: use of polymerase chain reaction (PCR) compared with parasitological and serological methods. *Acta Trop* 2002;81:21–31.

Barr SC. Canine Chagas' disease (American Trypanosomiasis) in North America. *Vet Clin North Am Small Animal Clin Pract* 2009;39:1055–1064.

Kjos SA, Snowden KF, Craig TM, et al. Distribution and characterization of canine Chagas disease in Texas. *Vet Parasitol* 2008;152:249–256.

Nieto PD, Boughton R, Dorn PL, et al. Comparison of two immunochromatographic assays and the indirect immunofluorescence antibody test for diagnosis of *Trypanosoma cruzi* infection in dogs in south central Louisiana. *Vet Parasitol* 2009;165:241–247.

Roellig DM, Ellis AE, Yabsley MJ. Oral transmission of *Trypanosoma cruzi* with opposing evidence for the theory of carnivory. *J Parasitol* 2009;95:360–364.

Cheyletiellosis

chapter **25**

DEFINITION/OVERVIEW

- A highly contagious parasitic skin disease of dogs, cats, and rabbits, caused by infestation with *Cheyletiella* spp. mites
- Signs of scaling and pruritus can mimic other more common diseases.
- Often referred to as "walking dandruff," because of the large mite size and excessive scaling
- Prevalence varies by geographic region owing to mite susceptibility to common flea-control insecticides.
- Human (zoonotic) lesions can occur.

ETIOLOGY/PATHOPHYSIOLOGY

- *Cheyletiella yasguri*—dogs (Fig. 25-1)
- *Cheyletiella blakei*—cats
- *Cheyletiella parasitivorax*—rabbits

SIGNALMENT/HISTORY

- Dogs and cats
- More common in young animals
- Cocker spaniels, poodles, and long-haired cats are frequent asymptomatic carriers.
- Cats may exhibit bizarre behavioral signs or excessive grooming.
- Pruritus—none to severe, depending on the individual's response to infestation
- Infestation may be suspected after lesions in humans have developed.
- Young animals and those in frequent contact with others are most at risk.
- Common sources of infestation—animal shelters, breeders, and grooming establishments

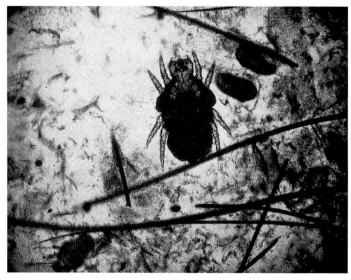

■ **Figure 25-1** *Cheyletiella yasguri* (dog). (From Rhodes KH: *The 5-Minute Veterinary Consult Clinical Companion: Small Animal Dermatology*. Baltimore, MD: Lippincott Williams & Wilkins, 2002.)

 CLINICAL FEATURES

- Scaling—most important clinical sign; diffuse or plaque-like; most severe in chronically infested and debilitated animals (Fig. 25-2)
- Lesions—dorsal orientation is commonly noted
- Underlying skin irritation—may be minimal
- Cats—may exhibit bilaterally symmetrical alopecia; head may be affected

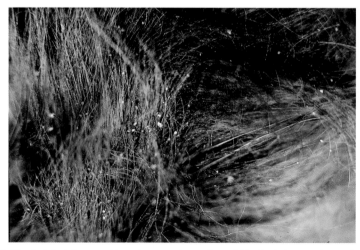

■ **Figure 25-2** Cheyletiellosis in a cat. Note the excessive scaling within the hair coat. (From Rhodes KH: *The 5-Minute Veterinary Consult Clinical Companion: Small Animal Dermatology*. Baltimore, MD: Lippincott Williams & Wilkins, 2002.)

DIFFERENTIAL DIAGNOSIS

- Cheyletiellosis should be considered in every animal that has scaling, with or without pruritus.
- Also consider—seborrhea, flea-allergic dermatitis, *Sarcoptes* spp. mite infestation, atopy, food hypersensitivity, and idiopathic pruritus

 ## DIAGNOSTICS

- Examination of epidermal debris with a lens or microscope—very effective in diagnosing infestation
- Collection of debris—flea combing (most effective), skin scraping, and acetate tape preparation
- *Cheyletiella* mites are large and can be visualized with a simple handheld magnifying lens; scales and hair may be examined under low magnification; staining is not necessary.
- Finding mite eggs is diagnostic.
- Response to insecticide preparations may be required to definitively diagnose suspicious cases in which mites cannot be identified.

 ## THERAPEUTICS

- Must treat all animals in the household.
- Clip long coats to facilitate treatment.
- Mainstay—6 to 8 weekly baths to remove scale, followed by rinses with an insecticide
- Lime-sulfur and pyrethrin rinses—cats, kittens, puppies, and rabbits
- Pyrethrin or organophosphates—dogs
- Routine flea sprays and powders—not always effective
- Environmental treatment with frequent cleanings and insecticide sprays—important for eliminating infestation
- Combs, brushes, and grooming utensils—discard or thoroughly disinfect before reuse
- Zoonotic lesions—self-limiting after eradication of the mites from household animals
- Alternatives (or additions) to topical therapy—amitraz and ivermectin
- Amitraz (Mitaban)—use on dogs only (four rinses at 2-week intervals)
- Fipronil spray—at 2-week intervals for four treatments; not to be used on rabbits
- Selamectin (Revolution)—apply every 2–4 weeks for three applications
- Imidacloprid/moxidectin (Advantage-Multi) topical formula
- Milbemycin oxime (Interceptor)—once a week for 4 weeks
- Moxidectin (Cydectin)—SC injection every 2 weeks for three treatment
- Doramectin (Dectomax)—SC injection every week for for three treatments

- Ivermectin—highly effective (300 μg/kg, SC, three times at 2-week intervals); dogs, cats, and rabbits >3 months old; pour-on forms have shown efficacy in cats (500 μg/kg two times at 2-week intervals)

 COMMENTS

- Ivermectin—several dog breeds (e.g., collies, shelties, Australian shepherds) have shown increased sensitivity and should not be treated.
- Ivermectin, fipronil, selamectin, imidacloprid/moxidectin, milbemycin, moxidectin, doramectin— not FDA-approved for use in dogs, cats, or rabbits; client disclosure and consent are paramount before administration
- Prevent ingestion of avermictins in sensitive dogs (MDR1 gene mutation).
- Fipronil is contraindicated in rabbits.
- Treatment failure—necessitates re-evaluation for other causes of pruritus and scaling
- Reinfestation may indicate contact with an asymptomatic carrier or the presence of an unidentified source of mites (e.g., untreated bedding).
- Zoonotic potential—A pruritic papular rash may develop in areas of contact with the pet.

Suggested Reading

Patel A, Forsythe P. *Small Animal Dermatology. Saunders Solutions in Veterinary Practice*. Philadelphia: Saunders Elsevier, 2008.

Chlamydiosis: Cats

chapter 26

DEFINITION/OVERVIEW

- A chronic respiratory tract infection of cats caused by an intracellular bacterium, characterized by conjunctivitis, mild upper respiratory tract signs, and mild pneumonitis

ETIOLOGY/PATHOPHYSIOLOGY

- *Chlamydia felis* (previously *psittaci*)—an obligate intracellular bacterium
- Replicates on the mucosa of the upper and lower respiratory tract epithelium, producing a persistent commensal flora—causes a local irritation with resulting mild upper and lower respiratory signs
- Ophthalmic—chronic conjunctivitis, often unilateral but may be bilateral
- Colonization—can colonize the mucosa of the GI tract (with or without signs) and reproductive tract (without signs)
- Incidence of clinical disease—sporadic
- May get outbreaks of respiratory disease—especially in multi-cat facilities
- Overall incidence—5% to 10% chronically infected
- Incubation period—7 to 10 days

SIGNALMENT/HISTORY

- Cats <1 year of age—usually clinically affected
- Carriers—any age
- Historically—Cats show upper respiratory tract signs with sneezing, watery eyes, coughing, occasionally difficulty breathing with anorexia, especially if concurrent infections are present.
- Commonly occurs as a coinfection with other respiratory pathogens

135

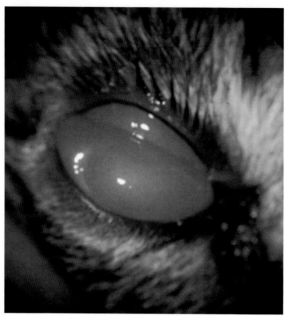

■ **Figure 26-1** Chemosis associated with conjunctivitis caused by *C. felis* (courtesy of Dr. R. Riis, Cornell University).

 ## CLINICAL FEATURES

- Conjunctivitis—often granular; initially unilateral, but usually becoming bilateral (Fig. 26-1)
- Lacrimation
- Photophobia
- Blepharospasm
- Rhinitis with nasal discharge—usually mild
- Pneumonitis—with the inflammatory process in the alveoli
- Airways—audible wheezes on auscultation

 ## DIFFERENTIAL DIAGNOSIS

- Feline viral rhinotracheitis—short incubation period (4–5 days), rapid onset of bilateral conjunctivitis, severe sneezing, and ulcerative keratitis
- Feline calicivirus infection—short incubation period (3–5 days); ulcerative stomatitis; and severe pneumonia
- Feline reovirus infection—very mild upper respiratory tract infection; short incubation and duration

- Bronchial pneumonia caused by bacteria such as *Bordetella bronchiseptica*—focal bronchoalveolar pattern on lung radiographs

DIAGNOSTICS

- CBC—neutrophilic leukocytosis
- Thoracic radiographs of animals with pneumonitis—mild diffuse interstitial pattern
- Conjunctival scrapings stained with Giemsa—intracytoplasmic inclusions
- Isolation of organism—conjunctival swabs submitted to laboratory for cell culture.
- PCR assay for *C. felis*—preferred; conjunctival swab sample
- Serum antibody assay—unvaccinated cats; indicates infection

THERAPEUTICS

- Generally as outpatient
- Inpatient only if complicated by concurrent infections causing anorexia or respiratory distress
- Physically clean discharge away from nostrils and eyes.
- Quarantine affected cats from contacting other cats (do not let affected cats outside).
- Both inactivated and modified live vaccines are available to reduce the severity of infection.
- Vaccines do not prevent infection, but do reduce severity and duration of illness.
- Give a single vaccination on the initial visit; revaccinate 1 year later; then give annual revaccination.
- American Association of Feline Practitioners classifies vaccination as noncore.
- For at risk cats, give a single vaccination at initial visit as early as 9 weeks of age, repeat in 3–4 weeks; revaccinate annually where *C. felis* is endemic.

Drugs of Choice

- Systemic antibiotics—doxycycline or tetracycline (Table 26-1)
- Ocular—ophthalmic ointments containing tetracycline (q8h)

TABLE 26-1 **Drug Therapy for Chlamydiosis in Cats**				
Drug	Dose (mg/kg)	Route	Interval (h)	Duration (weeks)
Doxycycline	5	PO	12	3–4
Tetracycline	22	PO	8	3–4

Precautions/Interactions

- Tetracyclines—discolor growing teeth
- Doxycycline—has been associated with esophagitis/strictures in cats; give with food
- Adverse vaccine reactions—mild clinical disease; small percentage of vaccinated cats

 COMMENTS

- Colonies—the entire colony may have to be treated
- Endemic breeding catteries—Treat all cats with doxycycline for at least 4 weeks, then vaccinate.
- Treatment may have to be continued for as long as 6 weeks.
- Inform clients of the causative organism, anticipated chronic course of disease, and need to vaccinate other cats before exposure.
- Prognosis—tends to be chronic, lasting for several weeks or months, unless successful antibiotic treatment is given
- Zoonosis—*C. felis* can infect humans
- Limited number of reports in humans—mild conjunctivitis transmitted from infected cats
- Role of *C. felis* as a pathogen during pregnancy—unclear
- Organism can colonize the reproductive mucosa—Severe conjunctivitis neonatorum can occur in neonatal kittens infected at or shortly after birth.
- *C. felis* does not cause sexually transmitted disease in humans (caused by *Chlamydia trichomatosis*).

Abbreviations

CBC, complete blood count; GI, gastrointestinal; IFA, immunofluoresence assay.

Suggested Reading

Greene CE, Sykes JE. Chlamydial infections. In: Greene CE, ed. *Infectious Diseases of the Dog and Cat*. Philadelphia: WB Saunders, 2006:245–252.

Gruffydd-Jones T, Addie D, Belák S, et al. *Chlamydophila felis* infection: ABCD guidelines on prevention and management. *J Fel Med Surg* 2009;11:605–609.

Richards JR, Elston TH, Ford RB, et al. The 2006 American Association of Feline Practioners Feline Vaccine Advisory Panel Report. *J Am Vet Med Assoc* 2006;229:1405–1441.

Sykes JE. Feline chlamydiosis. *Clin Tech Small Anim Pract* 2005;20:129–134.

Clostridial Enterotoxicosis

chapter 27

DEFINITION/OVERVIEW

- A syndrome characterized by diarrhea in dogs and cats associated with the production of enterotoxin by normal bacterial flora in the GI tract

ETIOLOGY/PATHOPHYSIOLOGY

- *Clostridium perfringens*—common enteric inhabitant generally found in the vegetative form living in a symbiotic relationship with the host
- Certain strains of *C. perfringens* (generally type A based on PCR analysis)—produce enterotoxin that binds to the enteric mucosa, alters cell permeability, and results in cell damage with subsequent local enterocyte death, but no systemic illness
- *C. perfringens* enterotoxin—probably associated with enteric sporulation
- Enterotoxin production—a number of intrinsic host-related factors influence enterotoxin production and pathogenicity of *C. perfringens*
- Pathogenicity of *C. perfringens*—may depend on the metabolic, mucosal, and immunologic integrity of the GI tract
- IgA deficiency—possibly
- Alkaline intestinal luminal environment—promotes *C. perfringens* sporulation and enterotoxin production
- Incidence—unknown
- Chronic large bowel diarrhea—suspected that up to 20% of cases of chronic large bowel diarrhea in dogs are *C. perfringens*–related
- Cats—infection less common than in dogs

SIGNALMENT/HISTORY

- Most animals tend to be middle-aged or older
- No sex or breed predilections
- Historically, large-bowel diarrhea with mucus
- Small amounts of fresh blood
- Tenesmus with increased frequency commonly reported

- Small-bowel diarrhea signs (large volume of watery stool) also reported
- Vomiting
- Flatulence
- Abdominal discomfort
- Stress factors to the GI tract, dietary change, concurrent disease, or hospitalization may precipitate signs.

 # CLINICAL FEATURES

- Signs usually associated with either:
  - An acquired acute, self-limiting large-bowel diarrhea lasting for 5–7 days
  - Chronic intermittent diarrhea
  - Signs associated with other GI or non–GI tract disease
- Chronic disease—often characterized by intermittent episodes occurring every 2–4 weeks that may persist for months to years
- The syndrome may develop from a nosocomial (hospital-acquired) infection, with signs developing during or shortly following hospitalization or kennel boarding.
- *C. perfringens*—occasionally associated with cases of parvovirus and acute hemorrhagic gastroenteritis

 # DIFFERENTIAL DIAGNOSIS

- All causes of diarrhea, including systemic or metabolic disease and specific intestinal disorders, should be considered.
- Other causes of acute enterocolitis are dietary indiscretion; IBD; neoplasia (especially GI tract lymphoma); drugs (antibiotics); toxins (lead); parasites (cryptosporidiosis, trichomoniassis, whipworms, giardiasis); infectious agents (parvovirus, FIP, salmonellosis, rickettsia, GI tract bacterial overgrowth, histoplasmosis, leishmaniasis, pythiosis); systemic organ dysfunction (renal, hepatic, pancreatic, cardiac); metabolic (hypoadrenocorticism, feline hyperthyroidism).

 # DIAGNOSTICS

- CBC and biochemical panel—usually normal except may reflect dehydration
- Diagnostic confirmation of. *C. perfringens* enterotoxicosis—as yet controversial
- Testing—no test appears to be completely accurate
- Anaerobic fecal cultures—generally identify high concentrations of *C. perfringens* organisms but occasionally will be negative

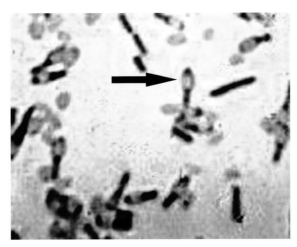

■ **Figure 27-1** Clostridial spores (*arrow*) in the feces of a dog with clostridial enterotoxicosis.

- Specific fecal spore cultures—will detect high concentrations of *C. perfringens* spores ($>10^6$ spores per gram of feces) in affected animals and correlate well with clinical disease but are rarely performed
- Fecal enterotoxin assay by ELISA (Tech Labs)—positive result in conjunction with clinical signs, fecal culture, and response to antibiotic therapy support *C. perfringens* as a contributing pathogen
- Assay—requires 1 g (pea-size sample) of feces, can be frozen
- False-positive and false-negative results—can occur
- PCR to identify *C. perfringens* enterotoxin—not commercially available but correlates well with clinical disease
- Reverse passive latex agglutination assay for enterotoxin—considered inaccurate

Diagnostic Feature

- **Fecal cytology—high numbers of *C. perfringens* endospores in the feces do not always correlate with clinical disease or fecal enterotoxin assay**
- Cytologic examination—performed by making a thin fecal smear on a microscope slide, air-drying or heat-fixing, and staining with Diff-Quick or Wright's stain
- *C. perfringens* spores—have a typical "safety-pin" appearance with an oval structure and a dense body at one end of the spore wall; >5 spores per high power oil immersion field is considered abnormal for spores (Fig. 27-1)

THERAPEUTICS

- Outpatient—most treated as outpatients
- Hospitalize—when diarrhea or vomiting is severe, resulting in dehydration and electrolyte imbalance

TABLE 27-1 Drug Therapy for Clostridial Enterotoxicosis

Drug	Dose (mg/kg)	Route	Interval (h)	Duration (days)
Metronidazole	10	PO	8–12	5–7
Tylosin (Tylan soluble powder)[a]	10–20	PO	12	5–7
Amoxicillin/clavulanic acid	22	PO	12	5–7
Ampicillin	22	PO	8–12	5–7
Clindamycin	10	PO	12	5–7

[a]Given with the food or formulated in capsules for long-term management (~3 g/tsp).

- Dietary manipulation—plays an important role in the treatment and management of cases with chronic recurring disease
- High-fiber diets—either soluble (or fermentable) or insoluble fiber, often result in clinical improvement
- High-fiber diets—reduce enteric clostridial numbers, acidify the distal intestine, thus limiting *C. perfringens* sporulation and enterotoxin production
- Commercial high-fiber diets—can be supplemented with psyllium ($1/2$ to 2 tsp/day) as a source of soluble fiber
- Diets low in fiber—supplement with either course bran (1–3 tbsp/day) as a source of insoluble fiber or psyllium added as a source of soluble fiber
- Prebiotic diets (containing fermetable substances such as fructo-oligosaccharides)—may be beneficial for changing GI flora

Drugs of Choice

- Acute self-limiting disease—5- to 7-day antibiotic course (e.g., oral ampicillin or amoxicillin, clindamycin, metronidazole, or tylosin) (Table 27-1)
- Tetracyclines—many *C. perfringens* are resistant, so not a good choice
- Acute cases—Most patients respond well to appropriate antibiotic therapy.
- Chronic reoccurring cases—often require prolonged antibiotic therapy
- Chronic cases—tylosin (Tylan Soluble powder; Elanco; 100-g container, ~3 g/tsp) best for long-term management
- High doses of antibiotics may not be necessary to prevent recurrence in chronic cases.
- Administration of oral antibiotics at submicrobial inhibitory concentrations may be effective in chronic cases.
- Low antibiotic levels may not actually reduce enteric *C. perfringens* numbers but may change the ecologic microenvironment, preventing sporulation and enterotoxin production.
- Probiotics (lactobacillus and others) may have antibacterial effects; anecdotal reports suggest some benefit in chronic cases.

COMMENTS

- Inform owners—acute disease is often self-limiting
- Inform owners—chronic cases may require prolonged therapy
- Infection—associated with environmental contamination, and disinfection is difficult
- Feeding high-fiber diets may decrease the incidence of nosocomial diarrhea.
- Most animals respond well to therapy, although chronic cases may require life-long therapy to control clinical signs.
- A failure in response suggests concurrent disease (such as parvovirus, acute HGE, or IBD), and further diagnostic evaluation is indicated.

Abbreviations

CBC, complete blood count; ELISA, enzyme-linked immunosorbent assay; FIP, feline infectious peritonitis; HGE, hemorrhagic gastroenteritis; GI, gastrointestinal; IBD, inflammatory bowel disease; PCR, polymerase chain reaction.

Suggested Reading

Albini S, Brodard I, Jaussi A. Real-time multiplex PCR assays for reliable detection of *Clostridium perfringens* toxin genes in animal isolates. *Vet Microbiol* 2008;127;179–185.

Marks SL, Kather EJ. Antimicrobial susceptibilities of canine *Clostridium difficile* and *Clostridium perfringens* isolates to commonly utilized antimicrobial drugs. *Vet Microbiol* 2003;94:39–45.

Marks SL, Kather EJ. Bacterial-associated diarrhea in the dog: a critical appraisal. *Vet Clin North Am Small Anim Pract* 2003;33:1029–1060.

Coccidioidomycosis

DEFINITION/OVERVIEW

- A systemic mycotic infection affecting dogs (usually <4 years old) and, rarely, cats

ETIOLOGY/PATHOPHYSIOLOGY

- *Coccidioides immitis*—grows several inches deep in the soil, where it survives high ambient temperatures and low moisture
- After a period of rainfall—organism returns to the soil surface, where it sporulates, releasing many arthroconidia that are disseminated by wind and dust storms
- Infection—by inhalation of arthroconidia
- Exposure to large doses of fungus in contaminated soil—associated with aggressive nosing about in soil and underbrush; dust storms after rainy season; earthquakes; land developments
- After inhalation—Fever, lethargy, inappetence, cough, and joint pain may be noticed before dissemination (10 days postinfection) to other organs.
- Asymptomatic infections—may occur
- Immunity—Some animals develop immunity without onset of clinical signs.
- Skin lesions—usually associated with dissemination; penetrating wounds have rarely been associated with skin lesions
- Signs of dissemination—may not be evident for several months after the initial infection
- Dissemination occurs—to long bones, joints, eyes, skin, liver, kidneys, CNS, cardio-vascular system (pericardium and myocardium), and testes

SIGNALMENT/HISTORY

- An uncommon disease, except in endemic areas
- Endemic regions are southwestern United States in the geographic Lower Sonoran Life Zone: Southern California, Arizona, and southwest Texas; less prevalent in New Mexico, Nevada, and Utah.

- Historically—anorexia, cough, fever unresponsive to antibiotics, lameness, weakness with paraparesis, back and neck pain, seizures, visual changes, and weight loss
- Most commonly diagnosed in dogs <4 years old but occurs in all age groups

 CLINICAL FEATURES

Dogs

- Pulmonary signs—cough, dyspnea, fever
- Disseminated disease—bone swelling, joint enlargement, lameness, cachexia, lethargy, and lymphadenopathy
- Neurologic signs—Both central and peripheral neurologic deficits may be present.
- Skin ulcers—with draining tracts
- Ocular signs—uveitis, keratitis, iritis, and retinitis

Cats

- Cachexia
- Draining skin lesions
- Dyspnea
- Lameness caused by bone involvement
- Uveitis

 DIFFERENTIAL DIAGNOSIS

- Pulmonary lesions—resemble those of other systemic mycoses (e.g., histoplasmosis, blastomycosis)
- Lymphadenopathy—lymphosarcoma, other systemic mycoses, and localized bacterial infections
- Bone lesions—primary or metastatic bone tumors or bacterial osteomyelitis
- Skin lesions—abscesses or other bacterial disease processes

 DIAGNOSTICS

- CBC—mild nonregenerative anemia, neutrophilic leukocytosis, monocytosis
- Serum chemistry profile—hyperglobulinemia, hypoalbuminemia, azotemia with renal involvement
- Urinalysis—low urine specific gravity; proteinuria with inflammatory glomerulonephritis

- Serologic tests for antibody to *C. immitis*—several technologies available, including AGID, ELISA, and latex agglutination, as well as the two classical tests based on two types of antigen:
  - TP—detects mainly IgM response, so positive titers appear early in disease (by 14 days postexposure); titers increase with dissemination or reactivation; may become negative 4–6 weeks postinfection
  - CF—detects mainly IgG response; good test for quantitative titers; the higher the complement fixation titer, the more likely it is that the disease is disseminated; positive titer can just indicate past exposure or healing or localized lesion; often positive in chronic cases when TP has become negative; higher CF titers ≥1 : 64 most often seen with disseminated or severe pulmonary disease; remain elevated months after successful treatment, then slowly decrease; false-negative result in immunosuppressed or anergic animals
- Serologic testing—Repeat serology titers in 4–6 weeks when low titers are accompanied by clinical signs.
- Radiology—lung (interstitial infiltrates) and bone lesions (osteolysis; Fig. 28-1)

Diagnostic Feature

- **Definitive method of diagnosis—microscopic identification of the large spherule form of C. immitis in lesion or biopsy material, lymph node aspirates, impression smears of skin lesions or draining exudates (Fig. 28-2)**
- Cultures—only performed by trained personnel in laboratories designed for the task
- Mycelial form is highly contagious.
- Biopsy of infected tissue—often preferred to avoid false-negative results, but tissues involved (lung) may be impractical to obtain (Fig. 28-3)
- Serologic testing—more logical approach in an animal with consistent clinical signs from an endemic region

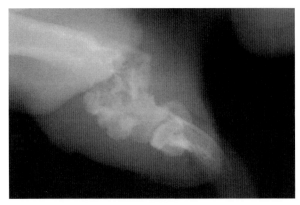

■ **Figure 28-1** Radiograph of a toe of a dog with coccidioidomycosis showing a proliferative lesion containing both lysis and bone production and extending into the joint, atypical for bone neoplasia.

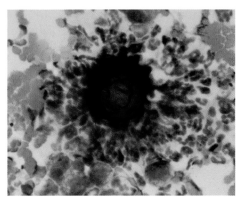

■ **Figure 28-2** Impression smear from a draining tract of a dog with coccidioidomycosis showing a spherule (usually between 10 and 80 mm, double walled, containing endospores) surrounded by neutrophils and macrophages (Wright's stain, 1000×).

 # THERAPEUTICS

- Generally treated as outpatients
- Concurrent clinical symptoms (e.g., seizures, pain, coughing) should be treated appropriately.
- Animals with a CF titer $>1:8$ should be monitored; if a repeat titer shows a rise after 4 weeks, institute drug therapy.

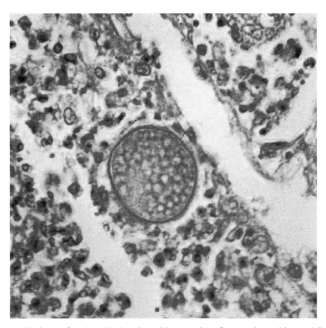

■ **Figure 28-3** Histopathology of C. *immitis* in a lung biopsy taken from a dog with coccidioidomycosis. Note the presence of the endospores, which differentiates the organism from blastomycosis organisms (PAS stain, 1000×).

- The necessity, expense, possible treatment failure, and possible side effects of the drugs used should be reviewed with the owner.
- Surgical removal of a focal granulomatous organ (lung lobe, eye, and kidney) may be indicated.

Drugs of Choice

- Fluconazole—drug of choice; crosses the blood/brain barrier; can be expensive in large-breed dogs
- Veterinary compounding pharmacies in Arizona and California have made fluconazole available more cheaply; however, not all compounding pharmacies are reliable, and treatment failures have been seen from compounded drugs.
- Ketoconazole—not as effective as fluconazole; give with food to improve absorption; continue for at least 1 year; monitor for side effects
- Itraconazole—produces no better clinical response than ketoconazole; fewer side effects but more expensive
- Amphotericin B—rarely recommended because of the high risk of renal damage and lack of availability of an oral preparation of the drug (Table 28-1)

Cats

- As per dogs, the azoles are preferred.

Precautions/Interactions

- Monitor—liver enzyme levels (rises in ALT) monthly when using azoles, especially ketoconazole, for extended periods

TABLE 28-1 Drug Therapy for Coccidioidomycosis in Cats and Dogs					
Drug	Species	Dose	Route	Interval (h)	Duration (months)
Fluconazole	D	5 mg/kg	PO	12	10–12[a]
	C	25–100/cat	PO	12–24	[a]
Ketoconazole	D	5–10 mg/kg	PO	12	[a]
	C	50 mg/cat	PO	12–24	[a]
Itraconazole	D	5 mg/kg	PO	12	[a]
	C	25–50/cat	PO	12–24	[a]
Amphotericin B	D	0.3–0.5 mg/kg	IV	48–2[b]	[c]

[a] Usually treat for 12 months or until clinical resolution and complement fixation titers <1:4.
[b] Give 3 days a week.
[c] Until a total cumulative dose of 8–11 mg/kg.
C, cats; D, dogs.

- Ketoconazole—teratogenic, so should be used in pregnant animals only if the potential benefit justifies the potential risk to offspring
- Amphotericin B—monitor for renal damage by frequent examination of urine sediment; discontinue treatment if granular casts are noted in the urine; consider lipid-encapsulated amphotericin B to decrease side effects.
- Pulmonary disease resulting in severe coughing—may temporarily worsen after therapy is begun, owing to inflammation in the lungs associated with killing of organisms
- Low-dose, short-term oral prednisone and cough suppressants may be required to alleviate the respiratory signs.

 COMMENTS

- Coccidioidomycosis is considered one of the most severe and life-threatening of the systemic mycoses with treatment of disseminated disease.
- Often requires at least 1 year of aggressive antifungal therapy
- Decision for termination of drug therapy is based on resolution of clinical disease, radiographic appearance of bone and lung lesions (progressive or not), and CF titers.
- Monitor CF titers 3–4 months, with animals being treated until their titers fall to <1:4.
- Animals displaying poor response to therapy should have a 2- to 4-hour postpill drug (fluconazole) level measured to ensure adequate absorption of the drug.
- Prognosis is guarded to grave.
- Many dogs improve after oral therapy, but relapses are common, especially if therapy is shortened.
- Overall recovery rate is approximately 60% (some report 90%) response to fluconazole therapy.
- In cats, the prognosis is not well documented, but rapid dissemination requires long-term therapy.
- Spontaneous recovery from disseminated coccidioidomycosis without treatment is extremely rare.
- No vaccine is available for dogs or cats
- Caution should be used if culturing draining lesions suspected of being infected with *C. immitis*; although the spherule-form of the fungus found in animal tissues is not directly transmissible to humans or other animals, the mycelial form is highly contagious.

Abbreviations

AGID, agar gel immunodiffusion; ALT, alanine aminotransferase; CBC, complete blood count; CF, complement fixation; CNS, central nervous system; ELISA, enzyme-linked immunosorbent assay; TP, tube precipitin.

Suggested Reading

Graupmann-Kuzma A, Valentine BA, Shubitz LF, et al. Coccidioidomycosis in dogs and cats: a review. *J Am Anim Hosp Assoc* 2008;44:226–235.

Greene RT. Coccidioidomycosis. In: Greene CE, ed. *Infectious Diseases of the Dog and Cat*, 2nd ed. Philadelphia: WB Saunders, 1998:391–398.

Tofflemire K, Betbeze C. Three cases of feline ocular coccidioidomycosis: presentation, clinical features, diagnosis, and treatment. *Vet Ophthalmol* 2010;13:166–172.

Coccidiosis

chapter 29

DEFINITION/OVERVIEW

- An enteric protozoan infection of dogs and cats traditionally confined to the GI tract and showing strict host specificity
- Does not include *Toxoplasma*, *Cryptosporidium*, *Sarcocystis*, *Besnoitia*, or *Hammondia* spp. (see specific chapters)

ETIOLOGY/PATHOPHYSIOLOGY

- *Isospora canis* mainly, but also *Isospora ohioensis*, *Isospora burrowsi*, and *Isospora neorevolta* (dogs) and *Isospora felis* and *Isospora revolta* (cats)—obligate intracellular coccidian protozoa potentially able to infect and cause diarrhea in puppies and kittens
- *Eimeria* spp.—not parasitic in dogs or cats; oocysts can appear in carnivore feces as a result of coprophagy or ingesting *Eimeria*-infected prey
- *Isospora* spp.—host specific
- Direct life cycles (fecal–oral transmission)—pass oocysts (relatively large at 32–53 mm, unsporulated) in feces
- Damage to the host's small intestinal enterocytes can cause watery diarrhea in the very young or immunosuppressed.
- Autoinfection—common, causing a continual recycling within the intestinal tract and loss of mucosal lining
- The direct role of *Isospora* spp. in causing disease—still in question because there are few studies elaborating pathogenesis
- Virtually every dog and cat becomes infected during its life (usually during the first month)—few show clinical disease

SIGNALMENT/HISTORY

- Puppies and kittens
- Most common in catteries, kennels—overcrowded situations

CLINICAL FEATURES

- Diarrhea—watery
- Diarrhea—can persist for weeks
- Diarrhea—can occasionally contain mucus or blood
- Anorexia, vomiting, leading to severe dehydration; death has been reported

DIFFERENTIAL DIAGNOSIS

- Other causes of diarrhea in young animals, including:
  - Dietary—indiscretion or poor nutrition
  - Parasites—giardiasis, cryptosporidiosis, trichomoniasis
  - Other infectious agents—parvovirus, FIP, FeLV, salmonellosis, rickettsia, *Campylobacter*, clostridia, or colibacillosis
- Consider also—systemic organ dysfunction (renal, hepatic, pancreatic, cardiac, peritonitis); drugs (antibiotics); toxins (lead, organophosphates)

DIAGNOSTICS

- CBC and biochemical panel—may reflect fluid and electrolyte loss from diarrhea
- Fecal examination—*Isospora* spp. oocysts, unsporulated and >30 mm long
- Oocysts—should be differentiated from those of other species:
  - Cat—*I. revolta* (unsporulated, <30 mm), *Besnoitia* and *Toxoplasma gondii* (unsporolated, 10–14 mm)
  - Dog—*Hammondia* spp. (unsporulated)
  - Both cats and dogs—*Sarcocystis* spp. and *Cryptosporidia* (both sporulated, 9–16 mm and <5 mm, respectively) (Figs. 29-1 and 29-2)

THERAPEUTICS

- Most animals will respond to coccidiostat therapy alone, without parenteral support
- Very young animals may need fluid support if diarrhea is extreme.
- Coccidiosis is rarely the sole cause of diarrhea; every effort should be made to identify other concurrent factors or infections.
- Examine for host stress factors and factors within the kennel—concurrent parasitism, weaning, poor diet, poor environmental conditions, or immunosuppression

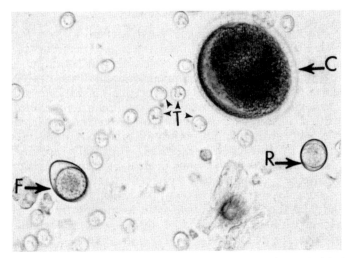

■ **Figure 29-1** Unsporulated oocysts of *Toxoplasma gondii* (*T*), *I. felis* (*F*), and *I. revolta* (*R*) with an egg of the helminth *T. cati* (*C*) in flotation of feline feces (unstained, 200×). (From Dubey JP: A review of *Sarcocystis* of domestic animals and of other coccidian of cats and dogs. *J Am Vet Med Assoc* 1976;169:1061–1078; used with permission).

Drugs of Choice

- Sulfadimethoxine (Albon; Pfizer Animal Health)—tablets, 5% oral suspension
- Trimethoprim-sulfadiazine (Tribrissen; Schering-Plough)—tablets, injectable
- Amprolium (Corid 9.6% oral solution; Merial)—off-label use for prevention or treatment (Table 29-1)

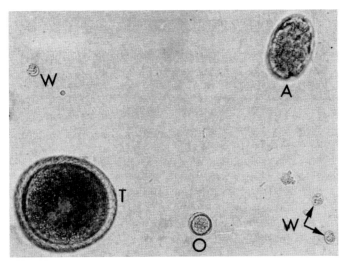

■ **Figure 29-2** Unsporulated oocysts of *I. ohioensis* (*O*) and *Hammonida heydornia* (*H*) compared with eggs of the nematodes *Toxocara canis* (*C*) and *Ancylostoma caninum* (*A*) in a flotation of canine feces (unstained, 200×). (From Dubey JP: A review of *Sarcocystis* of domestic animals and of other coccidian of cats and dogs. *J Am Vet Med Assoc* 1976;169:1061–1078; used with permission).

TABLE 29-1 Drug Therapy for Coccidiosis in Dogs and Cats

Drug	Species	Dose (mg/kg)	Route	Interval (h)	Duration (days)
Sulfadimethoxine (Albon)	B	50–60[a]	PO	24	14–21
Trimethoprim-sulfadiazine (Tribrissen)	B	30–60[b]	PO, SC	24[c]	6
Amproline (Corid)	D	100–200	PO[d]	24	7
	C	20–40[e]	PO	24	10
Diclazuril	C	25	PO	Once	
Ponazuril (Marquis Paste)	B	20	PO	24	1–3
	B	30	PO	Weekly	Repeat once
	B	50	PO	Once	
Toltrazuril	D	10–30	PO	24	1–3

[a] After first dose of 50–60 mg/kg, can halve dose until asymptomatic but not to exceed 3 weeks.
[b] If >4 kg body weight. Halve the dose if <4 kg body weight.
[c] Dose may be divided into two daily doses.
[d] Added to food or water.
[e] Can increase the dose to 300 mg/kg and give for 5 days.
B, both cats and dogs; C, cats; D, dogs.

- Ponazuril (Marquis Paste; Bayer Animal Health)—coccidiocidal; available in the United States for treating *Sarcocystis neurona* in horses; can be diluted for use in pups and kittens; in shelters or kennels with recurring problems, use ponazuril prophylactically by giving each kitten and puppy a dose at 2–3 weeks of age.
- Diclazuril and Toltrazuril-like ponazuril are coccidiocidal so likely to result in a clearing of infection where other drug regimes are coccidiostatic.

Precautions/Interactions

- TMS—can produce keratoconjunctivitis sicca; should not be used in dogs with a reduced Schirmer tear test; may occur 1 week after beginning drug; monitor Schirmer tear test weekly
- TMS—has been associated with folate acid–deficient anemias, hepatotoxicity, immune-mediated polyarthritis, retinitis, glomerulitis, vasculitis, thrombocytopenia, toxic epidermal necrolysis, and cutaneous drug eruptions
- Cats—TMS causes profound hypersalivation in cats; give as whole tablets, do not break; also, supplement cats with folic acid (2.5 mg/kg/day) to avoid development of megaloblastic anemia.

COMMENTS

- Coccidiosis outbreaks can occur even in well-managed kennels or catteries, especially when young animals are present in large numbers.
- Eradication—not usually possible

- Concentrate on controlling outbreaks by strict hygiene—live steam, ammonia or phenol-containing disinfectants
- Dry, hot conditions will kill cysts.
- Combination of sulfadimethoxine (55 mg/kg) and ormetoprim (11 mg/kg) daily for 23 days mixed with feed during pups' exposure to infective oocysts—shown to markedly reduce oocyst shedding and severity/incidence of diarrhea
- Ponazuril, diclazuril, and toltrazuril—use becoming more popular as seem to clear infections more completely than coccidiostatic alternatives
- Ponazuril—equine product easy for veterinarians to obtain and dilute for administration to puppies and kittens.

Abbreviations

CBC, complete blood count; FeLV, feline leukemia virus; FIP, feline infectious peritonitis; GI, gastrointestinal; TMS, trimethoprim-sulfadiazine.

Suggested Reading

Dubey JP, Lindsay DS, Lappin MR. Toxoplasmosis and other intestinal coccidial infections in cats and dogs. *Vet Clin Small Anim Pract* 2009;39:1009–1034.

30 *chapter*

Colibacillosis

DEFINITION/OVERVIEW

- Bacterial infection of dogs and cats causing a range of conditions, including septicemia in the very young, sometimes complicating other causes of enteritis (parvovirus), UTI, and so on
- Can be isolated as normal flora from the GI tract and prepuce and vagina of dogs and cats

ETIOLOGY/PATHOPHYSIOLOGY

- *Escherichia coli*—gram-negative Enterobacteriaceae, normal inhabitant of the GI tract of most mammals
- Under certain circumstances (immunosuppression; presence of other disease, such as GI disease or other pathogens)—can become systemic to affect other organs or contaminate other tissue/organ sites (urogenital system, skin, mammary gland)
- Virulence factors (various, depending on strains) exist—ability to cause septicemia probably due more to the immune status of host rather than virulence factors of bacterium
- A new type of E. *coli* has been found in Boxer dogs with IBD (granulomatous colitis) characterized by ability to adhere, to invade, and to replicate in macrophages resulting in a tremendous inflammatory response within the intestinal wall.

SIGNALMENT/HISTORY

- Mainly affects neonatal puppies and kittens <1 week of age, especially if they have not received colostrum
- Predisposition—overpopulated housing
- Older dogs and cats—mainly diarrhea, urogenital (cystitis, endometritis, pyelonephritis, prostatitis, mastitis), otitis, pneumonia, hepatobiliary disease, endocarditis, and, rarely, meningoencephalomyelitis
- Boxer dogs may be predisposed to large-bowel colitis.

CLINICAL FEATURES

Neonates (First 2 Weeks of Life)

- Sudden onset
- Vomiting
- Weakness
- Lethargy
- Diarrhea—often watery
- Hypothermia
- Loss of sucking reflex
- Cyanosis
- Usually multiple animals in litter affected
- Bitch/queen—may have poor health and nutritional status
- Unable to provide good care and colostrum to offspring
- Overcrowding and poor hygiene will precipitate fecal–oral spread of infection.

Puppies/Kittens and Adults

- Vomiting
- Diarrhea
- Rapid dehydration
- Fever with some strains
- Concurrent diseases (parvovirus, panleukopenia, parasitism) and use of antimicrobial agents that upset GI flora, or immunosuppression often precipitate disease

 DIFFERENTIAL DIAGNOSIS

- Dietary indiscretion, IBD; neoplasia (especially GI tract lymphoma); drugs (antibiotics); toxins (lead, organophosphates); parasites (giardiasis, cryptosporidiosis, trichomoniasis, whipworms); infectious agents (parvovirus, FIP, FeLV, salmonellosis, rickettsia, *Campylobacter*, clostridia, histoplasmosis, coronavirus); systemic organ dysfunction (renal, hepatic, pancreatic, cardiac, pyometra, peritonitis); metabolic (hypoadrenocorticism)

 DIAGNOSTICS

- CBC and biochemical panel—Usually neonates die very rapidly, not allowing too many changes.
- Hypoglycemia—usually present

- Adults may show consequences of electrolyte and fluid losses from diarrhea.
- Culture of *E. coli* from blood or other tissues (urine, aspirates) where not normally found—required to show that it is not a contaminant

 # THERAPEUTICS

- Acutely ill neonates must receive good nursing care in a heated environment.
- Parenteral fluids—containing glucose
- When stronger and able to take food orally, tube feeding with balanced milk substitute is indicated.
- Attention must be paid to warmth, elimination, and hydration.

Drugs of Choice

- Antibiotic use should be based on culture and sensitivity results, especially for UTI, and other non–life-threatening conditions (allowing time to get results back from lab).
- Empirically—use broad spectrum
- Amoxicillin
- TMS
- Fluoroquinolones such as enrofloxacin (Baytril; Bayer) for adult animals
- Cephalosporins such as cefixime (Suprax oral suspension; Lederle); cefaclor (Ceclor; Eli Lily); cefadroxil (Cefa-tabs; Fort Dodge Animal Health); third-generation injectable cephalosporins (Table 30-1)

Precautions/Interactions

- TMS can cause keratoconjunctivitis sicca—should not be used in dogs with a reduced Schirmer tear test

TABLE 30-1 Drug Therapy for *E. coli* Infections in Dogs and Cats if Culture and Sensitivity Results Are Not Available

Drug	Dose (mg/kg)	Route	Interval (h)	Duration (days)
Amoxicillin	10–20	PO, IV, SC	12	7
Trimethoprim-sulfa	30	PO	12	7–10
Enrofloxacin[a]	2.5–5	PO	12	7–10
Cefixime (Suprax)	5–10	PO	12	10
Cefaclor (Ceclor)	10	PO	8	7–10
Cefadroxil (Cefatabs)	22	PO	12	7

[a] For adult animals.

- TMS—associated with folate acid–deficient anemias, hepatotoxicity, immune-mediated polyarthritis, retinitis, glomerulonephritis, vasculitis, thrombocytopenia, toxic epidermal necrolysis, and cutaneous drug eruptions
- Do not use enrofloxacin in pregnant, growing, or neonatal animals.
- High doses of enrofloxacin may cause blindness in cats, particularly with concurrent ocular diseases.

 COMMENTS

- Enterobacteriaceae can change resistance to antibiotics over time—ideally, important to base antibiotic use on culture and sensitivity results

Abbreviations

CBC, complete blood count; FeLV, feline leukemia virus; FIP, feline infectious peritonitis; GI, gastrointestinal; IBD, inflammatory bowel disease; TMS, trimethoprim-sulfadiazine; UTI, urinary tract infection.

Suggested Reading

Johnson JR, Johnston B, Clabots CR, et al. Virulence genotypes and phylogenetic background of *Escherichia coli* serogroup O6 isolates from humans, dogs, and cats. *J Clin Microbiol* 2008;46:417–422.

Stenske KA, Bemis DA, Gillespie BE, et al. Prevalence of urovirulence genes cnf, hlyD, sfa/foc, and papGIII in fecal *Escherichia coli* from healthy dogs and their owners. *Am J Vet Res* 2009; 70:1401–1406.

Cryptococcosis

DEFINITION/OVERVIEW

- A systemic or localized fungal infection causing granulomas, usually in the nose, sinuses, and eyes of cats and brain, nasal passages, and sinuses of dogs

ETIOLOGY/PATHOPHYSIOLOGY

- *Cryptococcus neoformans*—an environmental yeast-like fungus able to form a heteropolysaccharide capsule in tissues
- Environment—found mainly in bird droppings and decaying vegetation (where it can survive for 2 years)
- Infection occurs by localization of the yeast in nasal passages after inhalation; some organisms may reach the terminal airways to establish lung infection (rare).
- Hematogenous dissemination to brain, eyes, lymph nodes, and other tissues may occur; local spread to the skin of the nose, eyes, and lymph nodes can occur.

SIGNALMENT/HISTORY

- Most common at 2–7 years of age
- Higher incidence in areas of southern California and Australia

Dogs

- Rare in North America; prevalence ~0.00013%
- Doberman pinschers, Labrador retrievers, and American cocker spaniels over-represented
- No sex predilection

Cats

- About 10 times more common than in dogs
- Siamese over-represented

- Occurs more commonly in males
- Patients concurrently infected with FeLV or FIV are at higher risk and suffer more extensive disease.

 ## CLINICAL FEATURES

- Lethargy
- Fever
- Signs vary depending on organ system affected

Dogs

- Organs mainly affected—brain, nasal passages, sinuses; also draining lymph nodes, eyes, periorbital tissue; rarely lungs and abdominal organs
- Usually neurologic signs—ataxia, seizures, paresis, blindness
- Lymphadenopathy
- Nasal discharge
- Skin mass or ulceration

Cats

- Organs mainly affected—nose, sinuses, facial skin, nasopharynx, brain, and eyes
- Firm mass over the bridge of the nose
- Masses—may ulcerate, develop weeping granulomatous tissue (Fig. 31-1)
- Nasal discharge—occasional sneezing, snuffling

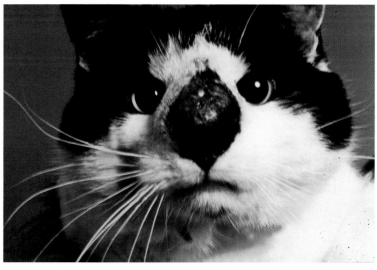

■ Figure 31-1 Ulcerated mass lesion over the bridge of the nose of a cat with cryptococcosis.

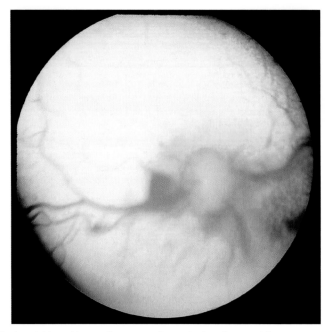

■ **Figure 31-2** Chorioretinitis and hemorrhage near the optic disc of a cat with cryptococcosis.

- Lymphadenopathy—especially submandibular, prescapular
- Nasopharyngeal mass lesions—snoring, stertor, inspiratory dyspnea
- Lower respiratory tract signs—rare
- CNS disease—cranial nerve involvement is common manifestation
- Ocular signs—common with CNS disease
- Blindness—due to exudative retinal detachment, granulomatous chorioretinitis (Fig. 31-2), panophthalmitis, anterior uveitis

 DIFFERENTIAL DIAGNOSIS

Dogs

- Neurologic disease—both focal and diffuse; tumors, rickettsial diseases, other fungal diseases, granulomatous meningoencephalomyelitis, toxins such as lead, distemper, neosporosis, toxoplasmosis, idiopathic epilepsy
- Nasal disease—immune mediated, especially when at the mucocutaneous junction; tumors, foreign body; other fungal infections; allergic rhinitis; and dental disease
- Lymphadenopathy—lymphosarcoma; other infections, such as with *Leishmania* spp.
- Ocular disease—other fungal infections, distemper, neoplasia, toxoplasmosis, rickettsial diseases

Cats

- Nasal disease—tumors, chronic rhinitis, sinusitis, or nasopharyngeal polyps
- Ulcerative skin lesions—bacterial infection, cat bite abscess, tumor (squamous cell carcinoma)
- Ocular disease—neoplasia (lymphoma), toxoplasmosis, FIP

 DIAGNOSTICS

- CBC—anemia of chronic disease (normocytic, normochromic); eosinophilia occasionally seen in some cats
- Serum biochemistry profile—usually normal; may show mild elevations in globulin proteins
- Imaging (radiographs, CT, MRI) of nasopharynx—may show cryptococcal granuloma as a soft tissue density that can on occasion erode dorsal nasal bones/turbinates. CT or MRI are best for identifying brain or intranasal lesions.
- Thoracic radiographs—diffuse mixed interstitial–alveolar pattern in animals with lung involvement
- Latex agglutination or ELISA—detect cryptococcal capsular antigen in serum, CSF, urine, or even nasal discharge; are very sensitive and reasonably specific tests
- Can get low false-positive titers (1 : 4)—due to reaction with talc from latex gloves or latex from rubber stoppers of blood collection tubes contaminating the sample
- Monitor capsular antigen titers—Because magnitude correlates with extent of infection, these titers can be used to monitor treatment efficacy.
- Cultures on Sabouraud's agar with antibiotics confirm diagnosis
- NOTE:—unlike in-house cultures of *Blastomyces* and *Histoplasma* organisms, *Cryptococcus* spp. do not present a zoonotic risk to staff.

Diagnostic Feature

- **Definitive diagnosis—Cytologic examination of aspirates of granulomas, nasal discharge material, lymph nodes, or CSF stained with Diff-Quick or Wright's stains (although New Methylene Blue and Gram's stain are the best) usually reveals pleomorphic yeast forms with clear mucopolysaccharide capsule (Fig. 31-3).**
- Biopsy, although definitive, is usually not required.

 THERAPEUTICS

- Surgically debulk mass lesions—especially if associated with respiratory distress (especially upper airway of cats), then administer systemic antifungal therapy.
- Nutritional support—especially cats after surgery (esophageal or PEG tube)
- Treat stable animals as outpatients—Neurologic cases may need in-hospital supportive care initially.

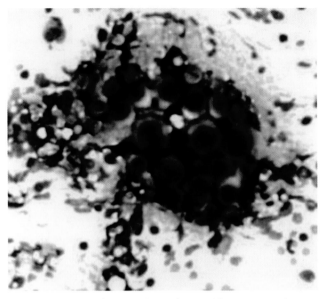

■ **Figure 31-3** Lymph node aspirate cytologic specimen of a cat with cryptococcosis. Note the pleomorphic yeast-like organisms surrounded by a halo (Wright's stain, 1000×).

Drugs of Choice

- Itraconazole (Sporanox; Janssen)—first choice in cases without ocular or neurologic involvement because it does not penetrate into these tissues; less expensive than fluconazole; give with fatty food (such as canned) to improve absorption
- Fluconazole (Diflucan; Pfizer)—first choice in cases with ocular or neurologic involvement because it does penetrate into these tissues
- Flucytosine (Ancobon; Roche)—best if used with trizoles (itraconazole or fluconazole) or amphotericin B when infection not responding well to single agent
- Amphotericin B deoxycholate (Fungizone; Squibb)—use if other therapies too expensive; often most successful when used with flucytosine; administer in conjunction with fluid therapy to protect against nephrotoxicity; using SC route in cats will reduce toxicity and is cost effective
- Amphotericin B may have some advantage in severe disease at an intravenous dose of 0.5 mg/kg every 48 hours given over 3–4 hours; then give subcutaneously on a chronic long-term basis.
- Amphotericin B lipid complex (Abelcet; Liposome Co.)—use in place of deoxycholate because it is less toxic but more expensive
- Terbinafine (Lamisil; Sandoz)—effective in cats with infections resistant to the triazoles; expensive (Table 31-1)

Precautions/Interactions

- Triazoles (itraconazole and fluconazole)—hepatotoxic (monitor for liver enzyme elevations monthly); can cause GI tract signs

TABLE 31-1 Drug Therapy for Cryptococcosis

Drug	Species	Dose (mg/kg)	Route	Interval (h)	Duration (months)
Itraconazole—100 mg capsules/ 100 mg/ml liquid	D C	5.0 10–15	PO PO	12 24	6–10 6–10
Fluconazole—50, 100, 150, 200 mg tablets	B	5–15	PO	24	6–10
Flucytosine[a]—250, 500 mg capsules	B	30	PO	8	1–9
Amphotericin B (deoxycholate)— 50 mg/vial powder for injection	C C D	0.1–0.5 0.5–0.8 0.25–0.5	IV SC IV	3 times/week 3 times/week 3 times/week	[b] [c] [b]
Amphotericin B (lipid)—100 mg/20 ml vial solution for injection	D	1.0	IV	3 times/week	[d]
Terbinafine—125, 250 mg tablets	B	5–10	PO	24	1–3

[a] Give with amphotericin B.
[b] Give to a total cumulative dose of 4–10 mg/kg.
[c] Add each dose to 400 ml of 0.45% saline/2.5% dextrose, to a total cumulative dose of 8–26 mg/kg.
[d] Can be given to a total cumulative dose of up to 12 mg/kg.
B, both cats and dogs; C, cats; D, dogs.

- Itraconazole—ulcerative dermatitis (usually develops toward treatment end but needs to be differentiated from cryptococcal lesions); do not give with the antihistamines terfenadine and astemizole, or with cisapride (fatal cardiac arrhythmias may occur)
- Fluconazole—water soluble, so excreted via kidneys; reduce dose in animals with renal insufficiency
- Flucytosine—can cause drug eruptions (depigmentation of lips or nose, ulceration, exudation, and crusting of skin), myelosuppression; avoid in neonates, pregnant animals, or in animals with renal insufficiency
- Amphoteracin B deoxycholate—nephrotoxic (monitoring urine for casts is the most sensitive method for detecting nephrotoxicity; creatine and BUN elevations are not as sensitive or specific but have been used to monitor nephrotoxicity)
- Amphotericin B lipid complex—much less toxic than deoxycholate but more expensive
- Terbinafine—reduce dosage by at least half in animals with reduced renal and hepatic function; may show GI tract signs

 COMMENTS

- Owner needs to be aware that triazole therapy is expensive and disease requires months of therapy—usual duration is 3–12 months.
- Drug choice—Generally, itraconazole is used in nonocular or non-neurologic disease, fluconazole when ocular and neurologic disease is present, and amphotericin B in

patients in situations in which financial restraints are present; the latter can be used inexpensively with SC administration on an outpatient basis.
- Assure owner that infection is not zoonotic.
- Inform owner that organism is acquired from the environment and that animal could be at increased risk, especially if immunosuppressed.
- Monitor liver enzymes monthly in patients receiving triazole antifungals.
- Use clinical signs and capsular antigen titers to monitor efficacy of therapy—check titers first, 2 months after onset of therapy (should be markedly reduced); generally, titers decline by 2- to 4-fold/month during successful treatment; if not responding to treatment, try another triazole or add flucytosine or terbinafine. Monitor antigen titers every 1–2 months during treatment and after stopping treatment; don't stop treatment until capsular antigen titers become negative (might be years in some animals). Anticipate treatment duration of 4–12 months; patients with CNS disease my require life-long treatment; median time of successful treatment with fluconazole is 4 months and 8 months with itraconazole.
- Cats with FIV or FeLV have a poorer prognosis.

Abbreviations

BUN, blood urea nitrogen; CBC, complete blood count; CNS, central nervous system; CSF, cerebrospinal fluid; CT, computed tomography; ELISA, enzyme-linked immunosorbent assay; FeLV, feline leukemia virus; FIP, feline infectious peritonitis; FIV, feline immunodeficiency virus; GI, gastrointestinal; MRI, magnetic resonance imaging; PEG, percutaneous endoscopic gastrostomy.

Suggested Reading

Malik R, Craig AJ, Wigney DI, et al. Combination chemotherapy of canine and feline cryptococcosis using subcutaneously administered amphotericin B. *Aust Vet J* 1996;73:124–128.
McGill S, Malik R, Saul N, et al. Cryptococcosis in domestic animals in Western Australia: a retrospective study from 1995–2006. *Med Mycol* 2009;47:625–639.
O'Brien CR, Krockenberger MB, Martin P, et al. Long-term outcome of therapy for 59 cats and 11 dogs with cryptococcosis. *Aust Vet J* 2006;84:384–392.
Quimby J, Lappin MR. Update on feline upper respiratory diseases: condition-specific recommendations. *Compend Contin Educ Vet* 2010;32:E1–E9.

Cryptosporidiosis

chapter 32

DEFINITION/OVERVIEW

- A coccidian protozoa causing diarrhea in dogs and cats; also infects humans and many other mammals, including calves, foals, and rodents

ETIOLOGY/PATHOPHYSIOLOGY

- Multiple species occur—including *Cryptosporidium canis* and *Cryptosporidium felis*
- Morphologically—species very similar
- Some species are host specific—others (e.g., *Cryptosporidium parvum*) infect multiple species
- *C. parvum*—main species to infect small animals
- Infection—occurs by ingestion of sporulated oocysts; sporozoites are released from oocysts to infect intestinal epithelial cells; multiply (asexually); merozoites released to infect other cells.
- PPP = 5–10 days in cats
- Immunocompetent animals—develop intestinal infection, which is usually asymptomatic; excrete oocysts in feces for about 2 weeks, then stop shedding
- Immunocompromised animals—usually have signs of enteritis, but can develop infections of respiratory tract, liver, biliary tree, and pancreas

SIGNALMENT/HISTORY

- No sex or breed predilection in either cats or dogs

Dogs

- Virtually all clinical cases occur in dogs <6 months of age.
- Older dogs can excrete cysts but not show signs unless complicated by intestinal disease (IBD or neoplasia such as GI tract lymphoma).

Cats

- Serologic examination results suggest approximately 15% exposure rate in cats in the United States.
- Virtually all clinical cases reported in immunocompromized cats
- More common in young and newborn kittens <6 months of age

CLINICAL FEATURES

- Most commonly, asymptomatic oocyst shedding
- Small-bowel diarrhea, although large-bowel diarrhea reported

DIFFERENTIAL DIAGNOSIS

- Anything that causes acute small-bowel diarrhea, including dietary indiscretion; IBD; neoplasia (especially GI tract lymphoma); drugs (antibiotics); toxins (lead); parasites (giardiasis, trichomoniasis, whipworms); infectious agents (parvovirus, FIP, salmonellosis, rickettsia, GI bacterial overgrowth, clostridia, histoplasmosis, leishmaniasis); systemic organ dysfunction (renal, hepatic, pancreatic, cardiac); metabolic (hypoadrenocorticism, hyperthyroidism of cats)
- NOTE: Patients with diarrhea and *Cryptosporidia* cysts in their feces invariably have an underlying disease process that could include a systemic cause for immunosuppression (neoplasia, FIP, FeLV, FIV, distemper, chronic corticosteroid use) or underlying intestinal tract disease (IBD, intestinal lymphoma, chronic antibiotic use).

DIAGNOSTICS

- CBC, biochemical panel, urinalysis, imaging—are usually normal unless altered by underlying disease process
- Identify oocysts in feces—sugar and zinc sulfate flotation (specific gravity, 1.18)
- Because the organism is so small, identification of the oocysts is often difficult and best accomplished by experienced laboratory staff.
- Routine salt flotation—often fails because oocysts are very small (4–8 mm) (Fig. 32-1)
- Preferred stain—modified acid-fast; oocysts stain orange–red (Fig. 32-2)
- Crystal violet will stain fecal material but not oocysts—making visualization clearer (negative staining).
- NOTE: When submitting feces to a laboratory, mix 1 part 100% formalin with 9 parts feces to inactivate oocysts and decrease health risk to laboratory staff.

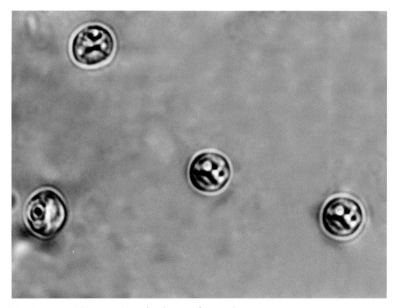

■ **Figure 32-1** *Cryptosporidium* cysts in a fecal smear from a dog.

- Direct fluorescent antibody kits (Merifluor; Meridian Diagnostics) are effective in cats and dogs but often only available in diagnostic laboratories.
- Antigen detection methods (ProSpecT, *Cryptosporidium* Mitrotiter Assay [Alexon]; Color-Vue *Cryptosporidium* [Seradyn])—are available and seem to detect *C. felis* and *C. canis*.
- PCR techniques—available in some commercial laboratories

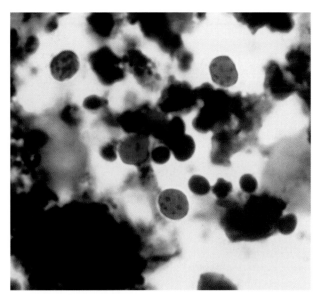

■ **Figure 32-2** *Cryptosporidium* cysts in the feces of a cat (modified acid fast stain, 1200×).

- PCR—approximately 10–100 times more sensitive for the diagnosis of cryptosporidiosis in cats than other techniques
- Intestinal biopsy or cytology may reveal organisms in epithelial cells but can produce false-negatives results.

 # THERAPEUTICS

- In immunocompetent animals, diarrhea is usually very mild and self-limiting.
- Wait 2 weeks, then check for oocyst shedding again (unless public health/zoonosis issues of primary concern).
- Underlying diseases—treat aggressively
- Mild diarrhea—treat on outpatient basis; withhold food for 24–48 hours; supplement with oral glucose-electrolyte solutions (Entrolyte; Pfizer).
- Severe diarrhea—NPO, parental fluids (isotonic with potassium added at least to 30 mEq/liter)

Drugs of Choice

- None of these drugs are registered for this use in small animals.

Paromomycin (Humatin; ParkDavis)

- Stops oocyst shedding in both cats and dogs
- Not absorbed from GI tract if intact
- If the drug is absorbed from the GI tract (possible in animals with hemorrhagic diarrhea, very young animals), it can cause renal failure and deafness (similar to other aminoglycosides).
- Toxicity responds to diuresis; monitor renal toxicity by monitoring urine for casts.

Tylosin (Tylan; Elanco)

- Has been used successfully in cats, but long treatment course required

Nitazoxanide (Alinia; Romark Labs)

- Registered for the treatment of cryptosporidiosis and giardiasis in humans
- Stops oocyst shedding in cats
- Dosing usually associated with vomiting, which can be ameliorated by antiemetics (chlorpromazine) (Table 32-1).

Precautions/Interactions

- Paromomycin will be absorbed across the blood–GI tract barrier in very young animals and animals with hemorrhagic diarrhea; because it is an aminoglycoside, its side effects of renal failure and deafness will be exacerbated in animals receiving parenteral aminoglycosides (gentamicin).
- Nitazoxanide—only been used in a limited number of cats with cryptosporidiosis and needs further evaluation; few side effects other than vomiting

TABLE 32-1 Drug Therapy for Cryptosporidiosis in Small Animals

Drug	Species	Dose (mg/kg)	Route	Interval (h)	Duration (days)
Paromomycin[a]—250 mg capsules	B	125–165	PO	12	5
Tylosin—100 g containers (<3 g/tsp)	C	11	PO	12	28
Nitazoxanide[b]—100 mg/5 ml suspension	C	25	PO	24	7–28

[a] Monitor closely for renal toxicity
[b] Only experimental to date
B, cats and dogs; C, cats.

COMMENTS

- Zoonosis—*C. canis* and *C. felis* are only rarely the cause of infection in man; the risk of infection from pet to owner is very low.
- Although some studies suggest that the incidence of cryptosporidiosis in HIV-positive people who own dogs is not increased, it would be prudent to make such owners aware of the infectivity of the organism.

Disinfection

- Resistant to commercial bleach (5.25% sodium hypochlorite) and chlorination of drinking water
- A 10% formaldehyde solution and 5% ammonia solution will kill oocysts, but requires 18 hours of exposure.
- Higher concentrations of ammonia (50%) will kill oocysts in 30 min.
- Moist heat (steam or pasteurization [>55°C]), freezing and thawing, or thorough drying are also effective.

Abbreviations

CBC, complete blood count; FeLV, feline leukemia virus; FIV, feline immunodeficiency virus; FIP, feline infectious peritonitis; GI, gastrointestinal; IBD, inflammatory bowel disease; HIV, human immunodeficiency virus; NPO, nothing per os; PCR, polymerase chain reaction; PPP, prepatent period.

Suggested Reading

Lucio-Forster A, Griffiths JK, Cams VA, et al. Minimal zoonotic risk of cryptosporidiosis from pet dogs and cats. *Trends Parasitol* 2010;26:174–179.

Cuterebriasis

DEFINITION/OVERVIEW

- A disease caused by the migration through tissues of the larvae of flies (genus *Cuterebra*) in dogs and cats

ETIOLOGY/PATHOPHYSIOLOGY

- *Cuterebra* spp. are obligatory parasites of rodents and lagomorphs (rabbits).
- The fly lays eggs on blades of grass or in the host's nest; the eggs hatch, and larvae crawl onto the skin of a passing host.
- The small maggot enters a body orifice, migrates through various internal tissues, and, eventually, migrates to the skin where it makes a warble.
- These small maggots (3–5 mm in length) are sometimes the parasite found to cause clinical disease.
- Once matured, the maggot (now up to 1 inch long) drops out of the host to pupate in the soil (Fig. 33-1).
- Cats and dogs infected in the same way as other hosts.
- Signs are associated with either the warble in the skin or migration of the larvae through tissues (nares, upper respiratory tract, skin of the face, ocular tissue, brain).

SIGNALMENT/HISTORY

- All ages and breeds of outdoor dogs and cats may be affected.
- Disease mainly seen during mid-summer to early autumn (northern states) or nearly year round (southern states) when flies are most active.

CLINICAL FEATURES

Skin Warble

- More common in dogs but also cats
- Appears as a single draining 2- to 5-mm cutaneous fistula (Fig. 33-2)

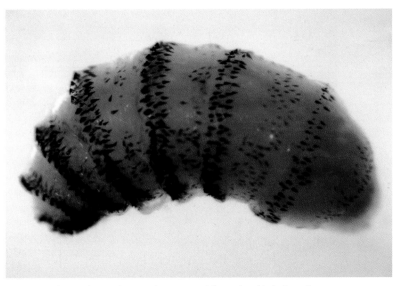

■ **Figure 33-1** Second-instar larva of *Cuterebra* removed from the skin lesion of a cat.

- Sometimes, a bot with protruding spiracles can be seen within the fistula.
- Before the bot penetrates the skin, the early developing warble can appear as a tender 1-cm swelling of the subcutis.

Tissue Migration

- Neurologic disease—most common form in cats
- Larvae migrate through the cribriform plate into the brain, causing acute onset of ataxia, circling, paralysis, blindness, and recumbency (Fig. 33-3).
- Nasal irritation—Migration may be preceded by 4–14 days of signs of nasal irritation.

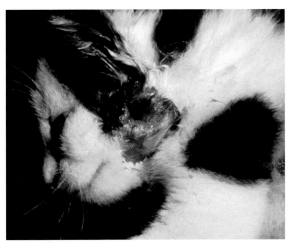

■ **Figure 33-2** A draining fistula or warble in the neck of a cat after a *Cuterebra* larva has been removed.

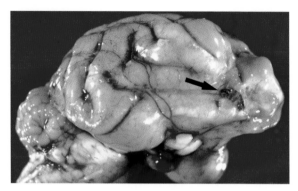

■ **Figure 33-3** A *Cuterebra* larva (*arrow*) on the frontal lobe of a cat's brain, where it was found at necropsy. Note the area of necrosis anterior to the larvae (courtesy of Dr. A. deLahunta, Cornell University).

- Respiratory—serous nasal discharge with sneezing as larvae migrate through nares; usually cats affected
- Swelling—can see unilateral facing swelling
- Larvae migration to nasopharynx and larynx—may see respiratory distress and stridor
- Migration into lungs—can cause eosinophilic respiratory disease
- Ophthalmic lesions—larvae migrate into globe or conjunctiva

 DIFFERENTIAL DIAGNOSIS

Skin Warble

- Mature warble is unmistakable because larvae with characteristic spiracles can be seen on the bot within the wound.
- Immature warble (before breaking through the skin) needs to be differentiated from subcutaneous foreign body, aggressive neoplasia, focal infectious lesion due to bacterial abscess, nocardia, fungal (blastomycosis).

Tissue Migration

- Neurologic—rabies, distemper, brain neoplasia, trauma, inflammatory neurologic disease, *Angiostrongylus* infection, toxoplasmosis, neosporosis, fungal diseases
- Respiratory
  - Cats—Causes of acute respiratory distress are feline asthma; lungworms; cardiomyopathy; upper respiratory tract viruses (herpes virus, calicivirus); nasopharyngeal foreign body or abscess; pleural effusion; pneumonia; diaphragmatic hernia; pulmonary edema (electric shock).
  - Dogs—Causes of acute respiratory distress are allergic bronchitis; pneumonia; cardiac disease; parasitic disease.
- Ophthalmic—foreign body; larval hypoderma

DIAGNOSTICS

- CBC—usually normal but may show mild neutrophilia and eosinophilia
- Aspirate cytologic examination of immature warble—neutrophils and eosinophils on proteinacious background
- CSF tap—usually normal but may show increased protein and mild increase in cell content
- MRI—demonstrates larval migration tract through brain; CT scan not as sensitive

Diagnostic Feature

- Identification of larvae in a cutaneous fistula

THERAPEUTICS

- Remove maggot from subcutaneous lesion—Increase size of hole through skin using a scalpel, grasp maggot with forceps and remove intact.
- Shaving hair around fistula tract—improves rate of healing
- Breaking maggot—may result in severe foreign body reaction but rarely occurs and may be alleviated by pretreatment with chlorpheniramine
- Manifestations of respiratory tract and neurologic disease—may be alleviated with the use of corticosteroids
- Neurologic disease—requires hospitalization and fluid and nutritional support during first week of recovery period

Drugs of Choice

- Ivermectin—thought to kill migrating larvae
- Prednisone—improves neurologic disease and reduces inflammation associated with larval migration through soft tissues, especially respiratory tract (nasopharynx)
- Chlorpheniramine—Antihistamines proposed to alleviate anaphylactic reaction if parasite is ruptured during removal or during kill off by ivermectin (Table 33-1).

TABLE 33-1 Drug Therapy for Cuterebriasis				
Drug	Dose (mg/kg)	Route	Interval (h)	Duration (days)
Ivermectin	0.2	SC, PO	24	3
Prednisone	1–2	PO	12	3–5
Chlorpheniramine	2–12	PO	8	5

Precautions/Interactions

- Check dogs for heartworm microfilaria before using ivermectin.
- Do not use these doses of ivermectin in ivermectin-sensitive collies or collie-cross dogs.

 COMMENTS

- Once larvae are removed from warble, fistula track heals quickly.
- Larval migration seems to induce poor immunity because cats can become infected often in the same year and subsequent years.
- Application of monthly heartworm preventives (avermectin-containing products), flea development control products (lufenuron-containing products), or topical flea and tick treatments may prevent the maggots from either developing in the dog or cat or may kill them before they have time to gain access to an orifice for entry, although anecdotal evidence suggests that some pets on these products still develop warbles in their skin.
- Most cats with neurologic cuterebriasis have improved function after treatment, but prognosis has to be guarded.

Abbreviations

CBC, complete blood count; CSF, cerebrospinal fluid; CT, computed tomography; MRI, magnetic resonance imaging.

Suggested Reading

Bordelon JT, Newcomb BT, Rochat MC. Surgical removal of a *Cuterebra* larva from the cervical trachea of a cat. *J Am Anim Hosp Assoc* 2009;45:52–54.
Bowman DD. *Georgis' Parasitology for Veterinarians*, 9th ed. Philadelphia: Saunders, 2009:31–33.
Bowman DD, Hendrix CM, Lindsay DS, et al. *Feline Clinical Parasitology*. Ames, IA: Iowa State University Press, 2002:430–439.
Glass EN, Cornetta AM, deLahunta A, et al. Clinical and clinicopathologic features in 11 cats with cuterebra larvae myiasis of the central nervous system. *J Vet Intern Med* 1998;12:365–368.

Cytauxzoonosis

chapter **34**

DEFINITION/OVERVIEW

- Fatal tick-borne protozoal disease of domestic and feral cats (especially bobcats) affecting the vascular system of the lungs, liver, spleen, kidneys, and brain, with development stages in the RBCs

ETIOLOGY/PATHOPHYSIOLOGY

- *Cytauxzoon felis*—distributed in cats mainly in the south central and southeastern United States (Kansas and Oklahoma); range in feral cats (bobcats) is more extensive including North Carolina and Pennsylvania.
- Large schizonts (tissue phase) develop in macrophages, causing them to line the lumen of veins of almost every organ, leading to occlusion of the vessels (especially in lungs).
- DIC—often the final outcome
- Merozoites bud from the schizonts in macrophages—rupture cell to infect other macrophages and RBCs (1–3 days before death)
- Vector—*Dermacentor variabilis*, but probably others also involved

SIGNALMENT/HISTORY

- No sex, age, or breed predisposition

CLINICAL FEATURES

- Some cats remain asymptomatic
- Usually severe debilitation at presentation
- Anemia (beginning 5–6 days postinfection).
- Depression
- Anorexia
- Dehydration

- High fever
- Icterus
- Splenomegaly
- Hepatomegaly

 ## DIFFERENTIAL DIAGNOSIS

- Other causes of regenerative anemia—immune-mediated hemolytic anemia, Heinz body anemia, *Haemobartonella* spp., *Babesia* spp., blood loss, or hemorrhage (GI tract neoplasia, intercavity hemorrhage, GI tract parasitism)

 ## DIAGNOSTICS

- CBC—regenerative anemia due to hemolysis and hemorrhage
- Parasitemia phase—leukopenia, left shift and toxic neutrophils, thrombocytopenia, normocytic, normochromic nonregenerative anemia may be present
- *Cytauxzoon* RBC forms—usually indicates late stage of disease (Fig. 34-1)
- Splenic and bone marrow aspirates—extraerythrocytic form

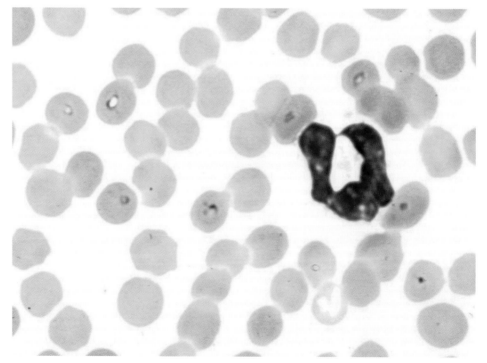

■ **Figure 34-1** Feline RBCs infected with *C. felis* piroplasms. Note the Howell–Jolly body for comparison in the RBC in the bottom right (Giemsa stain, 1000×).

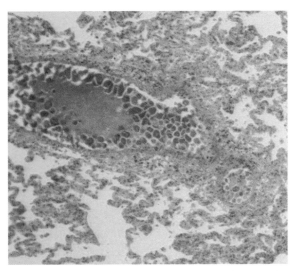

■ **Figure 34-2** Infected monocytes lining the walls of veins within a lung from a *C. felis*–infected cat (hematoxylin and eosin stain, 1000×).

- Biochemical profile and urinalysis—reflect DIC and changes due to severe anemia (organ hypoxia)
- In cats that die, histopathologic examination demonstrates marginalization of mononuclear cells in veins within most organs, but particularly lungs (Fig. 34-2).
- PCR—available but not commercially

 THERAPEUTICS

- Antibiotics—indicated if sepsis present (due to leukopenia)
- DIC—aggressive treatment, including:
  - IV isotonic fluids
  - Heparin (150 IU/kg, SC, q8h)
  - Plasma, and whole blood if anemia particularly severe

Drugs of Choice

- Atovaquane (15 mg/kg, PO, q8h) and azithromycin (10 mg/kg, PO, q24h) for 10 days – can be given via enteral feeding tube.
- Imidocarb dipropionate (Imizol [Schering-Plough]; Forray-65 [Hoechst Marion Roussel])
- Diminazene acetate (Berenil; Bayer; not available in United States) (Table 34-1)

Precautions/Interactions

- Imidocarb dipropionate—administer preanesthetic doses of atropine or glycopyrrolate

TABLE 34-1 Drug Therapy for *C. felis* in Cats

Drug	Dose (mg/kg)	Route	Interval (Hours)	Repeat Dose (Days)
Imidocarb dipropionate (Imazol)	2	IM	Once	3–7
Diminazene acetate[a] (Berenil)	2	IM	Once	3–7

[a] Not available in the United States.

- Imidocarb dipropionate—produces pain and swelling at the injection site as well as postinjection vomiting; other side effects can include periorbital edema, hypersalivation, diarrhea, signs similar to organophosphate toxicity
- Cats may become anorectic, febrile, and depressed after initial treatment with diminazene acetate.

COMMENTS

- The majority of cats will die if aggressive treatment is not begun immediately.
- Prevent tick transmission of disease by using products containing pyrethrin (collars, sprays) or fipronil (Frontline; Merial).

Abbreviations

CBC, complete blood count; DIC, disseminated intravascular coagulation; GI, gastrointestinal; PCR, polymerase chain reaction; RBCs, red blood cells.

Suggested Reading

Brown HM, Latimer KS, Erikson LE, et al. Detection of persistent *Cytauxzoon felis* infection by polymerase chain reaction in three asymptomatic domestic cats. *J Vet Diagn Invest* 2008;20:485–488.

Cohn LA, Birkenheuer JA, Brunker JD, et al. Efficacy of atovaquone and azithromycin or imidocarb dipropionate in cats with acute cytauxzoonosis. *J Vet Int Med* 2011;25:55–60.

Green CE, Latimer K, Hopper E, et al. Administration of diminazene or immidocarb dipropionate for treatment of cytauxzoonosis in cats. *J Am Vet Med Assoc* 1999;215:497–500.

Haber MD, Tucker MD, Marr HS, et al. The detection of *Cytauxzoon felis* in apparaently healthy free-roaming cats in the USA. *Vet Parasitol* 2007;146:316–320.

Holman PJ, Snowden KF. Canine hepatozoonosis and babesiosis, and feline cytauxzoonosis. *Vet Clin North Am Small Anim Pract* 2009;39:1035–1053.

Meinkoth J, Kocan AA, Whitworth L, et al. Cats surviving natural infection with *Cytauxzoon felis*: 18 cases (1997–1998). *J Vet Intern Med* 2000;14:521–525.

chapter 35

Demodicosis

DEFINITION/OVERVIEW

- An inflammatory parasitic disease of dogs and, rarely, cats that is characterized by an increased number of mites in the hair follicles, which often leads to furunculosis and secondary bacterial infection
- May be localized or generalized in dogs

ETIOLOGY/PATHOPHYSIOLOGY

Dogs

- Three species:
  - *Demodex canis*—a mite; part of the normal fauna of the skin; typically present in small numbers; resides in the hair follicles and sebaceous glands of the skin; transmitted from mother to neonate during first 2–3 days of nursing (Fig. 35-1)
  - *Demodex injai*—large, long-bodied mite found in the pilosebaceous unit; mode of transmission unknown; only associated with adult-onset disease with highest incidence noted in the terrier breeds often along the dorsal midline (West Highland white terrier and wire-haired fox terrier)
  - *Demodex cornei*—lives in the stratum corneum of the epidermis; mode of transmission unknown
- Pathology—develops when number of mites exceed that tolerated by the immune system
- Initial proliferation of mites—may be the result of a genetic or an immunologic disorder

Cats

- Poorly understood disorder
- Mites have been identified on the skin and within the otic canal
- Two species:
  - *Demodex cati*—often associated with immunosuppressive and metabolic disorders (e.g., diabetes)
  - *Demodex gotoi*—considered potentially contagious and associated with pruritic dermatitis

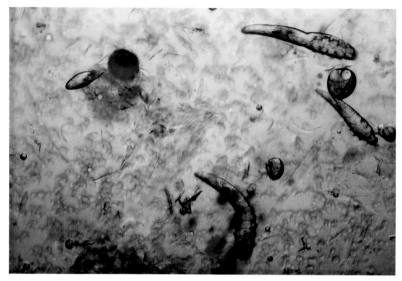

■ **Figure 35-1** *D. canis* mites in skin scraping. Note the different stages of the mite, including an egg (From Rhodes KH: *The 5-Minute Veterinary Consult Clinical Companion: Small Animal Dermatology*. Baltimore, MD: Lippincott Williams & Wilkins, 2002).

Dog/Cat

- Dead and degenerate mites may be found in noncutaneous sites (e.g., lymph node, intestinal wall, spleen, liver, kidney, urinary bladder, lung, thyroid gland, blood, urine, and feces) and are considered to represent drainage to these areas by blood and/or lymph.

 SIGNALMENT/HISTORY

- Dogs and rarely cats
- Localized—usually in young dogs; median age 3–6 months
- Generalized—both young and old animals

Dogs

- Exact immunopathologic mechanism unknown
- Studies indicate that dogs with generalized demodicosis have a subnormal percentage of IL-2 receptors on their lymphocytes and subnormal IL-2 production.
- Genetic factors, immunosuppression, and/or metabolic diseases may predispose animal.
- West Highland white and wire-haired fox terriers—greasy seborrheic dermatitis associated with *D. iniai*

Cats

- Potential increased incidence—Siamese and Burmese cat breeds
- Association—often with metabolic diseases (e.g., FIV, SLE, diabetes mellitus)

 CLINICAL FEATURES

Dogs

Localized

- Lesions—usually mild; consist of erythema and a light scale
- Patches—several may be noted; most common site is the face, especially around the perioral and periocular areas; may also be seen on the trunk and legs

Generalized

- Can be widespread from the onset, with multiple poorly circumscribed patches of erythema, alopecia, and scale (Fig. 35-2)
- As hair follicles become distended with large numbers of mites, secondary bacterial infections are common, often with resultant rupturing of the follicle (furunculosis) (Fig. 35-3).
- With progression, the skin can become severely inflamed, exudative, and granulomatous (Fig. 35-4).

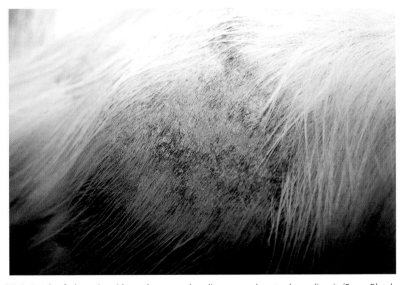

■ **Figure 35-2** Patch of alopecia with erythema and scaling secondary to demodicosis (From Rhodes KH: *The 5-Minute Veterinary Consult Clinical Companion: Small Animal Dermatology*. Baltimore, MD: Lippincott Williams & Wilkins, 2002).

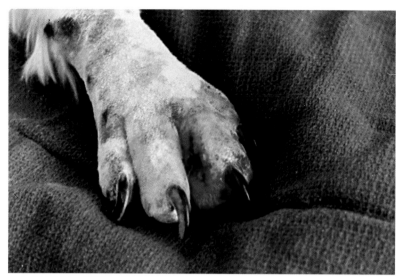

■ **Figure 35-3** Swelling of the digits caused by demodicosis and secondary furunculosis (From Rhodes KH: *The 5-Minute Veterinary Consult Clinical Companion: Small Animal Dermatology*. Baltimore, MD: Lippincott Williams & Wilkins, 2002).

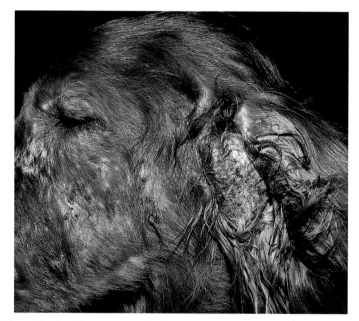

■ **Figure 35-4** Demodicosis with severe secondary bacterial infection of the facial and periauricular region (From Rhodes KH: *The 5-Minute Veterinary Consult Clinical Companion*: *Small Animal Dermatology*. Baltimore, MD: Lippincott Williams & Wilkins, 2002).

Cats

- Often characterized by partial to complete multifocal alopecia of the eyelids, periocular region, head, and neck
- Lesions are variably pruritic with erythema, scale, and crust; those caused by *D. gatoi* are often quite pruritic.
- Ceruminous otitis externa has been reported.
- *D. cati*—often associated with immunosuppressive disease

 ## DIFFERENTIAL DIAGNOSIS

Dogs

- Bacterial folliculitis/furunculosis
- Dermatophytosis
- Contact dermatitis
- Pemphigus complex
- Dermatomyositis
- SLE

Cats

- Allergic dermatitis
- Notoedres
- Dermatophytosis
- Psychogenic dermatitis

 ## DIAGNOSTICS

- May be useful for identifying underlying metabolic diseases in cats
- FeLV and FIV serologic examination—identify underlying metabolic diseases in cats
- Skin scrapings—diagnostic for finding large numbers of mites in the majority of cases
- Trichograms—may be an effective technique for mite identification
- Cutaneous biopsy—may be needed when lesions are chronic, granulomatous, and fibrotic (especially on the paw)

 ## THERAPEUTICS

- Localized—conservative; most cases (90%) resolve spontaneously with no treatment
- Evaluate—general health status of dogs with either the localized or the generalized form

- Generalized (adult dog)—frequent management problem; expense and frustration with the chronicity of the problem are issues; many cases are medically controlled, not cured; juvenile-onset considered an inheritable predisposition, therefore breeding of affected animals is not recommended

Drugs

Amitraz (Mitaban; Taktic-EC)

- A formamidine, which inhibits monoamine oxidase and prostaglandin synthesis; an α_2-adrenergic agonist
- Use weekly (the label states every other week) at $^1/_2$ vial (5 ml) per gallon of water until resolution of clinical signs and no mites are found on skin scrapings; do not rinse off; let air dry.
- Treat for 1 month after negative skin scrape.
- Apply a benzoyl peroxide shampoo before application of the dip as a bactericidal therapy and to increase exposure of the mites to the miticide through follicular flushing activity.
- The efficacy is proportional to the frequency of administration and the concentration of the dip.
- May be mixed with mineral oil (3 ml amitraz to 30 ml mineral oil) for application to focal areas, such as pododemodicosis
  - Rarely used in cats—0.015–0.025% applied to the entire body every 1–2 weeks (do not use on diabetic cats)
  - Dogs—0.03–0.05% applied weekly to every other week; total body/additional topical treatments for focal areas (pododermatitis) may be used every 1–3 days with 0.125% solution
  - Promeris—topical product applied every 2–4 weeks.
  - Preventic collar—anecdotal reports of success; change collar every 2–4 weeks; not FDA-approved for use
- Success with the 9% amitraz collar has not been established, although there are positive anecdotal reports.
- Between 11% and 30% of cases will not be cured; may need to try an alternative therapy or control with maintenance dips every 2–8 weeks.

Ivermectin (Ivomec; Eqvalan Liquid)

- A macrocyclic lactone with GABA agonist activity
- Daily oral administration of 0.3–0.6 mg/kg very effective, even when amitraz fails
- Treat for 60 days beyond negative skin scrapings (average 3–8 months)
- Ivermectin is contraindicated in collies, Shetland sheepdogs, old English sheepdogs, other herding breeds, and crosses with these breeds; sensitive breeds appear to tolerate the acaricidal dosages of milbemycin (see below)

Milbemycin (Interceptor)

- A macrocylic lactone with GABA agonist activity
- Dosage of 1–2 mg/kg, PO, q24h cures 50% of cases; 2 mg/kg, PO, q24h cures 85% of cases
- Treat for 60 days beyond multiple negative skin scrapings.

Moxidectin

- Anecdotal reports in dogs (400 μg/kg PO once weekly)
- Do not use in ivermectin-sensitive breeds.

Cats

- Exact protocols are not defined.
- Topical lime-sulfur dips or amitraz solutions applied weekly for 4–8 treatments often lead to good resolution of clinical signs.
- Ivermectin—use reported in cats (300 μg/kg)
- Doramectin—reported to be effective (0.6 mg/kg, SC, once weekly)

 COMMENTS

Amitraz

- Most common side effects—somnolence, lethargy, depression, anorexia seen in 30% of patients for 12–36 hours after treatment
- Other side effects—vomiting, diarrhea, pruritus, polyuria, mydriasis, bradycardia, hypoventilation, hypotension, hypothermia, ataxia, ileus, bloat, hyperglycemia, convulsions, and death
- The incidence and severity of side effects do not appear to be proportional to the dose or frequency of use.
- Humans can develop dermatitis, headaches, and respiratory difficulty after exposure.
- Antidote—yohimbine 0.11 mg/kg, IV

Ivermectin and Milbemycin

- Signs of toxicity—salivation, vomiting, mydriasis, confusion, ataxia, hypersensitivity to sound, weakness, recumbency, coma, and death
- Sensitive breeds may lack a gene (MDR1 mutation) that codes for a P-glycoprotein (drug-efflux pump) that predisposes to toxicity.

Possible Interactions

- Amitraz—may interact with heterocyclic antidepressants, xylazine, benzodiazepines, and macrocyclic lactones

- Ivermectin and milbemycin—cause elevated levels of monoamine neurotransmitter metabolites, which could result in adverse drug interactions with amitraz and benzodiazepines
- Multiple skin scrapings and evidence of clinical resolution are used to monitor progress.
- Avoid breeding animals with generalized form.

Comments

- Prognosis (dogs)—depends heavily on genetic, immunologic, and underlying diseases
- Localized—Most cases (90%) resolve spontaneously with no treatment; <10% progress to the generalized form.
- Adult onset (dogs)—often severe and refractory to treatment
- Adult onset—sudden occurrence is often associated with internal disease, malignant neoplasia, and/or immunosuppressive disease; approximately 25% of cases are idiopathic over a follow-up period of 1–2 years.
- No zoonotic protential

Abbreviations

FeLV, feline leukemia virus; FIV, feline immunodeficiency virus; GABA, γ-aminobutyric acid; IL, interleukin; SLE, systemic lupus erythematosus.

Suggested Reading

Scott DW, Miller WH, Griffin CE, eds. *Muller & Kirk's Small Animal Dermatology*, 5th ed. Philadelphia: WB Saunders, 1995:417–432.

chapter 36

Dermatophilosis

DEFINITION/OVERVIEW

- A crusting skin disease in dogs and a nodular subcutaneous and oral disease in cats
- Reported infrequently

ETIOLOGY/PATHOPHYSIOLOGY

- *Dermatophilus congolensis*—causative agent; gram-positive, branching filamentous bacterium classified as an actinomycete; common cause of crusting dermatoses in hoofed animals, which causes crusted skin lesions of affected large animals and persists in their environment within crusts and other debris shed from infected hoof stock
- Dogs, cats, and humans can rarely be secondarily infected.

SIGNALMENT/HISTORY

- Association with farm animals or free-roaming lifestyle often reported.
- Cats—episode of trauma; existence of a foreign body; lesions generally chronic; no systemic clinical signs, except when internal organs or large oral lesions develop
- Dogs, cats, and humans can be exposed directly from lesions on large animals or from environmental exposure.
- Infectious stage—requires wetting for activation; probably cannot penetrate intact epithelium; thus antecedent minor trauma or mechanical transmission by biting ectoparasites required
- Deeper infections—presumably acquired by traumatic inoculation of infectious material

CLINICAL FEATURES

- Dogs—lesions: papular; crusted; mainly on the skin of the trunk or head; circular to coalescent; similar to those in superficial pyoderma caused by *Staphylococcus*

pseudointermedius; resemble dermatophilosis in horses (adherent thick, gray–yellow crusts that incorporate hair and leave a circular, glistening shallow erosion when removed); pruritus variable
- Cats—subcutaneous, oral, or internal ulcerated and fistulated nodules or abscesses similar to lesions caused by other actinomycetes in this species; superficial pyogenic crusting disease of the face has been reported

 DIFFERENTIAL DIAGNOSIS

Dogs

- Staphylococcal pyoderma
- Acute moist dermatitis
- Dermatophytosis
- Pemphigus foliaceus
- Keratinization disorder

Cats

- Actinomycosis and nocardiosis
- Atypical mycobacterial granuloma
- Sporotrichosis
- Other subcutaneous fungal infection
- Deep mycotic infection

Cryptococcosis

- Foreign body
- Chronic bite/wound abscess
- Bacterial L-form infection
- *Rhodococcus equi* infection
- Cutaneous or mucosal neoplasm, especially squamous cell carcinoma

 DIAGNOSTICS

Dogs

- Cytologic examination of crusts—most important procedure; differentiates from more typical bacterial pyodermas
- Organism—distinctive morphology in cytologic and histologic preparations; resembles railroad tracks as the bacterium forms chains of small diplococci; chains often branching

- Cytologic diagnosis—from impression smears made of exudate from under crusts or by preparation of minced crusts; mince crusts finely in a drop of water and allow to macerate several minutes; then dry the preparation and stain with any Wright–Giemsa stain
- Histopathologic specimens—from crusts

Cats

- Histopathologic examination—biopsy of ulcerated nodules; procedure of choice
- Cytologic examination—exudate obtained from aspiration or swabbing of a draining tract
- Culture of biopsy specimens—may yield the organism; facilitated if the laboratory is alerted to the possible presence of *Dermatophilus* (aerobic, relatively slow growing, and easily obscured by contamination)
- Culture from crusts—requires the use of special selective medium; generally used to corroborate cytologic findings; isolation is possible but usually very difficult

 THERAPEUTICS

- Dogs—antibacterial shampoo and gentle removal (and disposal) of crusts; shampoo may contain benzoyl peroxide, ethyl lactate, chlorhexidine, or selenium disulfide; one or two applications suffice in most cases. Iodine or lime-sulfur may also be used.
- Cats—for pyogranulomas and abscesses: surgical debridement; exploration for foreign body; establishment of drainage for exudate; maintain effective drainage and postoperative wound care

Drugs

- Penicillin V—10 mg/kg, PO, q12h for 10–20 days; drug of choice
- Ampicillin—10–20 mg/kg, PO, q12h for 10–20 days
- Amoxicillin—10–20 mg/kg, PO, q12h for 10–20 days
- Tetracycline, doxycycline, or minocycline—standard dosage

 COMMENTS

- Dogs—re-examine after 2 weeks of treatment to ensure complete resolution of symptoms; give an additional 7 days of systemic therapy
- Cats—monitor biweekly for 1 month after apparent resolution of lesions, depending on their location
- Dogs—excellent prognosis

- Cats—Prognosis varies with the location of lesions and extent of surgical debridement; complete resolution can be achieved with timely diagnosis and appropriate surgical and medical therapy.
- Veterinarians and animal care workers—very seldom infected, even after traumatic exposure when working with farm animals known to be infected
- Dogs and cats—very unlikely to serve as a source for human infection; caution is warranted for exposure of immunocompromised individuals

Suggested Reading

Greene CE. Dermatophilosis. In: Greene CE, ed. *Infectious Diseases of the Dog and Cat.* Philadelphia: WB Saunders Elsevier, 2006:488–490.

Dermatophytosis: Keratinophilic Mycosis

chapter 37

DEFINITION/OVERVIEW

- A cutaneous fungal infection affecting the cornified regions of hair, nails, and occasionally the superficial layers of the skin
- Most commonly isolated organisms are *Microsporum canis*, *Trichophyton mentagrophytes*, and *Microsporum gypseum.*

ETIOLOGY/PATHOPHYSIOLOGY

- Exposure to or contact with a dermatophyte does not necessarily result in an infection.
- Infection may not result in clinical signs.
- Dermatophytes grow in the keratinized layers of hair, nail, and skin; do not thrive in living tissue or persist in the presence of severe inflammation—incubation period: 1–4 weeks
- Affected animal that does not show signs may remain in this inapparent carrier state for a prolonged period of time; some animals never become symptomatic.
- Corticosteroids can modulate inflammation and prolong the infection.
- Cats—*M. canis* is by far the most common agent.
- Dogs—*M. canis*, *M. gypseum*, and *T. mentagrophytes*; incidence of each agent varies geographically
- Reliance on clinical signs and incorrectly interpreted Wood's lamp examination results in overdiagnosis.

SIGNALMENT

- Cats—more common in long-haired breeds (Fig. 37-1)
- Clinical signs—more common in young animals
- Incidence—Although infection is ubiquitous, the incidence is higher in hot and humid regions.
- Lesions—may begin as alopecia or a poor hair coat
- History of previously confirmed infection or exposure to an infected animal or environment (e.g., a cattery)—a useful but not consistent finding

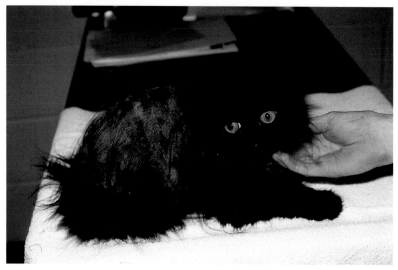

■ **Figure 37-1** Persian cat with *M. canis* infection. This breed is considered predisposed to dermatophytosis (courtesy of Dr. Carol Foil).

Risk Factors

- Immunocompromising disease or immunosuppressive medication
- High population density
- Poor nutrition
- Poor management practices
- Lack of an adequate quarantine period

 CLINICAL SIGNS

- Vary from an inapparent carrier state to a patchy or circular alopecia
- Classic circular alopecia common in cats; often misinterpreted in dogs (Fig. 37-2)
- Scales, erythema, hyperpigmentation, and pruritus are variable (Fig. 37-3).
- Paronychosis, granulomatous lesions, or kerions may occur.

 DIFFERENTIAL DIAGNOSIS

- Cats—miliary dermatitis and almost any other dermatitis
- Dogs—folliculitis, furunculosis, and most cases of alopecia
- Demodicosis and bacterial skin infection—epidermal collarettes more typical of a bacterial infection; grossly enlarged follicular ostia with furunculosis suggest

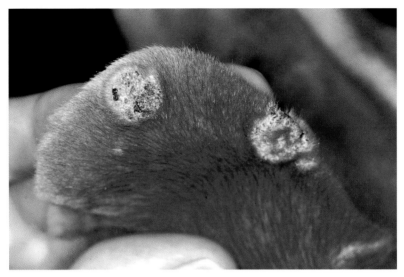

■ **Figure 37-2** Dermatophytosis (*M. canis*) in a dog. Circular patches of alopecia and scale are more characteristic in humans and cats (courtesy of Dr. Carol Foil).

demodicosis; these characteristics are not consistent; concurrent bacterial or mite infections can be seen with dermatophytosis; all three diseases can cause focal hyperpigmentation.

■ Immune-mediated skin diseases—severe inflammation associated with dermatophytosis affecting the face or feet

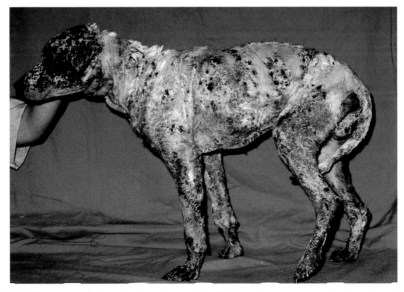

■ **Figure 37-3** Disseminated dermatophytosis caused by *Trichophyton mentagrophytes* (courtesy of Dr. Carol Foil).

DIAGNOSTICS

- Reliance on clinical signs and incorrectly interpreted Wood's lamp examination results in overdiagnosis.

Wood's Lamp Examination
- Not a useful screening tool
- Many pathogenic dermatophytes do not fluoresce.
- False fluorescence is common; medications, keratin associated with epidermal scales, and sebum may produce false-positive fluorescence.
- Lamp should warm up for a minimum of 5 minutes and then be exposed to suspicious lesions for up to 5 minutes.
- A true positive reaction associated with M. *canis* consists of apple-green fluorescence of the hair shaft.

Fungal Culture with Macroconidia Identification

- Best means of confirming diagnosis
- Hairs that exhibit a positive apple-green fluorescence under Wood's lamp examination are considered ideal candidates for culture.
- Pluck hairs from the periphery of an alopecic area; do not use a random pattern.
- Use a sterile toothbrush to brush the hair coat of an asymptomatic animal to yield better results.
- Test media change to red when they become alkaline; dermatophytes typically produce this color during the early growing phase of their culture; saprophytes, which also produce this color, do so in the late growing phase; thus, it is important to examine the media daily.
- Microscopic examination of the macroconidia necessary to confirm pathogenic dermatophyte and to identify genus and species; helps identify source of infection
- Positive culture indicates existence of a dermatophyte; however, it may have been there only transiently, as commonly occurs when the culture is obtained from the feet, which are likely to come in contact with a geophilic dermatophyte.

Microscopic Examination of Hair

- Examination after using a clearing solution can help provide a rapid diagnosis.
- Time-consuming and often produces false-negative results
- Use hairs that fluoresce under Wood's lamp illumination to increase the likelihood of identifying the fungal hyphae associated with the hair shaft.
- Wood's lamp examination is not a very useful screening tool; many pathogenic dermatophytes do not fluoresce; false fluorescence is common; lamp should warm up for a minimum of 5 minutes and then be exposed to suspicious lesions for up to 5 minutes; a true positive reaction associated with M. *canis* consists of apple-green

fluorescence of the hair shaft; keratin associated with epidermal scales and sebum will often produce a false-positive fluorescence.

Skin Biopsy

- Not usually needed
- Can be helpful in confirming true invasion and infection

 ## THERAPEUTICS

- Zoonosis—consider quarantine owing to the infective and zoonotic nature of the disease.
- Griseofulvin—most widely prescribed systemic drug; microsized formulation: 25–60 mg/kg, PO, q12h for 4–6 weeks; ultramicrosized formulation: 2.5–5.0 mg/kg, PO, q12–24h; pediatric suspension: 10–25 mg/kg, PO, q12h; GI upset is the most common side effect; alleviate by reducing the dose or dividing the dose for more frequent administration
- Griseofulvin—fatty meal improves absorption
- Ketoconazole—not labeled for use in dogs or cats in the United States; true efficacy unknown; dose: 10 mg/kg, PO, q24h or divided twice per day for 3–4 weeks; anorexia is most common side effect
- Ketoconazole—acid meal (add tomato juice) enhances absorption.
  - Itraconazole—similar to ketoconazole, but with fewer side effects, more effective, but expensive; dose of itraconazole capsules in dogs is 5–10 mg/kg, PO, q24h for 4–8 weeks; dose in cats is 10 mg/kg, PO, q24h for 4–8 weeks or until cured; dose of 20 mg/kg, q48h may be considered for both cats and dogs. In some cats, the dosage regimen is altered after 4 weeks of therapy to an every-other-week schedule for a total of 8–10 weeks of therapy; alternative schedule is one-week-on, one-week-off with apparent efficacy to reduce drug cost; available in 100 mg capsules and as 10 mg/ml liquid containing cyclodextrin; liquid preferred over compounded formulations due to absorption variability. Itraconazole has become many clinicians' preferred therapeutic choice for dermatophytosis in small dogs and cats (kittens as young as 6 weeks).
  - Topical therapy and clipping—recommended use with concurrent systemic therapy; may help prevent environmental contamination; often associated with an initial exacerbation of signs after the procedures are initiated; lime sulfur (1 : 16 dilution or 8 oz per gallon of water), enilconazole and miconazole (with or without chlorhexidine) are the most effective generalized topical agents; lime sulfur is odoriferous and can stain; enilconazole is not available in the United States for household use. Miconazole-containing solutions are available in both shampoo and "leave-on" preparations; use of an Elizabethan collar, particularly in cats, is recommended to prevent ingestion of these products. Chlorhexidine alone has been

shown to be ineffective, but there is recent research that shows that chlorhexidine may work synergistically with miconazole to increase its effectiveness.
- Vaccination—Product literature claims are based on clinical signs and Wood's lamp findings; may be useful as an adjuvant to systemic therapy; may be valuable for treating asymptomatic carriers, which can be frustrating to the client and veterinarian and can complicate the diagnosis and management; studies involving dermatophyte cultures as a measure of achieving a cure or prevention are necessary to ensure true efficacy.

Griseofulvin Precautions

- Bone marrow suppression (anemia, pancytopenia, and neutropenia)—can occur as an idiosyncratic reaction or with prolonged therapy
- Neutropenia—most common fatal reaction in cats; can persist after discontinuation of drug; weekly or biweekly CBC is recommended; can be life-threatening in cats with FIV infection
- Side effects—neurologic
- Do not use during the first two trimesters of pregnancy—It is teratogenic.

Ketoconazole Precautions

- Hepatopathy has been reported and can be quite severe.
- Inhibits endogenous production of steroidal hormones in dogs

Itraconazole Precautions

- Vasculitis and necroulcerative skin lesions were reported in 7.5% of dogs with blastomycosis that were treated with itraconazole doses of 5 mg/kg, q12h. Lesions were not noted in patients receiving 5 mg/kg, q24h.
- Hepatotoxicity has been reported in dogs in approximately 5–10% of cases being treated for blastomycosis.

 COMMENTS

- Dermatophyte culture is the only means of truly monitoring response to therapy; many animals will clinically improve but remain culture positive.
- Repeat fungal cultures toward the end of the treatment regimen and continue treatment until at least one culture result is negative.
- In resistant cases, the culture may be repeated weekly, using the toothbrush technique; continue treatment until 2–3 consecutive culture results are negative.
- Initiate a quarantine period and obtain dermatophyte cultures of all animals entering the household to prevent reinfection from other animals.
- Consider the possibility of rodents aiding in the spread of the disease.
- Avoid infective soil, if a geophilic dermatophyte is involved.

- Consider using griseofulvin for 10–14 days as a prophylactic treatment of exposed animals.
- Many animals will self-clear a dermatophyte infection over a period of a few months.
- Treatment for the disease hastens clinical cure and helps reduce environmental contamination.
- Some infections, particularly in long-haired cats or multianimal situations, can be very persistent.

Client Education

- Inform owner that many short-haired cats in a single-cat environment and many dogs will undergo spontaneous remission.
- Advise owner that treatment can be both frustrating and expensive, especially in multianimal households or recurrent cases.
- Inform owner that environmental treatment, including fomites, is important, especially in recurrent cases; diluted bleach (1 : 10) is a practical and relatively effective means of providing environmental decontamination; concentrated bleach and formalin (1%) are more effective at killing spores, but their use is not as practical in many situations; chlorhexidine was ineffective in pilot studies.
- Inform owner that, in a multianimal environment or cattery situation, treatment and control can be very complicated; referral to a veterinarian with expertise in this type of situation should be considered.

Abbreviations

CBC, complete blood count; GI, gastrointestinal

Suggested Reading

DeBoer DJ, Moriello KA. Cutaneous fungal infections. In: Greene CE, ed. *Infectious Diseases of the Dog and Cat*, 3rd edition. Philadelphia: WB Saunders, 2006:550–569.

Newbury S, Moriello K, Verbrugge M, Thomas C. Use of lime sulphur and itraconazole to treat shelter cats naturally infected with *Microsporum canis* in an annex facility: an open field trial. *Vet Dermatol* 2007;19:324–331.

Perrins N, Bond R. Synergistic inhibition of the growth in vitro of *Microsporum canis* by miconazole and chlorhexidine. *Vet Dermatol* 2003;14:99–102.

38 chapter

Ear Mites

DEFINITION/OVERVIEW

- *Otodectes cynotis* mites cause a hypersensitivity reaction that results in intense irritation of the external ear of dogs and cats.

SIGNALMENT/HISTORY

- Common in young dogs and cats, although it may occur at any age
- No breed or sex predilection

CLINICAL FEATURES

- Pruritus—primarily located around the ears, head, and neck; occasionally generalized
- Thick, red–brown or black crusts—usually seen in the outer ear
- Crusting and scales—may occur on the neck, rump, and tail
- Excoriations—often occur on the convex surface of the pinnae, owing to the intense pruritus

DIFFERENTIAL DIAGNOSIS

- Flea bite hypersensitivity
- Pediculosis
- Pelodera dermatitis
- Sarcoptic mange
- Notoedric mange
- Chiggers
- Allergic otitis dermatitis

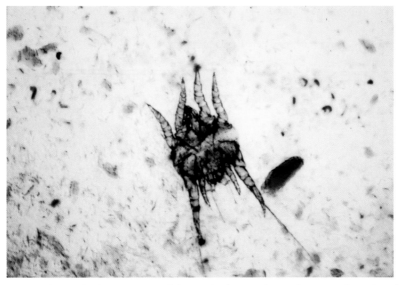

■ **Figure 38-1** *Otodectes* mite from an ear swab (From Rhodes KH: *The 5-Minute Veterinary Consult Clinical Companion: Small Animal Dermatology*. Baltimore, MD: Lippincott Williams & Wilkins, 2002).

 ## DIAGNOSTICS

- Skin scrapings—identify mites, if signs are generalized
- Ear swabs placed in mineral oil—usually a very effective means of identification (Fig. 38-1)
- Mites may be visualized in external ear canal
- Hypersensitive animals—diagnosis made by response to treatment

 ## THERAPEUTICS

- Very contagious—important to treat all in-contact animals
- Environment—thoroughly clean and treat
- Cleanse the ears thoroughly with mineral oil or a commercial ear cleaner to remove debris.
- Otic parasiticides should be used for 7–10 days to eradicate mites and eggs; effective topical commercial products contain: pyrethrins, thiabendazole, ivermectin, and rotenone; treatment during alternative weeks for two to three cycles also suggested to prevent reinfestation from eggs.
  - Selamectin (Revolution)—applied topically every 2–4 weeks
  - Imidacloprid/moxidectin (Advantage Multi/Advocate)—applied topically every 2–4 weeks

- Moxidectin—0.2–0.4 mg/kg every 1–2 weeks for 4 treatments; not FDA-approved for use
- Ivermectin—300 μg/kg every 1–2 weeks for 4 treatments; not FDA approved
- Milbemycin—1–2 mg/kg, PO, q24h in alternative weeks for two to three treatment cycles; not FDA approved
- Amitraz—topical; place 1 ml in 33 ml mineral oil directly into the ear; not approved for this use
- Pyrethrin-based flea spray—Treat entire animal weekly for 4–6 weeks if not using systemic ivermectin.
- Flea treatments should be applied to animal for elimination of ectopic mites.

 COMMENTS

- Environment—treat with a flea-type preparation 2 times, 2–4 weeks apart
- Ivermectin and moxidectin—Do not use in collies, shelties, their crosses, or other herding breeds; use only if absolutely necessary in animals <6 months of age; an increasing number of toxic reactions have been reported in kittens.
- Ivermectin and milbemycin may have adverse drug interactions with amitraz and benzodiazepines.
- Amitraz—reported to cause adverse reactions in cats when used topically for generalized infestations; thus, use with caution.
- Ear swab and physical examination—should be done 1 month after therapy commences
- Prognosis is good for most patients.
- Allergy—Rarely, the infestation will be cleared only to find an underlying allergy that keeps the otitis externa active.
- Humans—the mites will also bite humans (rare)

Suggested Reading

Medleau LA, Hnilica KA. *Small Animal Dermatology: A Color Atlas and Therapeutic Guide.* St. Louis, MO: Saunders Elsevier, 2006.
Scott DW, Miller WH, Griffin CE. *Muller & Kirk's Small Animal Dermatology,* 6th ed. Philadelphia: WB Saunders, 2001.

Ehrlichiosis

chapter **39**

DEFINITION/OVERVIEW

- A tick-borne disease of dogs and cats causing vasculitis, thrombocytopenia, hyperglobulinemia, and multisystem dysfunction

ETIOLOGY/PATHOPHYSIOLOGY

Dogs

- Recently reclassified—moved from the family *Rickettsiaceae* into the family *Anaplasmataceae*
- Within the family *Anaplasmataceae*—three pathogenic genera: *Ehrlichia*, *Anaplasma*, and *Neorickettsia*
- *Ehrlichia* spp.—divided into three groups:
  - *Ehrlichia canis*—ehrlichiosis found intracytoplasmically in circulating leukocytes
  - *Ehrlichia ewingii*—canine granulocytic ehrlichiosis; like *Anaplasma phagocytophila*, infects granulocytic cells in dogs, but differs in geographic distribution (mainly found in southeastern and south central United States)
  - *Ehrlichia chaffeensis*—like *E. canis*, tropism for mononuclear cells; mainly a human pathogen but can cause mild disease in dog
- *E. canis*—considered the main ehrlichiosis pathogen in North America, but in areas of high vector tick populations (southcentral states), infection with *E. ewingii* and *E. chaffeensis* is more common
- *Anaplasma* spp.—two organisms of importance:
  - *phagocytophila*—previously *E. equi*, *E. phagocytophila*, and HGE agent; infects mainly horses but also the granulocytic cells of dogs; mainly found in northeastern and upper Midwestern states and California
  - *Anaplasma platys*—previously *E. platys*; tropism for platelets; does not share serologic cross reactivity with *E. canis*
- *Neorickettsia* spp.—two organisms of importance:
  - *Neorickettsia risticii*—previously *E. risticii*; causes Potomac horse fever in horses but also infects dogs and cats; like other *Neorickettsia*, this organism is not transmitted by ticks; infections acquired by ingesting infected snails, free nematode

life stages, or aquatic insects with encysted metacercaria; grazing or drinking from standing water explains why horses become infected more often than dogs; infected dogs have negative *E. canis* titers

- *N. helminthoeca*—causes salmon poisoning disease in dogs (see Chapter 96)
- Pathophysiology for *E. canis*—*Rhipicephalus sanguineus* (brown dog tick) transmits disease to dogs in saliva (*Dermacentor variabilis* also).
- Immature *R. sanguineus* stages—infected when feed on a rickettsemic dog, and then maintain infection trans-stadially (enables transmission when tick feeds again as a nymph or adult)
- Adult *R. sanguineus* ticks—can transmit *E. canis* intrastadially as adults readily move between dogs as they intermittently feed and mate
- Incubation period—2 to 4 weeks after tick transmission
- Due to the wide variety of *Ehrlichia* spp. infecting dogs, and variations in pathogenicity of different strains of *E. canis*, there is a wide spectrum of disease presentation from inapparent to severe.
- Three stages of disease:
  - Acute—spreads from bite site to the spleen, liver, and lymph nodes (causes organomegaly), then subclinical, with mild thrombocytopenia; mainly endothelial cells affected; vasculitis; antiplatelet antibodies may exacerbate thrombocytopenia; variable leukopenia; mild anemia; severity depends on organism
  - Subclinical—organism persists; antibody response increases (hyperglobulinemia); thrombocytopenia persists
  - Chronic—impaired bone marrow production (platelets, erythroid suppression); marrow hypercellular with plasma cells
- Multisystemic disease—including bleeding tendencies (thrombocytopenia and vasculitis), lymphadenopathy, splenomegaly, CNS, ocular (anterior uveitis), and lung (rarely affected by vasculitis)
- *E. chaffeensis*—white-tailed deer is the primary reservoir host; *Amblyomma americanum* the tick vector (adults and nymphs); clinical signs—vomiting, epistaxis, lymphadenopathy, and anterior uveitis reported in naturally infected dogs; experimental infections demonstrate mild to inapparent signs
- Only PCR will differentiate *E. chaffeensis* infection from that of *E. canis*.
- *E. ewingii*—tick vector is also *Amblyomma americanum*; serologic cross-reactivity with *E. canis*; main clinical manifestation is neutrophilic polyarthritis with fever; splenomegaly, hepatomegaly, mild to moderate thrombocytopenia, and meningitis (ataxia, head tilt, paresis) also noted
- Fatal infections due to *E. ewingii* are rare—quick recovery with appropriate therapy
- *A. phagocytophila*—*Ixodes* spp. ticks (same as for Lyme disease) are the vectors; mild illness typified by fever, lethargy, and thrombocytopenia; polyarthritis occurs but is rare in comparison to infection with *E. ewingii*; most dogs present in autumn and are females; *E. canis* titers are usually negative.
- *A. platys*—transmission thought to be via *R. sanguineus* ticks; moderate to severe cyclic thrombocytopenia but bleeding rare; coinfections with *E. canis* occur to cause a more severe syndrome

- *N. risticii*—Lethargy, vomiting, bleeding disorders, and arthralgia are common signs.
- Blood transfusion—can be a source of infection for *E. canis* and *Anaplasma* spp. (and probably others) as infection survives blood storage; perinatal and transplacental transmission confirmed in people and cattle but not dogs

Cats

- Extremely rare
- *N. risticii* and *A. phagocytophilum*
- Serologic evidence suggests a species that cross-reacts with *E. canis* can cause illness.

SIGNALMENT/HISTORY

Dogs

- Worldwide distribution
- North America—mainly Gulf Coast and eastern seaboard; also Midwest and California
- Occurs throughout the year—insidious
- Breed predilection—chronic (*E. canis*) disease may be more severe in Doberman pinschers and German shepherd dogs
- Average age—5.22 years (range: 2 months to 14 years)
- Historically—may show lethargy, depression, anorexia and weight loss, fever, spontaneous bleeding, epistaxis, respiratory distress, ataxia, head tilt, and ocular pain (uveitis)

CLINICAL FEATURES

Dogs

- Duration of clinical signs from initial acute illness to presentation—usually >2 months.

Acute

- Bleeding diatheses—petechiation of mucous membranes such as conjunctiva (Fig. 39-1) or retinal hemorrhage (Fig. 39-2) as a result of thrombocytopenia
- Fever—with depression, anorexia, weight loss
- Lymphadenopathy—generalized
- Ticks—found in 40% of cases
- Respiratory signs—dyspnea (even cyanosis) and increased bronchovesicular sounds
- Diffuse CNS disease—meningitis
- Ataxia—with upper motor neuron dysfunction

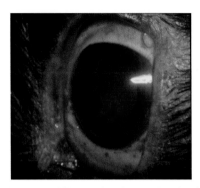

■ **Figure 39-1** Conjunctival petechiation and fibrin within the anterior chamber of a dog with acute *E. canis* (courtesy of Dr. R. Riis, Cornell University).

- CNS—vestibular dysfunction
- Hyperesthesia—generalized or local
- Most dogs recover without treatment, then enter a subclinical state.

Chronic

- In nonendemic areas
- Spontaneous bleeding
- Anemia
- Generalized lymphadenopathy
- Polyarthritis
- Scrotal and limb edema
- Splenomegaly
- Hepatomegaly
- Uveitis
- Hyphema
- Retinal hemorrhages and detachment with blindness
- Corneal edema
- Seizures—rare

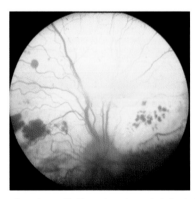

■ **Figure 39-2** Retinal hemorrhage in a dog with thrombocytopenia infected with *E. canis* (courtesy of Dr. R. Riis, Cornell University).

Cats

- Fever—with anorexia, lethargy, and weight loss
- Hyperesthesia—joint pain and irritability
- Polyarthritis—some cases
- Bone marrow hypoplasia or dysplasia—with pancytopenia and thrombocytopenia
- Splenomegaly, lymphadenopathy, dyspnea, pale mucous membranes

 DIFFERENTIAL DIAGNOSIS

Dogs

- RMSF (*Rickettsia rickettsii*)—usually seasonal between March and October; serologic testing for diagnosis; responds to same treatment as ehrlichiosis
- Immune-mediated thrombocytopenia—not usually associated with fever or lymphadenopathy; serologic testing best distinguishes; may treat for both until results are known
- SLE—ANA test usually negative with ehrlichiosis; serologic testing for diagnosis
- Multiple myeloma—serologic testing to differentiate and determine cause of hyperglobulinemia; bone marrow cytology and punched-out bone lesions on radiology
- Chronic lymphocytic leukemia—differentiate by lymphocytosis and cytology of bone marrow
- Brucellosis—serologic testing for diagnosis and to determine cause of scrotal edema

Cats

- Other causes of polyarthritis—feline syncytium-forming virus infection that may reflect coinfection with FIV (screen with antibody test; screen also for FeLV); septic joint disease (rare); immune-mediated polyarthritis
- Bone marrow dyscrasias with thrombocytopenia, pancytopenia—consider FeLV (panleukopenia syndrome, lymphoma); feline panleukemia; immune-mediated, drug-induced bone marrow suppression (estradiol cypionate, chloramphenicol, albendazole)

 DIAGNOSTICS

Dogs

Acute

- CBC—thrombocytopenia (before onset of clinical signs), anemia, leukopenia (due to lymphopenia and eosinopenia), leukocytosis, and monocytosis (as disease becomes more chronic)

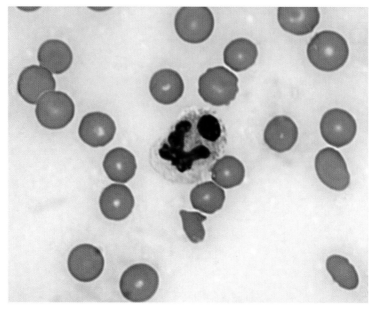

■ **Figure 39-3** A canine neutrophil containing a morula in a dog with acute ehrlichiosis (Wright–Giemsa stain, 1000×).

- Morulae—Intracytoplasmic inclusions in leukocytes are rare, especially in *E. canis* and *E. chaffeensis* infections (Fig. 39-3); morulae in neutrophils are more common in *A. phagocytophilum* and *E. ewingii* infections (morulae are indistinguishable between these ricketsial spp.).
- Nonspecific changes—mild increases in ALT, ALP, BUN, creatinine, and total bilirubin (rare)
- Hyperglobulinemia—progressively increases 1–3 weeks postinfection
- Hypoalbuminemia—usually from renal loss
- Proteinuria—with or without azotemia

Chronic

- CBC—pancytopenia typical; monocytosis and lymphocytosis may be present
- Serum biochemistry profile—hyperglobulinemia; magnitude of globulin increase correlates with duration of infection; usually polyclonal gammopathy, but monoclonal (IgG) gammopathies occur
- Hypoalbuminemia
- High BUN and creatinine—from primary renal disease, owing to glomerulonephritis and renal interstitial plasmacytosis

Serologic Testing

- IFA—most clinically useful and reliable method
- Highly sensitive—poor specificity with cross-reactivity between *E. canis* and *A. phagocytophila*, but not between *E. canis* and *A. platys*

- Titers—reliable 3 weeks after infection; >1 : 10 diagnostic; paired titers recommended because single titer can reflect past infection; high seroprevalence compared to disease prevalence
- Canine SNAP 3Dx and 4Dx Diagnostic Test (IDEXX Laboratories)—an in-house snap test that tests for antibodies against Lyme disease and *E. canis*, and heartworm antigen (3Dx) and *A. phagocytophilum* (4Dx); detects positive titers to *E. canis* at an equivalent IFA titer of >1 : 100; sensitivity of 95%; specificity of 100% (according to manufacturer); however, as with any serologic test, predictive value also depends not only on sensitivity and specificity but also prevalence; in low-prevalence areas, likely to get a high false-positive rate; *E. canis* analyte will detect antibodies for *E. chaffeensis*, and *A. phagocytophilum* analyte also reacts with antibodies against *A. platys*; assays can also be used in cats and other species; irrespective of assay, disease can occur before antibodies develop leading to false-negative results; similarly, antibodies can remain elevated in dogs after recovering with infection with no future consequences.
- Coombs'-positive anemia (rare)—may be present and confuse the diagnosis
- PCR—proving to be more sensitive than IFA; tests whole blood samples; should be used in conjunction with serololgic testing
- Test for other accompanying pathogens—*Babesiosis* spp., *Hemobartonellosis* spp. (erythrocytic mycoplasmal infections), *A. platys*, and *Hepatozoon canis*

PCR Testing

- During rickettsemia—PCR effective method of differentiating species of *Ehrlichia* and *Anaplasma*; available in most reference laboratories; may get cross-reactivity with *Wolbachia* spp. (in heartworm-positive dogs) so need speciation to definitively separate; negative PCR results, should not be used to rule-out infection

Cats

- CBC—nonregenerative anemia (not in all cats), leukopenia (in about a third of cats), and thrombocytopenia (in a quarter of cats)
- Morulae—found in about half of cases (none of the *E. canis*–infected cats had morulae)
- Isolation into monocyte culture—usually successful
- Serum biochemical profile—hyperglobulinemia with polyclonal gammopathy in some
- Serologic examination—All cats infected with *E. canis*–like organisms have positive ANA titer (highest reported at 1 : 640) and had negative results on conventional IFA serologic testing (some infected with other *Ehrlichia* spp. were positive).
- Cats infected with *E. canis*–like organisms—positive results on PCR of blood
- SNAP 3Dx and 4Dx assays (IDEXX) work equally well on cats as dogs.

THERAPEUTICS

- Inpatient—initial medical stabilization for anemia and/or hemorrhagic tendency resulting from thrombocytopenia (balanced electrolyte solution or blood transfusion if indicated)
- Outpatient—stable patients; monitor CBC and response to medication frequently

Drugs of Choice

- Doxycycline (treatment of choice in both dogs and cats)—see rapid (within 72 hours of onset of treatment) improvement of platelet count in acute cases
- Imidocarb dipropionate (Imazol; Schering-Plough Animal Health)—effective against both *E. canis* and babesiosis; reasonable alternative to doxycycline; pretreatment with atropine may lessen anticholinergic adverse effects (salivation, serous nasal discharge, diarrhea).
- Fluoroquinolones (enrofloxacin)—not effective against *Ehrlichia* spp., but may be effective against *Anaplasma* spp.
- Glucocorticoids (dogs only; cats treated with steroids do not eliminate infection when treated with doxycycline)—may be indicated when thrombocytopenia is life-threatening (thought to be a result of immune-mediated mechanisms); because immune-mediated thrombocytopenia is a principal differential diagnosis, may be indicated until results of serologic tests are available, and will not affect the outcome if final diagnosis is ehrlichiosis.
- Androgenic steroids (oxymetholone or nandrolone decanoate)—to stimulate bone marrow production in chronically affected dogs with hypoplastic marrows; oxymetholone or nandrolone decanoate (Table 39-1)

TABLE 39-1 **Drug Therapy for Ehrlichiosis in Dogs and Cats**					
Drug	Species	Dose (mg/kg)	Route	Interval (Hours)	Duration (Days)
Doxycycline	B	10	PO	24	28
Imidocarb	B	5	IM	Once[a]	—
Prednisone	D	1–2	PO	12	14[b]
Oxymetholone	D	2	PO	24	Until response
Nandrolone	D	1.5	IM	Weekly	Until response

[a] Repeat 2 weeks later; pretreat with atropine.
[b] Gradually decrease dose as thrombocytopenia improves; taper in 50% decrements every 2 weeks.
B, cats and dogs; D, dogs.

Precautions/Interactions

- Tetracycline (and derivatives)—Do not use in dogs <6 months old (permanent yellowing of teeth occurs); do not use with renal insufficiency (try doxycycline because it can be excreted via the gastrointestinal tract).
- Enrofloxacin—not effective against *E. canis*
- Glucocorticoids—Prolonged use at immunosuppressive levels may interfere with the clearance and elimination of *E. canis* after use of tetracycline.

 COMMENTS

- Concurrent infection with *Babesia* spp., *Haemobartonella* spp., *A. platys*, and *Hepatozoon canis*—worsens clinical syndrome
- Acute—Prognosis excellent with appropriate therapy.
- Chronic—Response may take 1 month; prognosis poor if the bone marrow is severely hypoplastic.
- Progression from acute to chronic—can be easily prevented by early, effective treatment; but many dogs remain seropositive and may relapse (even years later)
- Dogs remain susceptible to reinfection with *E. canis* and *E. chaffeensis* following successful resolution of primary infection after treatment.
- German shepherd dogs and Doberman pinschers—more chronic and severe form of disease
- Inform owner on how to control tick infestation—dips or sprays containing dichlorvos, chlorfenvinphos, dioxathion, propoxur, or carbaryl; acaricides including imidacloprid/permethrin and fipronil prevent infection (topical selamectin is less effective; use acaricides year round to prevent infestation with all stages of ticks; avoid tick-infested areas.
- Removing ticks by hand—use gloves; ensure mouth parts are removed to avoid a foreign body reaction
- Zoonotic potential—except for *A. platys*, the *Ehrlichia* and *Anaplasma* spp. that cause disease in pets can be zoontic to man; probably not directly infected from dogs; tick exposure thought to be necessary; *R. sanguineus* probably not the vector in humans

Abbreviations

ALP, alkaline phosphatase; ALT, alanine aminotransferase; ANA, antinuclear antibody; BUN, blood urea nitrogen; CBC, complete blood count; CNS, central nervous system; FeLV, feline leukemia virus; FIV, feline immunodeficiency virus; HGE, human granulocytic ehrlichial agent; IFA, indirect fluorescent antibody; PCR, polymerase chain reaction; RMSF, Rocky Mountain spotted fever; SLE, systemic lupus erythematosus.

Suggested Reading

Harrus S, Waner T. Diagnosis of canine monocytotropic ehrlichiosis (*Ehrlichia canis*): an overview. *Vet J* 2011;187;292–296.

Little SE. Ehrlichiosis and anaplasmosis in dogs and cats. *Vet Clin North Am Small Anim Pract* 2010;40:1121–1140.

Little SE, O'Connor TP, Hempstead J, et al. *Ehrlichia ewingii* infection and exposure rates in dogs from the southcentral United States. *Vet Parasitol* 2010;172:355–360.

Neer TM, Harrus S. Canine monocytotropic ehrlichiosis and neorickettsiosis (*E. canis, E. chaffeensis, E. ruminantium, N. sennetsu*, and *N. risticii* infections). In: Greene CE, ed. *Infectious Diseases of the Dog and Cat*. Philadelphia: WB Saunders, 2006:203–216.

Feline Calicivirus Infection

40

DEFINITION/OVERVIEW

- A common viral respiratory disease of cats characterized by upper respiratory tract signs; ulceration on the tongue, hard palate, lips, or tip of nose or around claws; pneumonia; and occasionally arthritis

ETIOLOGY/PATHOPHYSIOLOGY

- A small, nonenveloped single-stranded RNA virus
- Numerous strains occur in nature—varying degrees of cross-reactivity
- More than one serotype—most produce similar diseases
- A very virulent hemorrhagic strain (FCV-ari) described first in California in 1998 but has caused several outbreaks since—causes a hemorrhagic disease syndrome developing 1–5 days after exposure; extremely infectious
- Relatively stable—resistant to many disinfectants
- Transmission—cats may become infected from FCV carriers (some carries shed virus virtually continuously and thus are always infectious to other cats); directly from other cats with acute disease; fomites within the environment (cages, bowls, etc.)
- Routes of infection—nasal, oral, and conjunctival
- Once invades cells—rapid cytolysis with tissue damage and ulceration on mucosal surfaces
- Clinical disease—common in multi-cat facilities and breeding catteries
- Incubation period—clinical disease usually appears 3–4 days after exposure
- Neutralizing antibodies—appear about 7 days after exposure, resulting in rapid recovery
- Persistent infections (carrier states) are common—virus persists in tonsillar and oropharyngeal tissues, in some cats for life
- FCV carriers—tend to be low, medium, or high shedders in that they shed fairly constant amounts of virus; high shedders are very infectious to other cats
- Up to 25% of healthy cats may be shedding FCV at any one time—vaccinated cats can still be FCV shedders
- Routine vaccination—has reduced incidence of clinical disease but has not decreased the prevalence of the virus

SIGNALMENT/HISTORY

- Mainly affects young kittens >6 weeks of age
- Cats of any age may show clinical disease.
- Historically, presents with a sudden onset of anorexia
- Owner may report dyspnea, open-mouth breathing.
- Acute onset of lameness due to arthritis

 CLINICAL FEATURES

- Patients are generally alert and in good body condition.
- Fever, especially in those cats with secondary bacterial infections
- Ocular or nasal discharge with little or no sneezing may result in crusting around the face in young kittens (Fig. 40-1).
- Ulcers appear on the tongue and hard palate (Fig. 40-2), lips, or tip of nose (Fig. 40-3) or around claws.
- Ulcers may occur without any other signs; tongue ulcers are common; occasionally ulcers form on the hard palate and lips; rarely, ulcers can occur around nail beds, leading to pododermatitis and secondary bacterial infection.
- Intestinal ulceration usually does not cause clinical disease.

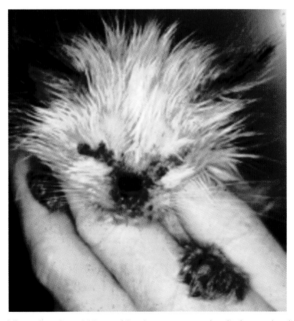

■ **Figure 40-1** Severe bilateral conjunctivitis resulting in a serous ocular discharge that has dried into crusts around the eyes and mouth of this young kitten with calicivirus infection (courtesy of Dr. R. Riis, Cornell University).

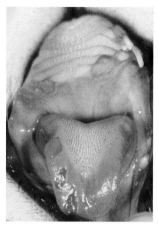

■ **Figure 40-2** Ulceration of the tongue and hard palate of a cat caused by calicivirus infection (courtesy of Dr. J. Richards, Feline Health Center, Cornell University).

- Ophthalmic signs are acute serous conjunctivitis with matting of the hair below the eyes, usually without keratitis or corneal ulceration (Fig. 40-4).
- Lameness, usually shifting, may or may not be associated with oral or respiratory signs; fever; dull and anorexia; full recovery after 24–48 hours; can occur secondary to FCV vaccination
- Infections may be complicated by secondary bacterial invasion, resulting in pneumonia.
- Hemorrhagic syndrome may occur; as well as the typical signs (oral ulceration, nasal and ocular discharge), which are often severe; cats develop a fever; cutaneous edema usually over the head and limbs; alopecia, crusting, and ulceration on the nose, pinnae, occasionally distal limbs; pulmonary edema and pleural effusion develop in some cats; vomiting, diarrhea, and icterus if GI and liver involvement occur; DIC terminally.

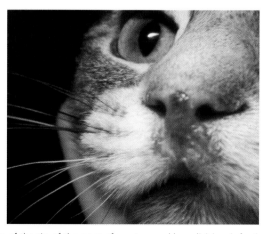

■ **Figure 40-3** Ulceration of the tip of the nose of a cat caused by calicivirus infection (courtesy of Dr. J. Richards, Feline Health Center, Cornell University).

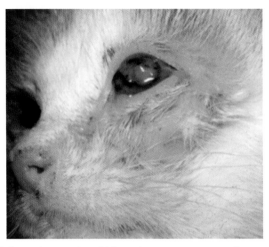

■ **Figure 40-4** Ocular discharge from conjunctivitis can become severe enough to cause the fur to matt below the eye and cause hair loss and irritation of the skin (courtesy of Dr. R. Riis, Cornell University).

 ## DIFFERENTIAL DIAGNOSIS

- Feline viral rhinotracheitis—short incubation period (4–5 days); rapid bilateral conjunctivitis; severe sneezing; and ulcerative keratitis
- Chlamydiosis—tends to have a longer incubation period (7–10 days); not characterized by ulcerative stomatitis or pneumonia (although can produce a mild pneumonitis); conjunctivitis mild
- Feline reovirus infection—very mild upper respiratory tract tinfection; short incubation period and duration of infection
- Bronchopneumonia caused by bacteria such as *Bordetella bronchiseptica*—occasionally, localized areas of density within the lungs on radiographs

 ## DIAGNOSTICS

- Diagnosis usually made based on history and clinical signs
- CBC, serum biochemical profile, urinalysis—normal; except in hemorrhagic syndrome, in which changes include hyperbilirubinemia, hypoalbuminemia, hyperglycemia, elevated CK, AST, and ALT
- Thoracic radiology—alveolar–interstitial lung pattern in cats with pneumonia
- Serologic titers on paired serum samples demonstrate a rise in neutralizing antibody titers against the virus—rarely performed
- Viral isolation—cultures of swabs from ocular and nasal discharge
- PCR—available through some diagnostic laboratories

THERAPEUTICS

- Unless severe pneumonia is present, treat as an outpatient to decrease the risk of contamination of the hospital.
- Recommend that owners isolate cats from others to prevent transmission.
- Careful cleaning of ocular nasal discharges and enticing with highly palatable foods will encourage cats to start eating again; feed soft food if oral ulcers present.
- Place a feeding tube until ulcers are healed sufficiently to allow cat to start eating.
- Acute arthritis rarely requires treatment except for pain medication.

Vaccination

- MLV or inactivated vaccines should be given when vaccinated against FHV (8–10 weeks of age or as early as 6 weeks) and booster every 3–4 weeks until at least 16 weeks of age.
- Breeding catteries—respiratory disease is a problem; vaccinate kittens at an earlier age
- American Association of Feline Practitioners—classifies FHV, FPV, and calicivirus as core vaccines; vaccinate all cats with these 3 agents on the initial visit as early as 6 weeks of age, repeat every 3–4 weeks until 16 weeks of age, and 1 year after the last kitten vaccine; revaccinate for calicivirus every 3 years.
- In breeding colonies with a severe problem, vaccinate kittens at an earlier age (4–5 weeks). either with an additional vaccination at 4–5 weeks of age or with an intranasal vaccine at 10–14 days of age; follow-up vaccinations every 3–4 weeks until 16 weeks of age . . .
- Annual booster vaccines recommended, although immunity undoubtedly lasts >1 year.
- American Association of Feline Practitioners recommends vaccination of all cats with core vaccines (against FHV, FPV, and calicivirus) on initial visit, after 12 weeks of age, and then 1 year later; booster for FCV should then be given every 3 years.
- Administer parenteral MLV vaccine carefully—Vaccine virus may induce clinical signs if it reaches the oral-respiratory mucosa (if cat licks injection sites, or if an aerosol is produced with the syringe).
- Intranasal MLV vaccination—induces quicker onset and better protection than parenteral MLV vaccination; however, intranasal vaccination may induce slight side effects including sneezing and ocular and nasal discharge; the best protection is achieved when both intranasal and parenteral vaccinations are given.
- Inactivated adjuvant vaccines—not as effective as MLV vaccines but have a place in virus-free catteries because there is no risk of spread or revision to virulence; some are licensed for use in pregnant queens.

- Vaccination—will not eliminate infection in a subsequent exposure but will prevent clinical disease caused by most strains of the virus; vaccination will not prevent shedding.
- Hemorrhagic syndrome—isolation; aggressive fluid therapy including colloid-containing fluids (hetastarch); treat for DIC with heparin and plasma.

Drugs of Choice

- Specific antiviral drugs are not available.
- Broad-spectrum antibiotics—usually indicated to prevent secondary bacterial infections. Antibiotics—amoxicillin (22 mg/kg, PO, q12h) or doxycycline (10 mg/kg, PO, q24h)
- Antibiotic eye ointment—reduce chance of secondary bacterial infections of the conjunctiva.
- Human ra-interferon (Roferon; Roche)—may improve cats but findings subjective (30 U/cat, PO, q24h for 7 days, repeated every other week)

Precautions/Interactions

- Proper vaccination protocol should be explained to clients, especially those owning catteries, where kittens require vaccination before becoming infected (often at 6–8 weeks of age) from an infected queen.
- MLV vaccines—not to be used in pregnant queens

 COMMENTS

- Monitor patients carefully—susceptible to developing interstitial pneumonia or secondary bacterial infections
- Prognosis—Clinical course is usually only 3–5 days in uncomplicated cases; rapid recovery usually occurs once neutralizing antibodies appear (~7 days after exposure).
- Prognosis excellent—unless severe pneumonia develops
- Recovered cats—persistently infected for long periods; many will continuously shed small quantities of virus in oral secretions

Abbreviations

ALT, alanine aminotransferase; AST, aspartate aminotransferase; CBC, complete blood count; CK, creatine kinase; DIC, disseminated intravascular coagulation; FCV, feline calicivirus; FHV, feline herpesvirus; FPV, feline parvovirus; GI, gastrointestinal; MLV, modified live vaccine; PCR, polymerase chain reaction; RNA, ribonucleic acid.

Suggested Reading

Gaskell RM, Dawson S, Radford A. Feline respiratory disease. In: Greene CE, ed. *Infectious Diseases of the Dog and Cat*. Philadelphia: WB Saunders, 2006:145–154.

Pesavento PA, Chang K-O, Parker JSL. Molecular virology of feline calicivirus. *Vet Clin North Am Small Anim Pract* 2008;38:775–786.

Radford AD, Addie D, Belák S, et al. Feline calicivirus infection: ABCD guidelines on prevention and management. *J Feline Med Surg* 2009;11:556–564.

Richards JR, Elston TH, Ford RB, et al. The 2006 American Association of Feline Practioners Feline Vaccine Advisory Panel Report. *J Am Vet Med Assoc* 2006;229:1405–1441.

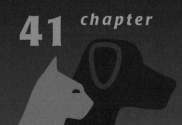

41 *chapter*

Feline Foamy (Syncytium-Forming) Virus Infection

DEFINITION/OVERVIEW

- A common viral infection of cats that causes rare disease

ETIOLOGY/PATHOPHYSIOLOGY

- Retrovirus (spumavirus)
- Worldwide distribution
- Estimated prevalence is 10–70% or greater
- Present in some nondomestic feline populations
- Infection linked statistically with chronic progressive polyarthritis
- Disease has not been reproduced by experimental infection
- Transmission primarily by bites from other cats
- Free-roaming cats are at greater risk of infection.
- Transmitted efficiently from infected queens to their offspring, probably in utero

SIGNALMENT/HISTORY

- Prevalence of virus—low in kittens; increases with age
- Males—more likely than females to be infected due to outdoor roaming habits
- Chronic progressive polyarthritis—occurs predominantly in males aged 1.5–5 years

CLINICAL FEATURES

- Most affected cats remain healthy.
- Coinfections of FeFV with FIV and FeLV—fairly common, probably because of shared transmission modes and risk factors
- Main syndrome—chronic progressive polyarthritis characterized by stiff gait, swollen joints, and lymphadenomegaly

- Two forms of polyarthritis tend to occur:
  - Osteoporosis with periarticular periosteal proliferation
  - Periarticular erosions, collapse of joint space, and joint deformities

 ## DIFFERENTIAL DIAGNOSIS

- Signs of chronic progressive polyarthritis—test for FIV, FeLV, and septic joint disease

 ## DIAGNOSTICS

- CBC, UA, and serum biochemical profile— normal
- Serologic testing for FeFV antibodies and virus isolation—not readily available and not particularly useful because correlation between FeFV infection and disease is so tenuous
- Joint fluid cytologic examination (chronic progressive polyarthritis)—may reveal high numbers of neutrophils and large mononuclear cells

 ## THERAPEUTICS

- Treat chronic progressive polyarthritis
- No vaccine available

Drugs of Choice

- Prednisolone
- Cyclophosphamide (Table 41-1)

TABLE 41-1 Drugs use to treat chronic progressive polyarthritis caused by Feline foamy (syncytium-forming) virus infection

Drug	Dose (mg/cat)	Route	Interval (hours)	Duration (weeks)[a]
Prednisolone	10–15	PO	24	4
Cyclophosphamide	7.5	PO	24[b]	4

[a]Treat for 4 weeks or until improvement of clinical signs then taper doses.
[b]Treat for 4 days each week.

Precautions/Interactions

- Immunosuppressive drugs—take care when using in patients coinfected with FIV or FeLV
- Cyclophosphamide—may cause myelosuppression and/or sterile hemorrhagic cystitis

 COMMENTS

- Infection with FeSFV alone—adverse consequences unlikely
- Chronic progressive polyarthritis—often difficult to control
- Prognosis—poor for long-term recovery

Abbreviations

CBC, complete blood count; FeLV, feline leukemia virus; FeFV, feline foamy virus; FIV, feline immunodeficiency virus; UA, urine analysis.

Suggested Reading

Greene CE. Syncytium-forming virus infection. In: Greene CE, ed. *Infectious Diseases of the Dog and Cat*. Philadelphia: WB Saunders, 2006:154–155.

chapter **42**

Feline Herpesvirus Infection

DEFINITION/OVERVIEW

- A viral infection of domestic and exotic cats characterized by sneezing, fever, rhinitis, conjunctivitis, and ulcerative keratitis

ETIOLOGY/PATHOPHYSIOLOGY

- FHV-1—causes an acute cytolytic infection of respiratory or ocular epithelium after oral, intranasal, or conjunctival exposure
- Affects:
  - Respiratory tract—rhinitis with sneezing and serous to purulent nasal discharge; tracheitis may occur; chronic sinusitis may be a sequela
  - Eyes—conjunctivitis with serous or purulent ocular discharge, ulcerative keratitis, or panophthalmitis
  - Reproductive tract—In utero infection due to infection of pregnant queens may result in severe herpetic infections in neonates.
  - Dermis—Herpes dermatitis may occur near the nasal openings.
- Common worldwide—especially in multi-cat households or facilities housing large numbers of cats (catteries, shelters) because of ease of transmission under crowded circumstances
- Perpetuated by latent carriers—harbor the virus in nerve ganglia, especially in the trigeminal ganglion

SIGNALMENT/HISTORY

- Kittens are the most susceptible, but cats of all ages can be affected.
- Kittens born to carrier queens are infected at about 5 weeks of age.
- Acute onset of paroxysmal sneezing.
- Blepharospasm and ocular discharge; brachycephalic breeds have more severe corneal disease and more likely to have corneal sequestra
- Anorexia from high fever, general malaise, or inability to smell
- Signs can be recurrent (carriers).
- Abortion

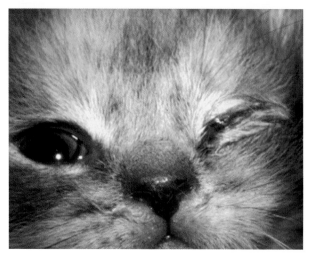

■ **Figure 42-1** Serous to mucopurulent ocular and nasal discharge in a kitten infected with rhinotracheitis virus (courtesy of Dr. Ron Riis, Cornell University).

 ## CLINICAL FEATURES

- Fever—up to 106°F (41°C)
- Rhinitis—serous, mucopurulent, or purulent nasal discharge; sinusitis may occur but requires radiographic imaging to confirm
- Conjunctivitis—serous, mucopurulent, or purulent ocular discharge (Fig. 42-1)
- Chronic rhinitis/sinusitis—chronic purulent nasal discharge
- Keratitis—ulceration, descemetocele, or panophthalmitis (Figs. 42-2 and 42-3)

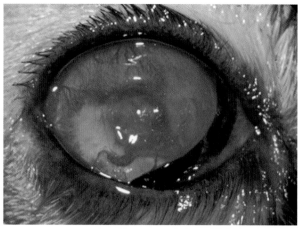

■ **Figure 42-2** Chronic keratitis and corneal ulceration in a cat infected with rhinotracheitis virus (courtesy of Dr. Ron Riis, Cornell University).

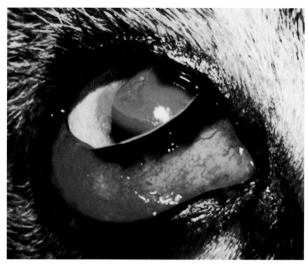

■ **Figure 42-3** Corneal ulceration as shown by uptake of fluorescene stain on a cornea of a cat infected with rhinotracheitis virus (courtesy of Dr. Ron Riis, Cornell University).

 # DIFFERENTIAL DIAGNOSIS

- Feline calicivirus infection—less sneezing, conjunctivitis, or ulcerative keratitis; may cause ulcerative stomatitis, pneumonia
- Feline chlamydiosis—more chronic conjunctivitis, which may be unilateral; pneumonitis; intracytoplasmic inclusions in conjunctival scrapings; responds to tetracyclines or chloramphenicol
- Bacterial infection (*Bordetella, Haemophilus,* or *Pasteurella* spp.)—less nasal and ocular involvement
- Bacterial infections—often respond to antibiotics

 # DIAGNOSTICS

- CBC—Transient leukopenia followed by leukocytosis may occur.
- Skull radiologic examination—shows no lesions during acute disease
- Open mouth and skyline radiographic views of the skull—may reveal presence of chronic disease in the nasal cavity and frontal sinuses (increased fluid densities and erosion of nasal turbinates)
- Skull radiographs—cannot be reliably distinguished from neoplasia, inflammatory polyps, or chronic rhinotracheitis infection
- IFA—nasal or conjunctival scrapings; viral detection
- Viral isolation—pharynxgeal swab sample

- Stained conjunctival smears—detect intranuclear inclusion bodies
- PCR testing from pharyngeal and conjunctival swabs will identify presence of the virus; more sensitive than other diagnostic modalities; may be transiently positive following MLV FHV-1 vaccination

THERAPEUTICS

- Outpatient—Keep patient indoors to prevent environmentally induced stress, which may lengthen the course of the disease.
- Inpatient—nutritional and fluid support to anorectic cats
- Isolate within hospital—to prevent contagion (especially during acute phase)
- Fluids—intravenous or subcutaneous to correct and prevent dehydration and to keep nasal secretions thin
- Diet—entice to eat by feeding foods of appealing tastes and smells
- Enteral feeding for anorectic cats—esophageal or PEG tube
- Nose—Clean off nasal secretions from around external nares.
- Routine vaccination with an MLV or inactivated virus vaccine—prevents development of severe disease
- MLV—does not prevent infection and local viral replication with virus shedding
- Vaccinations—at 8–10 weeks of age, at 12–14 weeks of age, and with boosters every 3 years
- Endemic multi-cat facilities or households—Vaccinate kittens with a dose of an intranasal vaccine at 10–14 days of age; then parenterally at 6, 10, and 14 weeks of age; isolate the litter from *all* other cats at 3–5 weeks of age; then use kitten vaccination protocol to prevent early infections.
- Vaccinations—queens at least 2 weeks before breeding

Drugs of Choice

- Broad-spectrum antibiotics—amoxicillin; for secondary bacterial infections
- Antibiotics—can use amoxicillin in combination with enrofloxacin
- Lysine (available at health food stores)—may have some virucidal effect
- Ophthalmic antibiotics—for keratitis
- Ophthalmic antivirals—vidarabine (Vira-A; Parke-Davis); or idoxuridine, trifluridine for herpetic ulcers; must be instilled every 2 hours for significant effect
- Systemic antiviral agents—Famciclovir—early reports indicate efficacy (at 15 mg/kg, q8-12h, PO); expensive
- Therapeutic vaccination—Conjunctival vaccination with an intranasal FHV-1 vaccine may improve chronic keratitis.
- Human recombinant interferon (Roferon; Roche):
  - Some efficacy in controlling the viral aspect of chronic infectious nasal discharge
  - To help prevent the effects of early exposure to FHV-1 in kittens (Table 42-1)

TABLE 42-1 Drug Therapy for Cats Infected with Feline Rhinotracheitis Virus

Drug	Dose (mg/kg)	Route	Interval (h)	Duration (weeks)
Amoxicillin	22	PO	12	2–4
Enrofloxacin	2.5–5	PO	12	1–2
Orbifloxacin	2.5–7.5	PO	24	1–2
Marbofloxacin	2.75–5.5	PO	24	1–2
Lysine	250 mg[a]	PO	24	4
Interferon (Roferon)—chronic	30 U[a]	PO	24	2[b]
Early exposure	2 U[a]	PO	24	5[c]

[a]Total dose.
[b]Follow by 1 week on, 1 week off.
[c]Begin dosing when 3–8 weeks of age.

Precautions/Interactions

- Do not use MLV in pregnant queens.
- Systemic corticosteroids may induce relapse in chronically infected cats.
- Ophthalmic corticosteroids may predispose to ulcerative keratitis.
- Idoxuridine ophthalmic may be painful in some cats; discontinue medication
- Nasal decongestant drops, 0.25% oxymetazoline HCl; decrease nasal discharge; contraindicated because some cats object and some experience rebound rhinorrhea
- Enrofloxacin has been associated with blindness in some cats at high doses; avoid use in kittens because it can produce arthropathies.
- Amoxicillin may cause anorexia, vomiting, and diarrhea in some cats.

 # COMMENTS

- Essential to monitor appetite closely—Hospitalize for tube feeding and fluid therapy if anorexia develops.
- Inform client of the contagious nature of the disease.
- Discuss with client—proper vaccination protocols and early vaccination of cats in multi-cat facilities and households
- Inform client—Early weaning and isolation from all other cats, except littermates, may prevent infections.
- Warn owners—Chronic rhinosinusitis with lifetime sneezing and nasal discharge, herpetic ulcerative keratitis, and permanent closure of the nasolacrimal duct with chronic ocular discharge are consequences of chronic infection.

- Warn owners—Pregnant cats that develop disease may transmit FHV-1 to kittens in utero, resulting in abortion or neonatal disease.
- Prognosis—acute disease; usually 7–10 days before spontaneous remission, if secondary bacterial infections do not occur
- Prognosis generally good—if fluid and nutritional therapy are adequate

Abbreviations

CBC, complete blood count; FHV-1, feline herpesvirus type 1; IFA, immunofluorescense assay; MLV, modified live virus; PCR, polymerase chain reaction; PEG, percutaneous endoscopic gastrostomy.

Suggested Reading

Gaskell RM, Dawson S, Radford A, et al. Feline herpesvirus. *Vet Res* 2007;38:337–354.
Maggs DJ. Update on pathogenesis, diagnosis, and treatment of feline herpesvirus type 1. *Clin Tech Small Anim Pract* 2005;20:94–101.
Malik R, Lessels NS, Webb S, et al. Treatment of feline herpesvirus-1 associated disease. *J Feline Med Surg* 2009;11:40–48.
Thiry E, Addie D, Belak S, et al. Feline herpesvirus infection: ABCD guidelines on prevention and management. *J Feline Med Surg* 2009;11:547–555.

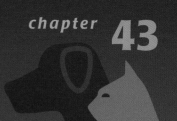
Feline Immunodeficiency Virus

DEFINITION/OVERVIEW

- A viral infection causing immunodeficiency in domestic cats

ETIOLOGY/PATHOPHYSIOLOGY

- Retrovirus (lentivirus)—same genus as HIV, the causative agent of AIDS in humans
- Infection disrupts immune system function—Immune dysfunction occurs due to cytokine alterations, nonspecific hyperactivation of B and T lymphocytes, immunologic anergy, and apoptosis fo T cells.
- Acute infection—Virus spreads from the site of entry (usually a cat bite) to the lymph tissues and thymus via dendritic cells, first infecting T lymphocytes then macrophages.
- CD41 and CD81 cells—Virus selectively and progressively decreases CD41 (T helper) cells.
- CD41 : CD81 ratio becomes inverted (from ∼2 : 1 to <1 : 1)—develops slowly over time
- An absolute decrease of CD41 T cells—seen after several months of infection
- Early infection and activation of $CD4^+CD25^+$ regulatory T cells may limit effective immune response to infection.
- Patients—remain clinically asymptomatic until cell-mediated immunity is disrupted
- Humoral immune function—altered in advanced stages of infection
- Macrophages—main reservoir of virus in affected cats; transport virus to tissues throughout the body; defects in function (e.g., increased production of TNF)
- Other cells infected—astrocyte and microglial cells in the brain (resulting in neuronal loss), megakaryocytes and mononuclear bone marrow cells
- Coinfection with FeLV—may increase the expression of FIV in many tissues, including kidney, brain, and liver
- Distribution—worldwide
- North America—Incidence is 1.5–3% in the healthy cat population, 9–15% in cats with clinical illness.

SIGNALMENT/HISTORY

- Prevalence of infection—increases with age; mean age 5 years at time of diagnosis
- Males mainly—More aggressive, roaming behavior increases likelihood of being bitten by another cat.
- Diverse historical findings—owing to immunosuppressive nature of infection
- Associated disease—cannot be clinically distinguished from FeLV-associated immunodeficiencies
- Recurrent minor illnesses—especially with upper respiratory and GI signs

CLINICAL FEATURES

- Depend on occurrence of opportunistic infections
- Lymphadenomegaly—mild to moderate
- Gingivitis
- Stomatitis
- Periodontitis—25–50% of cases
- Upper respiratory tract—rhinitis, conjunctivitis, keratitis (~30% of cases); often associated with feline herpesvirus and calicivirus infections
- Chronic renal failure and immune-mediated glomerulonephritis; gastrointestinal–panleukopenia-like syndrome may occur.
- Persistent diarrhea—in 10–20% of cases; bacterial or fungal overgrowth, parasite-induced inflammation; direct effect of FIV infection on the GI tract epithelium
- Chronic, nonresponsive, or recurrent infections of the external ear and skin—from bacterial infections or dermatophytosis
- Fever and wasting—especially in later stage; possibly from high levels of TNF
- Ocular disease—anterior uveitis, pars planitis, glaucoma
- Neoplasia—lymphosarcoma or other neoplasia
- Neurologic abnormalities—disruption of normal sleep patterns, behavioral changes (pacing and aggression), peripheral neuropathies

DIFFERENTIAL DIAGNOSIS

- Primary bacterial, parasitic, viral, or fungal infections
- Toxoplasmosis—neurologic and ocular manifestations may be the result of *Toxoplasma* infection, FIV infection, or both
- Nonviral neoplastic diseases

DIAGNOSTICS

- CBC—usually normal, but may show anemia, lymphopenia, neutropenia
- Neutrophilia—in response to secondary infections
- Serum biochemistry profile—occasionally hypergammaglobulinemia; variety of other abnormalities depending on organ system involved
- ELISA—routine screening test detects antibodies to FIV
- Confirm positive ELISA results—additional testing, especially in healthy, low-risk cats or when diagnosis would result in euthanasia
- Western blot (immunoblot)—confirmatory testing of ELISA-positive samples
- Kittens—when <6 months old, may have positive test result owing to passive transfer of antibodies from an FIV-positive queen
- Kittens—A positive test does not indicate infection; retest at 8–12 months to determine infection.
- PCR—useful in vaccinated cats or kittens with maternal antibody; currently not commercially available; newly developed discriminant ELISA may be useful in determining true FIV infection status
- CD41 : CD81 evaluation—helps determine extent of immunosuppression
- Virus isolation or detection—experimental only

 THERAPEUTICS

- Outpatient sufficient for most patients
- Inpatient—with severe secondary infections until condition is stable; parenteral fluid and nutritional support
- Manage secondary and opportunistic infections
- Periodontitis—frequent dental cleaning, tooth extraction, gingival biopsy may be required

Drugs of Choice

- AZT or zidovudine (Retrovir or Retrovis; Glaxo SmithKline)—direct antiviral agent; most effective against acute infection; neurologic FIV-related disease may show improvement; monitor for bone marrow toxicity (dose: 5–15 mg/kg, PO, q12h)
- Immunomodulatory drugs—may alleviate some clinical signs:
  - Human recombinant α-interferon (Roferon; Roche)—may increase survival rates and improve clinical status
  - *Propionibacterium acnes* (ImmunoRegulin; Neogen)
  - Acemannan (Carrisyn; Carrington Labs)—freeze-dried extract from aloe vera plant
  - *Staphylococcus* protein A (Prozyme; Pharmacia Biotech)

TABLE 43-1 Drugs Used to Manage Cats with Feline Immunodeficiency Virus Infections

Drug	Dose (mg/kg)	Route	Interval (h)	Duration (days)
AZT (Retrovir)	5–15	PO	12	[a]
Human ra-interferon (Roferon)	30[b]	PO	24	7[c]
Propionibacterium acnes (Immunoregulin)	0.5[d]	IV	Once or twice	Weekly
Acemannan (Carrisyn)	100[e]	PO	24	28
Staphylococcus protein-A	0.01	IP	Twice, 1st week	[f]
Metronidazole (Flagyl)	7–15	PO	12	14
Clindamycin (Antirobe)	11	PO	12	14
Diazepam (Valium)	0.2	IV	Once or twice	—
Oxazepam (Serax)	2.5[e]	PO	Once or twice	2
Midazolam (Versed)	0.02–0.05	IV	As needed	—
Cyproheptadine (Periactin)	2[e]	PO	12	As needed

[a]Until a response is seen.
[b]International unit total dose per cat.
[c]Repeat every other week.
[d]Milliliter total dose per cat.
[e]Milligram total dose per cat.
[f]After first week, treat once monthly.

- Gingivitis and stomatitis—may be refractory to treatment
- Antibacterial or antimycotic drugs—useful for overgrowth of bacteria or fungi; prolonged therapy or high dosages may be required; for anaerobic bacterial infections, use metronidazole (Flagyl; Pfizer) or clindamycin (Antirobe Pharmacia and Upjohn).
- Corticosteroids or gold salts—judicious but aggressive use may help control immune-mediated inflammation
- Anorexia—appetite stimulation:
  - Short term—diazepam (Valium; Roche); oxazepam (Serax; Wyeth-Ayerst); midazolam (Versed; Roche); cyproheptadine (Periactin; Merck) (Table 43-1)
  - Long term—anabolic steroids or megestrol acetate; efficacy in FIV-positive cats unknown
- Topical corticosteroids—for anterior uveitis; long-term response may be incomplete or poor; pars planitis often regresses spontaneously and may recur
- Glaucoma—standard treatment
- Yearly vaccination for respiratory and enteric viruses with inactivated vaccines is recommended.

Precautions/Interactions

- Griseofulvin—avoid or use with extreme caution in FIV-positive cats; may induce severe neutropenia; neutropenia is reversible if the drug is withdrawn early enough but secondary infections associated with the condition can be life-threatening.
- MLV vaccines—although unlikely, may have the potential to cause disease in immunosuppressed cats
- Systemic corticosteroids—use with caution especially at high doses as may lead to further immunosuppression
- Long-term use of megestrol acetate—may lead to development of diabetes mellitus

 COMMENTS

- Inform client—Infection is slowly progressive and healthy antibody-positive cats may remain healthy for years.
- Advise client that cats with clinical signs will have recurrent or chronic health problems that require medical attention.
- Discuss the importance of keeping cats indoors—to protect them from exposure to secondary pathogens and to prevent spread of FIV
- Quarantine and test incoming cats—before introducing into multi-cat households
- Zoonosis—no known zoonotic potential
- FIV-positive queens—reported abortions and stillbirths; transmission to kittens is infrequent if the queen is antibody-positive before conception.
- Prognosis—within the first 2 years after diagnosis or 4.5–6 years after the estimated time of infection, about 20% of cats die but >50% remain asymptomatic.
- In late stages of disease (wasting and frequent or severe opportunistic infections), life expectancy is ≤1 year.
- Vaccination—dual subtype (A&D), inactivated whole virus vaccine (Fel-O-Vax FIV; Fort Dodge Animal Health)
    - Efficacy of 60–80% after three doses
    - Cannot distinguish between vaccinated and FIV-infected cats with antibody assays
- Yearly vaccination for respiratory and enteric viruses—inactivated vaccines are recommended

Abbreviations

AIDS, acquired immunodeficiency syndrome; AZT, azidothymidine; CBC, complete blood count; ELISA, enzyme-linked immunosorbent assay; FeLV, feline leukemia virus; FIV, feline immunodeficiency virus; GI, gastrointestinal; HIV, human immunodeficiency virus; MLV, modified live virus; PCR, polymerase chain reaction; TNF, tumor necrosis factor.

Suggested Reading

Barr MC, Phillips TR. FIV and FIV-related diseases. In: Ettinger SJ, Feldman EC, eds. *Textbook of Veterinary Internal Medicine*, 5th ed. Philadelphia: WB Saunders, 2000:433–438.

Levy JK. CVT update: feline immunodeficiency virus. In: Bonagura JD, ed. *Kirk's Current Veterinary Therapy XIII: Small Animal Practice*. Philadelphia: WB Saunders, 2000:284–288.

Levy J, Crawford C, Hartmann K, et al. Feline retrovirus management guidelines. American Association of Feline Practitioners. *J Feline Med Surg* 2008;10:300–316.

Feline Infectious Peritonitis

chapter 44

DEFINITION/OVERVIEW

- A viral disease of cats characterized by insidious onset, persistent nonresponsive fever, pyogranulomatous tissue reaction, accumulation of exudative effusions in body cavities, and high mortality

ETIOLOGY/PATHOPHYSIOLOGY

- Two genomic types of FcoV—FCoV-1 (causes perhaps 85% of infections) and FCoV-2 (similar to canine coronavirus)
- Distinguishing between forms—There has been great effort to distinguish between the low-virulent or avirulent enteric strains (FECV) and the virulent strains.
- FECV and FIP virus—occur in both type 1 and type 2 forms
- Spectrum of disease within each type—avirulent viruses (producing asymptomatic infections) to fatal FIP
- Fecal shedding of virus—important in transmission
- FIP virus—replicates locally in epithelial cells of the upper respiratory tract or oropharynx and intestinal tract
- Immune-mediated disease—antiviral antibodies are produced and virus/antibody complex is taken up by macrophages
- The virus is transported within monocytes/macrophages throughout the body—localizes at various vein walls and perivascular sites
- Local perivascular viral replication and subsequent pyogranulomatous tissue reaction—produce the classic lesion
- Multisystemic—pyogranulomatous or granulomatous lesions in the omentum, on the serosal surface of abdominal organs (e.g., liver, kidney, and intestines), within abdominal lymph nodes, and in the submucosa of the intestinal tract
- Respiratory—lesions on lung surfaces
- Pleural effusion—in the wet form
- Nervous—vascular lesions can occur throughout the CNS, especially in the meninges
- Ophthalmic—lesions may include uveitis and chorioretinitis
- FIP virus can infect fetuses—resulting in fetal death or neonatal disease
- Distribution—worldwide

- Prevalence of antibodies against FCoV—high in most populations, especially in multi-cat facilities
- Incidence of clinical disease—low in most populations, especially in single-cat households
- Because of the difficulty in diagnosis, control, and prevention, outbreaks within breeding catteries may be catastrophic.
- In endemic catteries—risk of an FCoV antibody–positive cat eventually developing FIP is usually <10%.

 # SIGNALMENT/HISTORY

- Susceptibility—Some families or lines of cats appear more susceptible.
- Highest incidence in kittens—3 months to 2 years of age
- Incidence decreases—sharply after cats reach 2 years of age
- Incidence increases—again in cats >10 years of age, with geriatric cats having slightly increased incidence
- Onset—insidious onset
- Weight loss and decrease in appetite—gradual
- Growth—stunting in kittens
- Gradual increase in the size of the abdomen—giving a potbellied appearance
- Persistent fever—fluctuating and unresponsive to antibiotics

 # CLINICAL FEATURES

- Vary widely
- Depend on—virulence of the strain, effectiveness of the host immune response, organ system affected
- Two classic forms:
  - Wet or effusive form—targets the body cavities
  - Dry or noneffusive form—targets a variety of organs
- Depression
- Poor condition
- Stunted growth
- Weight loss
- Dull, rough hair coat
- Icterus
- Abdominal and/or pleural effusion (Fig. 44-1)
- Palpation of the abdomen—abdominal masses (granulomas or pyogranulomas) within the omentum, on the surface of viscera (especially the kidney), and within the intestinal wall

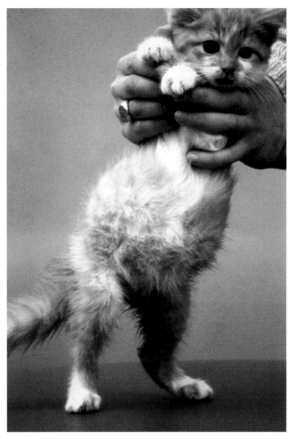

■ **Figure 44-1** Young kitten with enlarged abdomen from ascitic fluid typical of feline infectious peritonitis infection (courtesy of Dr. Fred Scott, Professor Emeritus, Cornell University).

- Mesenteric lymph nodes—may be enlarged
- Ocular—Anterior uveitis, keratic precipitates, fibrin in the anterior chamber, cataract formation, color change to the iris, and irregularly shaped pupil can all be presentations (Figs. 44-2, 44-3, and 44-4).
- Neurologic—brain stem, cerebrocortical, or spinal cord

DIFFERENTIAL DIAGNOSIS

- Fever of unknown origin—when other causes of fever are ruled out
- Cardiac disease causing pleural effusion—typically has low specific gravity and cell count
- Lesions of lymphoma, especially in the kidney, on palpation
- CNS tumors—most cats will have positive test for FeLV

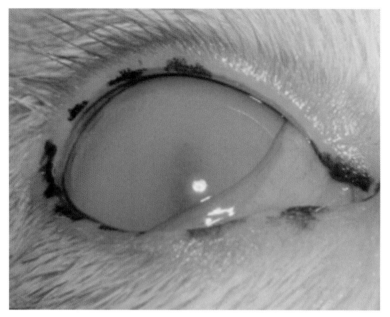

■ **Figure 44-2** Acute fibrin accumulation within the anterior chamber of a cat with acute-onset feline infectious peritonitis (courtesy of Dr. Ron Riis, Cornell University).

- FeLV-negative cats—biopsy the lesion (if accessible) for histopathology and immuno-histochemistry for diagnosis of FCoV
- Respiratory disease—FCV, FHV, chlamydiosis, or various bacteria
- Pansteatitis (yellow fat disease)—classic feel and appearance of fat within the abdominal cavity; pain on abdominal palpation; often a fish-only diet

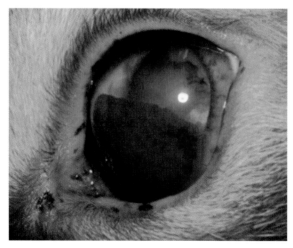

■ **Figure 44-3** Anterior uveitis with fibrin and keratic precipitate accumulation within the anterior chamber of a cat with feline infectious peritonitis (courtesy of Dr. Ron Riis, Cornell University).

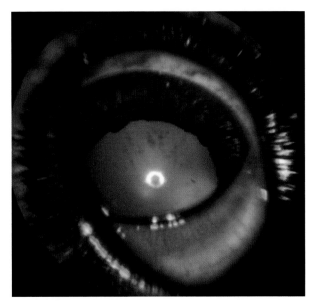

■ **Figure 44-4** Cataract formation with anterior uveitis in a cat with feline infectious peritonitis (courtesy of Dr. Ron Riis, Cornell University).

- Panleukopenia producing enteritis—leukopenia; positive fecal canine parvovirus antigen assay
- Hepatic involvement—cholangiohepatitis, lymphoma (and other neoplasia), infectious

 DIAGNOSTICS

- CBC
  - Leukopenia—common early in the infection
  - Later leukocytosis with neutrophilia and lymphopenia
  - Mild to moderate anemia may occur
- Serum biochemical profile—variety of abnormalities possible depending on organ involvement
- High total plasma globulin—common
- Hyperbilirubinemia and hyperbilirubinuria—often
- Serum antibody tests—immunoassays, viral neutralization assays
- Detect antibodies against FCoV—positive tests not diagnostic, indicate only previous infection or vaccination; correlation between height of titer and eventual confirmation of infection not high
- PCR assays—detect viral antigen; accuracy of positive tests correlating with clinical disease is still being evaluated

- RT-PCR assay of effusions and tissue—better positive predictive value for identifying cats with FIP
- Both PCR reactions—available at commercial laboratories
- Immunohistochemistry (immunoperoxidase) assays—detect FCoV within specific cells of biopsy samples or histopathologic sections of tissues from cats with fatal diseases
- Immunohistochemistry—excellent for confirming cause of specific lesions, especially inflammatory abdominal disease, which often is not diagnosed as FIP
- Fluid obtained via thoracocentesis and abdominocentesis—pale to straw colored, viscous, flecks of white fibrin often seen, will clot upon standing, specific gravity usually high (1.030–1.040), high protein concentrations (>3.5 g/dl)
- Laparoscopy or exploratory laparotomy—to observe specific lesions of the peritoneal cavity; to obtain a biopsy sample for histopathologic or immunohistochemistry confirmation

Diagnostic Feature

- **The triad of hyperglobulinemia, FCoV serum antibody titer >160, and lymphopenia—very high predictive value for diagnosing FIP in a patient with consistent clinical signs**

THERAPEUTICS

- Inpatient or outpatient—depends on stage and severity of disease, and owner's willingness and ability to provide good supportive care
- Therapeutic paracentesis—may relieve pressure on respiration from excessive ascites or pleural effusions
- Diet—important to encourage the affected cat to eat

Drugs of Choice

- Treatment—no treatment routinely effective
- Patients with generalized and typical signs—almost invariably die
- Most FCoV-positive cats—have subclinical infection or mild, localized granulomatous disease that is not diagnosed as FIP
- Immunosuppressive drugs (e.g., prednisolone and cyclophosphamide)—limited success
- Corticosteroids (subconjunctival injection)—may help ocular involvement
- Interferon—effective in vitro; limited success in vivo; a recombinant interferon reported to have some success in Japan
- Antibiotics—ineffective because generally not associated with secondary bacterial infections
- Antiviral drugs—none proven to be efficacious

- MLV intranasal vaccine—available against FIP virus; efficacy low; cannot rely on vaccination alone for control; may produce antibody-positive cats, complicating monitoring in catteries or colonies; should only be considered for seronegative cats that are at extremely high risk of exposure to FCoV; FIP vaccine is not generally recommended by the AAFP vaccine guidelines.

Precautions/Interactions

- N/A

 COMMENTS

- Inform client of all the various aspects of disease, including the grave prognosis.
- Inform client of the high prevalence of FCoV infection but low incidence of actual clinical disease.
- Less than 10% of FCoV antibody–positive cats <3 years of age eventually develop clinical disease.
- In mother/offspring—main method of transmission appears to be from asymptomatic carrier queens to their kittens at 5–7 weeks of age, after maternally derived immunity wanes.
- Break cycle of transmission—early weaning at 4–5 weeks of age and isolating litter from direct contact with other cats, including the queen
- Routine disinfection of premises, cages, and water/food dishes—readily inactivates virus and reduces transmission
- Introduce only FCoV antibody–negative cats to catteries or colonies that are free of virus.
- Restrict household cats to indoor environments.
- Clinical course—lasts a few days to several months
- Prognosis is grave once typical signs occur—mortality nearly 100%

Abbreviations

CBC, complete blood count; CNS, central nervous system; FCoV, feline coronavirus; FCV, feline calicivirus; FECV, feline enteric coronavirus; FeLV, feline leukemia virus; FHV, feline herpes virus; FIP, feline infectious peritonitis; MLV, modified live virus; PCR, polymerase chain reaction; RT-PCR, reverse transcriptase polymerase chain reaction.

Suggested Reading

Addie D, Belák S, Boucraut-Baralon C, et al. Feline infectious peritonitis. ABCD guidelines on prevention and management. *J Feline Med Surg* 2009;11:594–604.

Addie DD, Jarrett O. Feline coronavirus infections. In: Greene CE, ed. *Infectious Diseases of the Dog and Cat*. Philadelphia: WB Saunders, 2006:88–102.

Brown MA, Troyer JL, Pecon-Slattery J, et al. Genetics and pathogenesis of feline infectious peritonitis virus. *Emer Infect Dis* 2009;15:1445–1452.

Pederson NC. A review of feline infectious peritonitis virus infection: 1963–2008. *J Feline Med Surg* 2009;11:225–258.

Richards JR, Elston TH, Ford RB, et al. The 2006 American Association of Feline Practioners Feline Vaccine Advisory Panel Report. *J Am Vet Med Assoc* 2006;229:1405–1441.

Feline Leukemia Virus Infection

chapter 45

DEFINITION/OVERVIEW

- A viral infection that causes immunodeficiency and neoplastic disease in domestic cats

ETIOLOGY/PATHOPHYSIOLOGY

- Retrovirus—gammaretrovirus
- Early infection consists of five stages—(1) viral replication in tonsils and pharyngeal lymph nodes; (2) infection of a few circulating B lymphocytes and macrophages that disseminate the virus; (3) replication in lymphoid tissues, intestinal crypt epithelial cells, and bone marrow precursor cells; (4) release of infected neutrophils and platelets from the bone marrow into the circulatory system; and (5) infection of epithelial and glandular tissues, with subsequent shedding of virus into the saliva and urine.
- Adequate immune response—stops progression at stage 2 or 3 (4–8 weeks after exposure) and forces the virus into latency
- Persistent viremia (stages 4 and 5)—usually develops 4–6 weeks after infection, but may take 12 weeks
- Tumor induction—occurs when the DNA provirus integrates into cat chromosomal DNA in critical regions (oncogenes)
- Feline sarcoma viruses (mutants of FeLV)—arise by recombination between the genes of FeLV and host
- Virus-host fusion proteins—responsible for the efficient induction of fibrosarcomas
- Multiple systems affected—hemic/lymphatic/immune (anemia; blood cell dyscrasias; neoplasias originating in the bone marrow; immunosuppression, possibly resulting from neuroendocrine dysfunction; absolute decrease in CD41 and CD81 subsets of T cells; decreased CD41:CD81 ratio), nervous (degenerative myelopathy, neuropathy, neoplasias), other body systems (immunosuppression, with secondary infections or development of neoplastic disease)
- Cat-to-cat transmission—bites, close casual contact (grooming), shared dishes or litter pans

- Perinatal transmission—fetal and neonatal death of kittens from 80% of affected queens
- Transplacental and transmammary transmission—occurs in at least 20% of surviving kittens from infected queens
- Neonatal kittens—most susceptible to persistent infection (70–100%)
- Older kittens—<30% susceptible by 16 weeks of age

SIGNALMENT/HISTORY

- Distribution—worldwide
- North America—2–3% incidence in healthy cats; 3–4 times greater in cats exhibiting clinical illness
- Prevalence—highest between 1 and 6 (mean of 3) years of age
- Male:female ratio—1.7:1
- Most patients—live outdoor or in multi-cat households
- Onset of FeLV-associated disease—usually occurs over a period of months to years after infection
- Associated diseases—non-neoplastic or neoplastic
- Most of the non-neoplastic or degenerative diseases result from immunosuppression or bone marrow disease
- Clinical signs of FeLV-induced immunodeficiency—cannot be distinguished from those of FIV-induced immunodeficiency
- FIV and FeLV—may occur concurrently

CLINICAL FEATURES

- Depend—on the type of disease (neoplastic or nonneoplastic) and occurrence of secondary infections
- Lymphadenomegaly—mild to severe
- Upper respiratory tract—rhinitis, conjunctivitis, and keratitis
- Persistent diarrhea—bacterial or fungal overgrowth, parasite-induced inflammation, direct effect of infection on crypt cells
- Oral—gingivitis, stomatitis, periodontitis
- Skin—chronic nonresponsive or recurrent infections of the external ear and skin
- Fever
- Wasting
- Lymphoma (lymphosarcoma)—most common associated neoplastic disease; thymic and multicentric lymphomas highly associated; miscellaneous lymphomas (extranodal origin) most frequently involve the eye and nervous system
- Erythroid and myelomonocytic leukemias—predominant nonlymphoid leukemias

- Fibrosarcomas—in patients coinfected with mutated sarcoma virus, most frequently in young cats
- Peripheral neuropathies—progressive ataxia
- FeLV-positive queens—abortions, stillbirths, and fetal resorptions common

 ## DIFFERENTIAL DIAGNOSIS

- FIV
- Other infections—bacterial, parasitic, viral, or fungal
- Nonviral neoplastic diseases

 ## DIAGNOSTICS

- CBC—anemia (often severe, lymphopenia or lymphocytosis is possible, neutropenia—may be in response to secondary infections, thrombocytopenia and immune-mediated hemolytic anemia)—may occur secondary to immune complexes
- RBC macrocytosis
- *Haemobartonella* spp. (RBC mycoplasmal) infections—often secondary
- IFA—identifies FeLV p27 antigen in leukocytes and platelets in fixed smears of whole blood or buffy coat preparations
- Positive IFA result indicates—productive infection in bone marrow cells
- 97% of IFA-positive cats—remain persistently infected and viremic for life
- IFA—p27 antigen can usually be detected by 4 weeks after infection, but may take up to 12 weeks to develop a positive test.
- IFA for leukopenic cats—use buffy coat smears rather than whole blood smears
- IFA on bone marrow samples—may be positive when negative on peripheral blood
- ELISA—detect soluble FeLV p27 antigen in whole blood, serum, plasma, saliva, or tears
- ELISA—more sensitive than IFA at detecting early or transient infections
- A single positive ELISA test cannot predict which cats will be persistently viremic; retest in 12 weeks (many veterinarians test with IFA at this point).
- False-positive ELISA results—more common when whole blood rather than serum or plasma is used; positive tests with saliva or tears should be checked with whole blood (IFA) or serum (ELISA)
- A few cats have persistently ELISA-positive test results and IFA-negative results—FeLV proviral genetic material has been detected in circulating blood cells from some of these cats; demonstrates infection despite no detectable viremia
- Neither test detects FeLV-vaccinated cats—because the vaccine induces antibodies against gp70 antigen, not p27 antigen

- Bone marrow aspiration or biopsy—with erythroblastopenia (nonregenerative anemia), bone marrow often hypercellular owing to an arrest in differentiation of erythroid cells; true aplastic anemia with hypocellular bone marrow may be seen; some cases of anemia result from myeloproliferative disease; myelofibrosis in some

 # THERAPEUTICS

- Outpatient for most cats
- Inpatient—may be required with severe secondary infections, anemia, or cachexia until condition stable
- Blood transfusions—emergency support; multiple transfusions may be necessary; passive antibody transfer reduces level of FeLV antigenemia in some cats; thus immunization of blood donor cats with FeLV vaccines is useful
- Management of secondary and opportunistic infections—primary consideration
- Supportive therapy (e.g., parenteral fluids and nutritional supplements)—may be useful

Drugs of Choice

- AZT or Zidovudine (Retrovir or Retrovis; Glaxo SmithKline)—direct antiviral agent; clinical improvement but does not clear virus; monitor for bone marrow toxicity
- Immunomodulatory drugs—alleviate some clinical signs:
  - Human recombinant α-interferon (Roferon; Roche)—may increase survival rates and improve clinical status
  - *Propionibacterium acnes* (ImmunoRegulin; Neogen)
  - Acemannan (Carrisyn; Carrington Labs)—freeze-dried extract from aloe vera plant
  - *Staphylococcus* protein A (Prozyme; Sigma)
  - *Haemobartonella* spp. (RBC mycoplasmal) infections—suspect in all cats with regenerative hemolytic anemias; oxytetracycline (Terramycin; Pfizer) or doxycycline (Vibramycin; Pfizer); short-term use of oral glucocorticoids in severe cases (Table 45-1)
- Lymphosarcoma—managed successfully with standard combination chemotherapy protocols; periods of remission average 3–4 months; some cats may remain in remission for much longer.
- Myeloproliferative disease and leukemias—more refractory to treatment
- Yearly vaccination—for respiratory and enteric viruses with inactivated vaccines recommended
- Vaccines against FeLV—most commercial vaccines induce virus-neutralizing antibodies specific for gp70; reported efficacy ranges from <20% to almost 100%, depending on the trial and challenge system; test cats for FeLV before initial vaccination; if prevaccination testing is not done, clients should be aware that the cat may already be infected.

TABLE 45-1 Drugs Used to Manage Cats with Feline Leukemia Virus Infections

Drug	Dose (mg/kg)	Route	Interval (h)	Duration (days)
AZT (Retrovir)	5–15	PO	12	[a]
Human ra-interferon (Roferon)	30[b]	PO	24	7[c]
Propionibacterium acnes (Immunoregulin)	0.5[d]	IV	Once or twice	Weekly
Acemannan (Carrisyn)	100[e]	PO	24	28
Staphylococcus protein-A	0.01	IP	Twice, 1st week	[f]
Oxytetracycline	15	PO	8	10
Doxycycline	5–10	PO	24	10

[a]Until a response is seen.
[b]International unit total dose per cat.
[c]Repeat every other week.
[d]Milliliter total dose per cat.
[e]Milligram total dose per cat.
[f]After first week, treat once monthly.

- FeLV vaccines—Administer SC distally on the hind limb due to possibility of producing a vaccine-induced fibrosarcoma.
- One FeLV vaccine (Purevax; Merial) is adjuvant-free in a canarypox vector (reducing risk of fibrosarcoma formation); administered in a small volume (0.25 ml) using a transdermal vaccination system (removing needle use and disposal).
- Vaccination—kittens at 8–9 weeks and 12 weeks of age; boost at 1 year of age; revaccinate every 2–3 years

Precautions/Interactions

- MLV—may cause disease in immunosuppressed cats
- Systemic corticosteroids—Use with caution because of the potential for further immunosuppression.
- AZT—can cause anemia, which is reversible with discontinuation of the drug

 COMMENTS

- Discuss importance of keeping cats indoors and separated from FeLV-negative cats to protect them from exposure to secondary pathogens and to prevent spread of FeLV.
- Should be aggressive in dental tooth extraction if needed
- Prevent contact with FeLV-positive cats; quarantine and test incoming cats before introduction into multi-cat households.

- More than 50% of persistently viremic cats succumb to related diseases within 2–3 years after infection.
- Zoonotic potential is probably low, but controversial; studies report conflicting results of antibodies to FeLV in humans and of correlation between certain human leukemias and exposure to cats.

Abbreviations

AZT, azidothymidine; CBC, complete blood count; DNA, deoxyribonucleic acid; ELISA, enzyme-linked immunosorbent assay; FLeV, feline leukemia virus; FIV, feline immunodeficiency virus; IFA, immunofluorescent antibody; MLV, modified live virus; RBC, red blood cell.

Suggested Reading

Dunham SP, Graham E. Retroviral infections in small animals. *Vet Clin North Am Small Anim Pract* 2008;38:879–901.

Levy J, Crawford C, Hartmann K, et al. American Association of Feline Practitioners. Feline retrovirus management guidelines. *J Feline Med Surg* 2008;10:300–316.

Lutz H, Addie D, Boucraut-Baralon C, et al. Feline leukaemia. ABCD guidelines on prevention and management. *J Feline Med Surg* 2009;11:565–574.

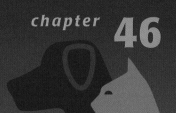

chapter 46

Feline Lungworm (*Aelurostrongylus*)

DEFINITION/OVERVIEW

- A helminth infection in cats causing a spectrum of disease from asymptomatic to severe respiratory distress with weight loss

ETIOLOGY/PATHOPHYSIOLOGY

- *Aelurostrongylus abstrusus*—a metastrongyloidae parasite
- Adult worms—curl within the lung parenchyma, producing small grayish-white subpleural nodules
- Adults worms—lay eggs within the alveoli of the lungs, where they develop to L1 larvae that hatch and ascend the trachea to be swallowed and eventually appear in the feces
- L1 larvae—enter snails and slugs, where they develop to L3, which are infective to cats
- Cats—also probably become infected by eating paratenic hosts (birds and rodents) or intermediate hosts (slugs, snails)
- Dogs—Copraphagia, and not infection, probably explains the occassional finding of larvae in dog feces.
- PPP = 5–6 weeks

SIGNALMENT/HISTORY

- Outdoor cats that hunt birds and rodents have a higher incidence.

CLINICAL FEATURES

- Most cats—asymptomatic
- Coughing—most consistent sign
- Respiratory distress—occasional sign

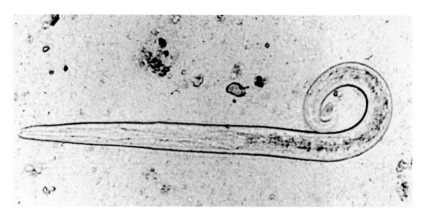

■ **Figure 46-1** L1 larvae of *A. abstrusus* in feces of a cat (Baermann's technique). Note the kinked tail and long esophagus typical of this larva.

- Severe infections—can produce lethargy and weight loss, especially in young cats
- Pleural effusion—rare consequence of infection

 # DIFFERENTIAL DIAGNOSIS

- Allergic (asthma), other parasitic (heartworm disease), and cardiac disease
- Although less likely, trauma (diaphragmatic hernia), pleural disease (pyothorax, chylothorax), neoplasia, and inflammatory diseases should be considered.
- Differentiated from other possible causes by finding L1 larvae in feces

 # DIAGNOSTICS

Diagnostic Feature

- **L1 larvae in the feces—Baermann's technique is very reliable (Fig. 46-1).**
- L1 larvae—may also be found in a transtracheal wash, along with many eosinophils
- CBC—Eosinophilia is consistently present.
- Thoracic radiographs—show bronchial pattern with alveolar infiltrates and some increased interstitial densities (Fig. 46-2)

 # THERAPEUTICS

- Many cases will spontaneously regress after 2–3 months without treatment.
- Treatment is very effective in resolving clinical signs and larval shedding in the feces.

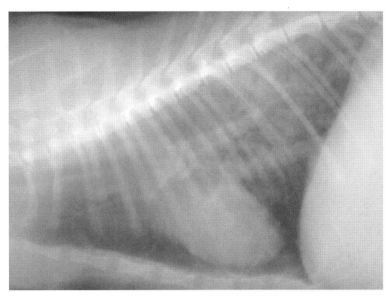

■ **Figure 46-2** Lateral thoracic radiograph showing diffuse interstitial alveolar pattern in a cat with lungworm infestation.

- Thoracic radiographic changes may worsen after treatment as the lesions consolidate and become more obvious (Fig. 46-3).
- Glucocorticoids may help alleviate clinical signs but may also interfere with parasitologic cure.
- Bronchodilators may alleviate clinical signs.

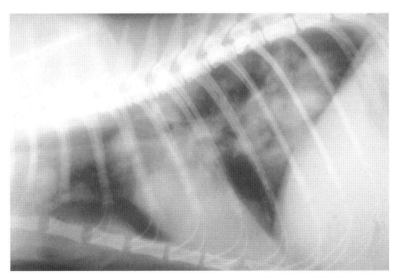

■ **Figure 46-3** Lateral thoracic radiograph showing more consolidated interstitial alveolar pattern in a cat 1 week after treatment for lungworm. Even though clinical signs and larvae in the feces disappear, radiographic lesions look worse immediately post-treatment.

TABLE 46-1 **Drug Therapy for Feline Lungworm (_A. abstrusus_)**				
Drug	Dose (mg/kg)	Route	Interval (h)	Duration (days)
Ivermectin	0.4	PO, SC	Once[a]	
Emodepside 2.1%/Praziqunatel 8.6%		Topical	Once	
Selamectin	6	Topical	Monthly	
Moxidectin (with imidocloprid)	1	Topical	Monthly	
Abamectin	0.3	SC	Once[a]	
Fenbendazole	20	PO	24	5[b]

[a]Repeat injection in 2 weeks time
[b]Repeat this course of fenbendazole after 7 days.

Drugs of Choice

- Ivermectin—very effective
- Fenbendazole—effective but difficult to administer in cats (Table 46-1)
- Moxidectin, abamectin, and selamectin—all effective
- Profender Spot-on (Bayer)—also very effective

    # COMMENTS

Precautions/Interactions

- The use of glucocorticoids may interfere with parasitologic cure.
- Thoracic radiographic changes look much worse up to a week post-treatment, even though clinical signs abate.
- Prognosis for complete cure in treated animals is excellent.

Abbreviations

CBC, complete blood count; PPP, prepatent period.

Suggested Reading

Conboy G. Helminth parasites of the canine and feline respiratory tract. _Vet Clin North Am Small Anim Pract_ 2009;39:1109–1126.

Traversa D, Milillo P, Di Cesare A, et al. Efficacy and safety of emodepside 2.1%/praziquantel 8.6% spot-on formulation in the treatment of feline aelurostrongylosis. _Parasitol Res_ 2009;105:S83–S89.

Feline Panleukopenia

chapter 47

DEFINITION/OVERVIEW

- An acute, enteric, viral infection of cats characterized by sudden onset, depression, vomiting and diarrhea, severe dehydration, and a high mortality rate

ETIOLOGY/PATHOPHYSIOLOGY

- FPV—infects only mitotic cells, causing acute cell cytolysis of rapidly dividing cells
- Affects organs containing rapid dividing cells—mainly the hemic/lymphatic/immune (severe panleukopenia; atrophy of the thymus), and GI systems (intestinal crypt cells of the jejunum and ileum)
- Death of crypt cells—results in shortened blunt villi with poor absorption of nutrients, acute enteritis with vomiting and diarrhea, dehydration, and secondary bacteremia
- In utero infection in nonimmune queens—leads to fetal death, fetal resorption, abortion, stillbirth, or fetal mummification
- Infections of neonatal kittens—affect the rapidly dividing granular cells of the cerebellum and retinal cells of the eye, causing cerebellar hypoplasia with ataxia and retinal dysplasia
- Distribution—worldwide
- The most severe and important feline infectious disease in unvaccinated populations—Routine vaccination provides almost total control of this disease.
- Extremely contagious and stable virus—survives for years on contaminated premises
- CPV-2a and CPV-2b—recently isolated from cats with feline panleukemia
- Properties of CPV—like those for FPV

SIGNALMENT/HISTORY

- History of recent exposure (e.g., adoption from shelter)
- Newly acquired kitten
- Kittens 2–6 months of age are most susceptible (once passively transferred maternal immunity is lost).

- No vaccination history or last vaccinated when <12 weeks of age
- Sudden onset of vomiting, diarrhea, depression, and complete anorexia
- Owner may suspect poisoning.
- Cat may have disappeared or hidden for 1 day or more before being found.
- Owner may report cat hangs head over water bowl or food dish but does not eat or drink.

CLINICAL FEATURES

- Depression—may be mild to severe
- Typical "panleukopenia posture"—sternum and chin resting on floor, feet tucked under body, and top of scapulae elevated above the back
- Dehydration—appears rapidly, may be severe
- Vomiting and diarrhea—may occur; less likely to occur in older cats
- Body temperature—usually mild to moderately elevated or depressed in the early stages of disease
- Body temperature—becomes severely subnormal as affected cat becomes moribund
- Abdominal pain—may be elicited on palpation
- Small intestine—either turgid and hoselike or flaccid
- Retina—retinal degeneration (discrete focal gray areas with dark margins) in kittens with neurologic signs or seen as an incidental finding in clinically normal cats (Fig. 47-1)
- Subclinical or mild infections—few or no clinical signs common, especially in adults

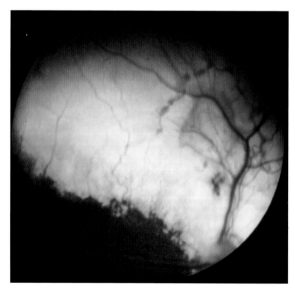

■ **Figure 47-1** Focal areas of retinal degeneration seen in a cat after recovery from panleukopenia virus infection (courtesy of Dr. R. Riis, Cornell University).

- Ataxia from cerebellar hypoplasia (kittens infected in utero or neonatally)—signs evident at 10–14 days of age and persist for life: hypermetria; dysmetria; incoordination with a base-wide stance and an elevated "rudder" tail; alert, afebrile, and otherwise normal; retinal dysplasia sometimes seen

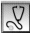 # DIFFERENTIAL DIAGNOSIS

- Panleukopenia-like syndrome of FeLV infection—chronic infection; chronic enteritis; chronic panleukopenia; often anemia; patient positive for FeLV antigen in the blood and/or saliva
- Salmonellosis—usually subclinical infection; severe gastroenteritis; total WBC counts usually high
- Acute poisoning—similar to acute or fulminating disease; severe depression; subnormal temperature; total WBC count not severely depressed
- Many diseases of cats can cause mild clinical signs that are hard to differentiate from those of mild feline panleukemia—Total WBC count is always low during the acute infection with feline panleukemia, even in subclinical infections.

 # DIAGNOSTICS

- CBC—panleukopenia (most consistent finding); leukocyte counts usually between 500 and 3000 cells/dl during the acute disease
- Serum biochemical profile—reflects dehydration and electrolyte loss from vomiting and diarrhea

Diagnostic Feature

- **CPV antigen fecal immunoassay (CITE Canine Parvovirus Test Kit; IDEXX Labs)— not licensed for feline panleukemia; will detect FPV antigen in feces**
- Chromatographic test strip—feces for FPV and CPV
- Unknown whether vaccination with MLV vaccine against FPV will cause a false-positive test result 5–15 days postvaccination, as can happen for CPV in dogs
- Serologic testing—paired serum samples (acute and convalescent); detects rising antibody titer
- Viral isolation—from feces or affected tissues (e.g., thymus, small intestine, spleen)
- Electron microscopy of feces—detects parvovirus particles, presumably FPV

 # THERAPEUTICS

- Main principles of treatment:
  - Rehydration
  - Re-establishment of electrolyte balance

- Supportive care until the patient's immune system produces antiviral antibodies that neutralize the virus
  - Protection against secondary bacterial infection
- Inpatient—severe cases; hydration and replacement electrolyte therapy
- Plasma transfusions—if plasma protein <4 g/dl
- Whole blood transfusions—rarely required because cats do not get that anemic
- Outpatient—mild cases

Drugs of Choice

- Broad-spectrum antibiotics (ampicillin/gentamicin combination)—to counter secondary bacterial infection from GI tract flora
- Vaccination—completely preventable by routine vaccination of kittens; vaccination after the development of clinical signs is contraindicated
- Vaccinations—MLV or inactivated parenteral vaccines and MLV intranasal vaccine
- Immunity—long duration, perhaps even for life
- Vaccinate kittens as early as 6 weeks of age, then every 3–4 weeks until16 weeks of age.
- Recent AAFP vaccine guideline recommendations have changed the last kitten vaccine to be given when kitten is at least 16 weeks of age, instead of 12 weeks of age; maternally derived immunity in some kittens may not have waned until 16 weeks of age.
- Boosters—after 1 year; repeat not more frequently than every 3 years.

Precautions/Interactions

- Chronic enteritis—due to vilus blunting and overgrowth with fungal infection or other pathogens not usually affected by antibiotics (protozoa, fungal, yeast)
- Teratogenic effects (cerebellar hypoplasia resulting in ataxia for life)—virus infection of fetus
- Monitor renal function closely if administering gentamicin—do not administer to dehydrated animals
- Do not use MLV in pregnant cats.

 ## COMMENTS

- Inform client that all current and future cats in the household must be vaccinated against FPV before exposure—The virus will remain infectious on the premise for years unless environment can be adequately disinfected.
- Disinfection—can be achieved with 1:32 dilution of household bleach
- Recovered cats are immune against FPV infection for life—do not require further vaccination

- Prognosis—most cases acute, lasting only 5–7 days; if death does not occur during the acute disease, recovery is usually rapid and uncomplicated.
- Recovery—may take several weeks for the patient to regain weight and body condition
- Prognosis—guarded during the acute disease, especially if the total WBC count is <2000 cells/dl

Abbreviations

CBC, complete blood count; CPV, canine parvovirus; FeLV, feline leukemia virus; FPV, feline parvovirus; GI, gastrointestinal; MLV, modified live virus; WBC, white blood cell.

Suggested Reading

Greene CE, Addie DD. Felineparvovirus infection. In: Greene CE, ed. *Infectious Diseases of the Dog and Cat.* Philadelphia: WB Saunders, 2006:78–88.

Lappin MR, Veir J, Hawley J. Feline panleukopenia virus, feline herpesvirus-1, and feline calicivirus antibody responses in seronegative specific pathogen-free cats after a single administration of two different modified live FVRCP vaccines. *J Feline Med Surg* 2009;11:159–162.

Richards JR, Elston TH, Ford RB, et al. The 2006 American Association of Feline Practioners Feline Vaccine Advisory Panel Report. *J Am Vet Med Assoc* 2006;229:1405–1441.

Truyen U, Addie D, Belák S, et al. Feline panleukopenia. ABCD guidelines on prevention and management. *J Feline Med Surg* 2009;11:538–546.

Fleas and Flea Control

DEFINITION/OVERVIEW

- Flea allergy dermatitis—hypersensitivity reaction to antigens in flea saliva, with or without evidence of fleas and flea dirt
- Flea infestation—large number of fleas and a large amount of flea dirt, with or without a flea allergy dermatitis

ETIOLOGY/PATHOPHYSIOLOGY

- FBH—caused by a low molecular weight hapten and two high molecular weight allergens that help initiate the allergic reaction
- High molecular weight allergens—increase binding to dermal collagen; when bound, form a complete antigen necessary for eliciting FBH
- Flea saliva—contains histamine-like compounds that irritate skin
- Intermittent exposure favors FBH; continuous exposure is less likely to result in hypersensitivity.
- Both IgE and IgG antiflea antibodies have been noted
- Hypersensitivity reactions—immediate and delayed have been noted
- Late-phase IgE-mediated response—part of FBH reaction; occurs 3–6 hours after exposure
- Cutaneous basophil hypersensitivity—part of FBH reaction; an infiltration of basophils into the dermis; mediated either by IgE or IgG; subsequent exposures cause the basophils to degranulate; manifests as immediate and delayed hypersensitivity

SIGNALMENT/HISTORY

- Dogs and cats
- FBH—any breed; most common in atopic breeds
- FBH—rare <6 months of age; average age range, 3 to 6 years, but may be seen at any age
- FBH—intermittent exposure to fleas increases the likelihood of development; commonly seen in conjunction with atopy

Historical Findings

- Compulsive biting
- Chewing (corncob nibbling)
- Licking—primarily in the back half of the body, but may include the antebrachial regions
- Cats—scratching around the head and neck
- Signs of fleas and flea dirt

 CLINICAL FEATURES

- Depends somewhat on the severity of the reaction and the degree of exposure to fleas—seasonal vs. year-round)
- Finding fleas and flea dirt is beneficial, although not essential, for the diagnosis of FBH—Sensitive animals require a low exposure and tend to overgroom, making identification of the parasites difficult.
- Dogs—lesions concentrated in a triangular area of the caudal-dorsal-lumbosacral region; caudal aspect of the thighs, lower abdomen, inguinal region, and cranial forearms usually involved; primary lesions are papules; secondary lesions (e.g., hyperpigmentation, lichenification, alopecia, and scaling) common in uncontrolled FBH; secondary folliculitis and furunculosis may be seen; firbopruritic nodules rare
- Cats—several patterns are seen; most common is a miliary crusting dermatitis in a wedge-shaped pattern over the caudal dorsal lumbosacral region and often around the head and neck; other presentations are alopecia of the inguinal region with or without inflammation or eosinophilic plaques and other forms of eosinophilic granuloma complex
- Exposure to other animals and previous flea treatment should be ascertained.

 DIFFERENTIAL DIAGNOSIS

- Food allergy
- Atopy
- Sarcoptic mange
- Cheyletiellosis
- Any pruritic skin disease

 DIAGNOSTICS

- Cats—hypereosinophilia may be detected
- Skin scrapings—negative
- Flea combings—fleas or flea dirt, but often nothing is found

- RAST and ELISA—variable accuracy; both false-positive and false-negative results reported
- Diagnosis—usually based on historical information and distribution of lesions
- Fleas or flea dirt—supportive but often quite difficult to find, especially in cats
- Identification of *Dipylidium caninum* segments—supportive
- Intradermal allergy testing with flea antigen—positive immediate reactions in 90% of flea-allergic animals; delayed reactions (24–48 hours) sometimes observed in allergic animals that show no immediate reaction
- The most accurate test may be response to appropriate treatment.

Biopsy

- Superficial perivascular dermatitis
- Eosinophilic intraepidermal microabscesses strongly suggest FBH.
- Eosinophils as a major cellular component of the dermis is supportive of FBH.
- Histopathologic evaluation cannot accurately differentiate FBH from atopy, food allergy, or other hypersensitivities.

 THERAPEUTICS

- Corticosteroids—anti-inflammatory dosages for symptomatic relief while the fleas are being controlled
- Antihistamines—symptomatic relief
- Dinotefuran/Pyriproxyfen—rapid-acting topical product for cats; canine product contains high dose permethrin and should not be used on cats.
- Fipronil (GABA antagonist)—monthly spot treatment for cats and dogs and spray treatment for dogs; activity against fleas and ticks; resistant to removal with water; excellent safety and efficacy profile
- Imidacloprid—monthly spot treatment for cats and dogs; excellent safety and efficacy profile
- Metaflumizone—blocks the influx of sodium required to propagate nerve impulses; results in reduced feeding, loss of coordination, paralysis, and death of the flea; studies have shown excellent flea and flea egg reduction up to 7 weeks with a high margin of safety; canine product contains amitraz and should not be used on cats
- Nitenpyram—neonicotinoid flea adulticide; orally administered; rapid onset, but short acting; removes over 95% of adult fleas from dogs and cats within 4–6 hours of oral administration but has residual activity for 48–72 hours
- Spinosad—monthly oral treatment approved for use in dogs only; mode of action is at nicotinic acetylcholine D α receptors with some effects on GABA resulting in nerve excitation paralysis and death of the flea; spinosad is felt to be safe in conjunction with all other flea control products and heartworm preventives.
- Sprays—usually contain pyrethrins and pyrethroids (synthetic pyrethrins) with an insect growth regulator or synergist; generally effective <48–72 hours; advantages

are low toxicity and repellent activity; disadvantages are frequent applications and expense.

■ Indoor treatment—fogs and premises sprays; usually contain organophosphates, pyrethrins, and/or insect growth regulators; apply according to manufacturer's directions; treat all areas of the house; can be applied by the owner; advantages are weak chemicals and generally inexpensive; disadvantage is labor intensity; premises sprays concentrate the chemicals in areas that most need treatment.

■ Professional exterminators—advantages are less labor intensive, relatively few applications, sometimes guaranteed, disadvantages are strength of chemicals and cost; specific recommendations and guidelines must be followed.

■ Inert substances—boric acid, diatomaceous earth, and silica aerogel; treat every 6–12 months; follow manufacturer's recommendations; very safe and effective if applied properly

■ Outdoor treatment—concentrated in shaded areas; sprays usually contain pyrethroids or organophosphates and an insect growth regulator; powders are usually organophosphates; product containing nematodes (*Steinerma carpocapsae*) is very safe and chemical-free

Precautions

■ Insecticidal sprays and dips should not be used on dogs and cats ≤3 months of age, unless otherwise specified on the label.

■ Spinosad can potentiate neurologic side effects of high-dose ivermectin (used in treatment of generalized demodicosis).

■ Pyrethrin/pyrethroid-type flea products—adverse reactions include depression, hypersalivation, muscle tremors, vomiting, ataxia, dyspnea, and anorexia

■ Organophosphates—Adverse reactions include hypersalivation, lacrimation, urination, defecation, vomiting, diarrhea, miosis, fever, muscle tremors, seizures, coma, and death.

■ All pesticides must be applied according to label directions.

■ Toxicity—If any signs are noted, the animal should be bathed thoroughly to remove any remaining chemicals and treated appropriately.

■ Rodents and fish are very sensitive to pyrethrins.

Possible Interactions

■ Organophosphate treatments—Do not use more than one form at a time.

■ Spinosad should not be used with high-dose ivermectin (used in generalized demodex); safe when combined with heartworm prevention dosage.

■ Topical organophosphates—Avoid in cats, very young animals (<3 months of age), and sick or debilitated animals.

■ Straight permethrin sprays or spot-ons—Do not use in cats.

■ Cythioate—contraindicated in heartworm-positive dogs and greyhounds

■ Piperonyl butoxide—Do not use in concentrations >1% in cats.

Alternative Drugs

- Powders—usually contain organophosphates or carbamates; advantage is high residual effectiveness; disadvantages are dry skin and toxicity; organophosphates and carbamates should be avoided in cats.
- Dips, sprays, powders, and foams—dips usually contain organophosphates and synthetic pyrethrins and should not be used more than once per week; follow manufacturer's instructions for safest and best results; after repeated use, these agents can be drying or irritating; newer, safer spot treatments have essentially replaced these products.

 COMMENTS

- Inform owners—There is no cure for FBH.
- Advise owners—Flea-allergic animals often become more sensitive to flea bites as they age.
- Inform owners—Controlling exposure to fleas is currently the only means of therapy; hyposensitization has not worked satisfactorily.
- Pruritus—A decrease means the FBH is being controlled.
- Fleas and flea dirt—Absence is not always a reliable indicator of successful treatment in very sensitive animals.
- Year-round warm climates—year-round flea control.
- Seasonally warm climates—begin flea control in May or June.
- Allergy—Approximately 80% of atopic dogs are also allergic to flea bites.
- Organophosphates—use with utmost caution in old animals; not recommended for use in very young animals (<3 months of age)
- In areas of moderate to severe flea infestation—Humans can be bitten by fleas; usually papular lesions are located on the wrists and ankles.
- Corticosteroids and organophosphates—Do not use in pregnant bitches and queens.
- Carefully follow the label directions for each individual product to determine its safety.
- People can be bitten by fleas, usually causing popular lesions on the wrists and ankles.

Abbreviations

ELISA, enzyme-linked immunosorbent assay; FBH, flea bite hypersensitivity; GABA, gamma-aminobutyric acid; Ig, immunoglobulin; RAST, radioallergosorbent test.

Suggested Reading

Sousa CA, Halliwell RE. The ACVD task force on canine atopic dermatitis (XI): the relationship between arthropod hypersensitivity and atopic dermatitis in the dog. *Vet Immunol Immunopathol* 2001;81:233–237.

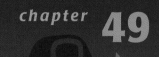

Giardiasis

DEFINITION/OVERVIEW

- Enteric protozoan infection that can cause small-bowel diarrhea in dogs and cats, but usually asymptomatic

ETIOLOGY/PATHOPHYSIOLOGY

- Several species—*Giardia lamblia* (humans), *Giardia canis* (dogs), and *Giardia felis* (cats), but cross-infection occurs
- Zoonosis—*G. canis* is not considered zoonotic, but *G. lamblia* cysts that infect humans have been identified in dogs (although rarely) and are considered zoonotic.
- Transmission—ingestion of cysts, which are usually water-borne, but also autotransmission (cysts survive well adhered to the perianal region and in a pet's contaminated environment) common
- Flagellated tachyzoites released (from cysts)—in GI tract attach to small intestinal enterocytes
- Causes malabsorption syndrome—sugars, vitamin B_{12}, folate, triglycerides
- Specific histologic changes—not identified, but blunting of intestinal villi can ensue
- Cysts—found in feces, but also trophozoites (especially in animals with diarrhea)
- Cysts—survive for months in moist cool environment outside host
- Trophozoites—do not survive outside host and are not infective
- PPP = 5–12 days (dogs) and 5–16 days (cats)

SIGNALMENT/HISTORY

- Clinical signs—mainly seen in young dogs and cats
- Older animals—rarely show signs unless there is an underlying problem (overcrowding stress, diet, concurrent GI tract disease)
- Prevalence
  - Dogs—varies greatly from 10% in client-owned single-single household pets, to 100% in kennels
  - Cats—usually between 1% and 10%

CLINICAL FEATURES

- Usually excrete cysts with no signs
- Diarrhea often small bowel (young animals); rancid odor, soft, frothy, pale, and steatorrheic
- May show intermittent or chronic diarrhea with occasional vomiting

 ## DIFFERENTIAL DIAGNOSIS

- Anything that causes acute small-bowel diarrhea, including dietary indiscretion; IBD; neoplasia (especially GI tract lymphoma); drugs (antibiotics); toxins (lead); parasites (cryptosporidiosis, trichomoniasis, whipworms); infectious agents (parvovirus, FIP, salmonellosis, rickettsia, GI bacterial overgrowth, clostridia, histoplasmosis, leishmaniasis, other rare infections—pythiosis); systemic organ dysfunction (renal, hepatic, pancreatic, cardiac); metabolic (hypoadrenocorticism, hyperthyroidism of cats)

 ## DIAGNOSTICS

- Finding cysts (Fig. 49-1) in an animal with diarrhea—does not always mean the diarrhea is caused by *Giardia*
- Testing—can be divided into in-house diagnostics (direct smear, fecal floatation without centrifugation, SNAP *Giardia* antigen fecal test (IDEXX labs), and laboratory tests (floatation with centrifugation, IFA, PCR, ELISA kits)
- Direct fecal smear—to identify trophozoites (reasonably sensitive in cats with diarrhea) or cysts; a drop of feces mixed with a drop of Lugol's iodine kills the trophozoites and stains them brown so morphology can be examined (under 403 magnification)
- Differentiate *Giardia* trophozoites (Fig. 49-2) from *Tritrichomonas fetus* (only other organism it can be confused with in cats)—*T. fetus* has a smoother rolling motion, no concave ventral disc, a single nucleus, and an undulating membrane.
- ZSCT—still considered the "gold standard" although other tests (IFA) clearly as good; three tests performed on sequential fecal samples is nearly 100% sensitive.
- Sucrose concentration techniques—distort cysts
- Commercial ZSCT (if do not include centrifugation)—lower specificity in comparison to techniques that include concentration by centrifugation; a poor in-house test for *Giardia*
- Commercial ELISA kits (ProSpecT/Giardia ELISA kit; Alexon)—have a false-negative rate of 31.6% and high specificity (95.7%) compared to ZSCT; can use frozen or formaldehyde-fixed feces

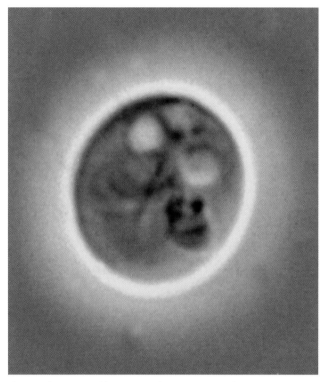

■ **Figure 49-1** *Giardia* cyst characterized by two circular structures within.

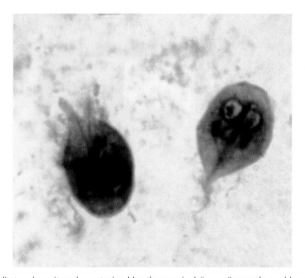

■ **Figure 49-2** *Giardia* trophozoites characterized by the comical "eyes," mouth, and long flagella.

- Commercial direct immunofluorescence test (Merifluor Cryptosporidium/Giardia Direct Immunofluorescence Assay; Meridian Diagnostics)—may be more sensitive and specific for detecting low cyst numbers, and for use in stored feces compared with the ZSCT
- SNAP *Giardia* antigen test (IDEXX Labs)—easy to use; identifies a cyst wall protein
- PCR—offered by some laboratories but seems to be no more reliable than other less costly tests
- Multiple reports comparing the various tests demonstrate one truth—that no single test is 100% accurate. Flotation (with centrifugation) and antigen tests (IFA or ELISA including the SNAP) used in combination on multiple samples is probably the most accurate.

Diagnostic Feature

- **ZSCT is still considered the gold standard of *Giardia* diagnosis, but ELISA and immunofluorescence assays are gaining in popularity and efficacy.**
- Duodenal aspiration—rarely identifies *Giardia* over and above ZSCT
- Peroral nylon string test (Entero-test [HDC Corp;)—not safe or effective in diagnosing *Giardia* infection in dogs

 # THERAPEUTICS

- If diarrhea is severe, treat supportively.
- Many recent studies suggest that, when controlling diarrhea in animals with giardiasis, antigiardiacidal drug treatment must be coupled with measures to clean cysts from the animal's environment and coat.
- QUAT (Roccal [Winthrop Labs]; Totil [Calgon Corp])—inactivate cysts within 1 minute of contact at room temperature; must clean up organic material first; can use on coat of animals as a rinse (allowing contact for 1 minute, then thoroughly rinse off) after washing the coat with a pet shampoo first to remove organic matter, then dry coat well (cysts very susceptible to drying).

Vaccination

- *Giardia* vaccine (GiardiaVax for cats and dogs; Fort Dodge Animal Health)—made of chemically inactivated trophozoites
- Pups and kittens (7-week-old and naïve to *Giardia* exposure)—receiving one vaccine and a booster 3 weeks later, were immune to a *Giardia* challenge 6 and 12 months later
- Older dogs—vaccination reduced the duration of cyst shedding and the number of cysts shed.

- The vaccine has been used as an immunotherapeutic agent in dogs; 13 dogs that failed to be cured of giardiasis using chemotherapeutic measures showed clinical cures and cessation of fecal cyst shedding between 3 and 10 weeks postvaccination (some required up to 3 vaccines); suggests that vaccine might have a place in the treatment of some chronically infected dogs in which chemotherapy and hygiene control methods have failed.
- Vaccination—In some studies, vaccination failed to prevent reinfection.
- Vaccination—anecdotal reports of asymptomatic infected dogs developing clinical symptoms of diarrhea after receiving the vaccine
- Vaccination for cats—vaccinated 4, 6, and 10 weeks after experimentally infected failed to clear the infection, suggesting that the vaccine may not be efficacious in those cats already infected
- Vaccine—little utility as a general vaccine for the control of giardiasis in the general population of dogs because most are exposed to the organism before vaccination

Drugs of Choice

- No drug is registered for use against *Giardia* in North America.
- Fenbendazole and combination of febantel-praziquantel-pyrantel (Drontal Plus; Bayer) are preferred because of the lack of side effects and high efficacy; these drugs are the most commonly used agents.
- Fenbendazole (Panacur; Hoechst-Roussel Agri-Vet)—over 90% efficacy; can be used in pregnant animals, unlike other benzimadazoles
- Febantel-praziquantel-pyrantel (Drontal Plus; Bayer)—contains similar efficacy to fenbendazole in dogs; active ingredient is febantel (which is converted to fenbendazole and oxfendazole), which might also have a synergistic action with praziquantel
- Oxfendazole (Dolthene; Merial Laboratories)—in Europe, has been shown very effective when combined with control methods
- Oxfendazole suspension—available in United States (Synanthic Bovine Dewormer Suspension 9.06%; Fort Dodge Animal Health); not registered for use in dogs
- Albendazole (Valbazen Cattle Dewormer; Pfizer Animal Health)—potentially toxic; may cause myelosuppression in both dogs and cats
- Metronidazole (Flagyl; Pfizer)—67% efficacious in dogs, but also has efficacy against other GI tract flora and possible immunologic effects on cell populations in the bowel
- Metronidazole benzoate (only available for formulation in the United States)—recently found to be 100% efficacious in cats (Table 49-1)
- Tinidazole (Tindamax or Fasigyn)—closely related to metronidazole; has recently been approved for use in man with giardiasis; little experience of its use in dogs, but is effective
- Ronidazole (Ridzol)—same class as tinidazole; used to treat Blackhead in turkeys; little experience but probably effective
- Ipronidaszole, quinacrine, and furazolidone—some have good efficacy but high side effects

TABLE 49-1 Drug Therapy for Giardiasis in Small Animals

Drug	Species	Dose (mg/kg)	Route	Interval (h)	Duration (d)
Fenbendazole (Panacur)	D	50	PO	24	3
	C	50	PO	24	5[a]
Febantel-praziquantel-pyrantel (Drontal Plus)	D	[b]	PO	24	3
Metronidazole (Flagyl)	D	20	PO	12	5
Metronidazole benzoate	C	25	PO	12	7[c]
Oxfendazole (Dolthene)	D	11.3	PO	24	3
Albendazole[d] (Valbazen)	D	25	PO	12	2
	C	25	PO	12	5

[a]Efficacy, 50%.
[b]Dose of each drug—febantel (26.8–35.2 mg/kg), praziquantel (5.4–7 mg/kg), and pyrantel (26.8–35.2 mg/kg).
[c]Efficacy, 100%.
[d]May cause myelosuppression.
C, cats; D, dogs.

Precautions/Interactions

- Albendazole, but not fenbendazole, is suspected of being teratogenic and, therefore, should not be given to pregnant animals.
- At higher doses, albendazole can cause myelosuppression in both dogs and cats.
- Metronidazole at higher doses (>30 mg/kg) can produce neurologic signs, including anorexia and vomiting, with deterioration to pronounced generalized ataxia and vertical positional nystagmus.

COMMENTS

- Apparent failure of drugs to clear infections is probably because autoinfection can occur immediately after drugs stopped, and, with a PPP of 5 days, cyst excretion can occur in dogs within 5 days of stopping drugs.
- Zoonosis—*Giardia* assemblages that infect man have also been found in dogs and cats; it is impossible to say in an individual case whether the animal has a zoonotic assemblage present (needs complex genetic studies of the organism), but the infection rate of zoonotic assemblages of cats and dogs is very low.
- There is a strong argument for not treating asymptomatic dogs because the risk of zoonosis is very low (some believe it to be nonexistent) and animals often get reinfected once treatment stops.
- Control of diarrhea and chronic giardiasis is more likely achieved when drugs are used in association with hygiene methods, particularly in kennel situations.

Abbreviations

CBC, complete blood count; ELISA, enzyme-linked immunosorbent assay; FIP, feline infectious peritonitis; GI, gastrointestinal; IBD, inflammatory bowel disease; IFA, immunofluorescent assay; PCR, polymerase chain reaction; PPP, prepatent period; QUAT, quaternary ammonium-containing disinfectants; ZSCT, zinc sulfate concentration technique.

Suggested Reading

Ballweber LR, Xiao L, Bowman DD, et al. Giardiasis in dogs and cats: update on epidemiology and public health significance. *Trends Parasitol* 2010;26:180–189.

Payne PA, Artzer M. The biology and control of *Giardia* spp. and *Tritrichomonas foetus*. *Vet Clin North Am Small Anim Pract* 2009;39:993–1007.

Rishniw M, Liotta J, Bellosa M, et al. Comparison of 4 *Giardia* diagnostic tests in diagnosis of naturally acquired canine chronic subclinical giardiasis. *J Vet Intern Med* 2010;24:293–297.

Heartworm Disease–Cats

DEFINITION/OVERVIEW

- Parasitic disease of cats affecting the heart and lungs

ETIOLOGY/PATHOPHYSIOLOGY

- *Dirofilaria immitis*—adults infect pulmonary arteries
- Unlike in dogs—worms are physically smaller, have a shorter life span (~2 years); lower worm burden (1–3 worms/cat)
- Microfilaria—uncommon (<20%)
- Prevalence—one-tenth that of unprotected dogs
- Clinical signs usually develop as a result of 2 periods during infection with heartworms:
  - Arrival of heartworms in the pulmonary vasculature 3–4 months postinfection; causes acute vascular and parenchymal inflammation; often misdiagnosed as asthma; known a Heartworm Associated Respiratory Disease (HARD); clinical signs present even in cats that eventually clear infection
  - Adult worms present in pulmonary artery begin to die causing pulmonary inflammation and thromboembolism; can lead to acute fatal lung injury.
- Caval syndrome is very rare in the cat; however, 1 or 2 worms may be enough to cause tricuspid regurgitation with a resultant heart murmur.
- Pulmonary hypertension—rare in cats because infections in cats are usually light and of short duration; right ventricular hypertrophy and failure are less common in cats than dogs.

SIGNALMENT/HISTORY

- No age or breed predisposition
- Males—more commonly infected
- Historically—Cats present with coughing, dyspnea, and vomiting.
- Sudden death—occurs due to acute respiratory failure from PTE
- Vomiting and respiratory signs—predominate in chronic disease

CLINICAL FEATURES

- Usually normal
- Increased bronchovesicular sounds with murmur or gallop rhythm—should increase suspicion of primary cardiac disease

 DIFFERENTIAL DIAGNOSIS

- Asthma—different radiographic signs; heartworm antibody/antigen negative
- Cardiomyopathy—differentiate on radiography and cardiac ultrasound
- Chylothorax—heartworm disease can be associated
- *Aelurostrongylus abstrusus* infection—larvae in feces
- *Paragonimus kellicotti* infection—eggs in feces
- Other causes of chronic vomiting—IBD, GI tract lymphoma, fur balls, food allergy, diaphragmatic hernia

 DIAGNOSTICS

- CBC:
  - Mild nonregenerative anemia
  - Eosinophilia inconsistent
  - Basophilia should increase suspicion.
- Hyperglobulinemia—occasionally
- Microfilaria (Modified Knotts, filter test)—low sensitivity, high specificity
- Heartworm antigen tests (ELISA or immunochromatographic tests)—detect circulating adult HWAg; more specific than antibody tests; a positive antigen test result is strong evidence of heartworm disease but low worm burdens (fewer than five worms) and single-sex infections can result in false-negative results; negative result does not rule out heartworm disease; risk of false-positive results increases with low prevalence (most of United States), so positive results in low-prevalence areas should be confirmed by other diagnostic criteria or second test.
- Heartworm antibody tests (ELISA or immunochromatographic tests)—detect circulating antibodies to immature and adult heartworms; can be positive as early as 2 months postinfection; the most sensitive tests for feline heartworm disease but sensitivity varies greatly between tests and depends on the duration of infection; a positive result documents exposure but does not always indicate mature or current infection (positive predictive value, 25%); the more intense the antibody response (higher titer or ABU level), the more likely it is that it is an adult infection; can detect male-only and immature infections; strength of test is to rule out infection; antibody levels decrease with time as the parsite matures; infected cats with clinical signs are

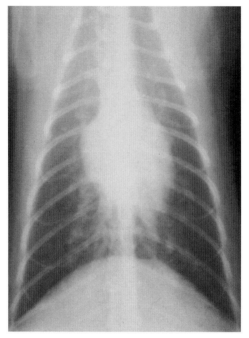

■ **Figure 50-1** Thoracic radiograph of a cat with heartworm disease showing enlarged blunted, tortuous pulmonary arteries, and patchy perivascular pulmonary infiltrates.

more likely to be antibody-positive than infected asymptomatic cats; antibody tests should be used in association with antigen tests to increase the power of diagnosis.

■ Radiographic/angiographic examination—will show enlarged pulmonary artery (if >1.6 times the width of the 9th rib, highly suggestive of infection); blunted, tortuous pulmonary arteries; patchy perivascular pulmonary infiltrates (Fig. 50-1); pulmonary arterial truncation, obstruction and linear filling defects often best viewed with nonselective angiography (Fig. 50-2).

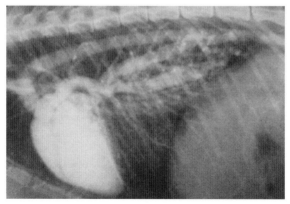

■ **Figure 50-2** Thoracic radiograph during nonselective angiography of a cat with severe heartworm disease showing dilated and truncated pulmonary arteries and mild thromboembolism.

- Echocardiographic examination—more sensitive in cats than dogs; will show dilated main pulmonary artery, see worms in heart or main pulmonary artery often as "double-lined echodensity" (most commonly, the right pulmonary artery); expertise and high index of suspicion increases sensitivity of test especially in infections greater than 5 months old.

THERAPEUTICS

- Administration of adulticide is controversial in cats—none are approved
- Severe and fatal PTE—frequently occurs after treatment
- Spontaneous "cure"—probably much more common in cats than dogs (shorter heartworm life span)
- Stabilize symptomatic cases—treat clinical signs

Drugs of Choice

- Initial stabilization—oxygen, theophylline (25 mg/kg, PO, q24h in evening; sustained release formulation)
- Prednisolone (1–2 mg/kg, PO, q24h for 10–14 days; then reduce gradually to every other day for 2 weeks the discontinued after an additional 2 weeks; use periodically if respiratory signs reoccur)—reduces severity of PTE
- Ivermectin (24 µg/mg monthly for 2 years)—reported to reduce worm burdens by 65% compared with untreated cats; watch for PTE development and treat aggressively with steroids.

Precautions/Interactions

- Thiacetarsamide (Caparsolate) and melarsomine (Immiticide)—not indicated in cats
- If an adulticide is used—PTE likely to occur 5–10 days after administration; mortality rate around 30%
- Aspirin therapy—no documented benefit
- Doxycycline—not assessed in cats to date

COMMENTS

- Serial evaluation of clinical response, thoracic radiographs, and heartworm antigen and antibody tests are most informative.
- With judicious use of prednisone—possible to control the symptoms while waiting for the heartworms to die naturally

- Prevention—use depends on prevalence in a particular area; formulations currently approved for cats include:
  - Ivermectin (Heartgard for Cats; Merial)—24 mg/kg, PO, every 30 days
  - Selamectin (Revolution for Cats; Pfizer)—6–12 mg/kg topically, every 30 days
    - Moxidectin (Advantage Multi for Cats; Bayer Animal Health)—1 mg/kg topically, every 30 days
  - Milbemycin oxime (Interceptor; Novartis)—2 mg/kg, PO, every 30 days

Abbreviations

ABU, antibody unit; CBC, complete blood count; ELISA, enzyme-linked immunosorbent assay; GI, gastrointestinal; HWAg, heartworm antigen; IBD, inflammatory bowel disease; PTE, pulmonary thromboembolism.

Suggested Reading

American Heartworm Society. 2005. Current feline guidelines. Available at: http://www.heartworm society.org/veterinary-resources/feline-guidelines.html.

Heartworm Disease: Dogs

chapter 51

DEFINITION/OVERVIEW

- Parasitic infection of the pulmonary arteries of dogs causing respiratory (pulmonary hypertension, embolization, allergic pneumonitis, eosinophilic granulomas), cardiac (myocardial hypertrophy and, in some animals, congestive heart failure due to high right ventricle afterload), and renal (immune complex glomerulonephropathy) disease

ETIOLOGY/PATHOPHYSIOLOGY

- *Dirofilaria immitis*—Adults (female worms up to 30 cm long) live in the pulmonary arteries of dogs, leading to endothelial damage and myointimal proliferation.
- Pulmonary artery damage—results in lobar arterial enlargement, tortuosity, and obstruction, causing pulmonary hypertension and thrombosis
- Severity of disease—directly related to the number of worms, duration of infection, and host response
- Female adult worms—release L1 (microfilaria) into circulation (can live there for 2 years)
- L1 in circulation—may infect mosquitoes feeding; develop to L3 in mosquito and injected back into dog to migrate to heart
- PPP = 6–7 months
- Prevalence—varies with geographic location, but widespread throughout North America, even into Alaska
- Prevalence—virtually 100% in unprotected dogs living in highly endemic regions
- Prevalence—common along the Atlantic and Gulf coasts and Ohio and Mississippi River basins
- Numerous pockets of infection in otherwise low-prevalence regions—usually where mosquito vector is ubiquitous

SIGNALMENT/HISTORY

- Medium- to large-breed dogs that spend a lot of time outdoors—most susceptible
- Endemic regions—all unprotected dogs at risk

- Most affected animals—between 3 and 8 years old
- Historically—Most infected dogs are asymptomatic or exhibit minimal signs such as occasional coughing (Class I).

 # CLINICAL FEATURES

- Class I—no abnormalities in an infected dog
- Class II—cough, exercise intolerance, weight loss, pulmonary changes on thoracic radiography, PCV between 20 and 25
- Class III—cachexia, exercise intolerance, syncope, tachycardia, ascites (right-sided heart failure), hepatomegaly, pulmonary and cardiac changes on thoracic radiography, PCV <20
- Hemoptysis—occasionally occurs; indicates severe pulmonary thromboembolic complications
- Vena cava syndrome—occurs when vena cava is obstructed by adult worms; hemoglobinuria due to acute hemolytic crisis (shock)

 # DIFFERENTIAL DIAGNOSIS

- Other causes of pulmonary hypertension and thrombosis—for example, hyper adrenocorticism
- Other causes of pulmonary disease—allergic lung disease, COPD, neoplasia, parasitic lung disease, foreign body, pneumonia; thoracic radiologic examination and heartworm antigen tests should differentiate from heartworm disease
- Other causes of ascites—dilated cardiomyopathy and other causes of heart failure, hypoproteinemia, hepatic disease, caudal caval or portal vein thromboembolism, neoplasia, pericardial effusion

 # DIAGNOSTICS

- CBC:
  - Anemia—mild in Class II, severe in Class III
  - Eosinophilia and basophilia (variable)—together, are a sensitive indicator of heartworm disease
  - Leukocytosis and thrombocytopenia—associated with thromboembolism
- Serum biochemical profile and urinalysis:
  - Hyperglobulinemia—inconsistent finding
  - Proteinuria—common in animals with severe and chronic infection; may be caused by immune-complex glomerulonephritis or amyloidosis
  - Hemoglobinuria—acute hemolytic crisis during vena cava syndrome

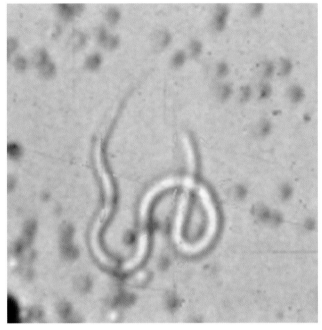

■ **Figure 51-1** Although rarely found because of the advent of monthly heartworm preventive agents, a blood smear may reveal *D. immitis* microfilaria in a dog with heartworm disease (wet preparation, 400×).

- Heartworm antigen tests—highly specific, sensitive serologic tests that identify adult female *D. immitis* antigen; widely available; standard tests for screening
- Antigen tests—take 7 months after infection to develop a positive status; do not use in pups under 7 months, and test 7 months after the end of the previous transmission season.
- Annual testing—unnecessary if dog receiving monthly macrolide chemoprophylaxis appropriately (2- to 3-year testing interval sufficient)
- Microfilaria identification tests—include the modified Knott's test, filter tests, and direct smear (Fig. 51-1); 20–25% of infected dogs will be missed if rely on these tests alone
- Thoracic radiologic examination—should always perform not only as a diagnostic aid but also to predict class of infection and extent of thromboembolism
- Thoracic radiologic examination—allows comparison between radiographs taken during treatment and recovery (Figs. 51-2 and 51-3)
- Thoracic radiographic signs:
  - Main pulmonary artery segment—enlargement
  - Lobar arterial enlargement and tortuosity—vary from absent (Class I) to severe (Class III)
  - Parenchymal lung infiltrates of variable severity (surround lobar arteries)—may extend into most or all of one or multiple lung lobes when thromboembolism occurs

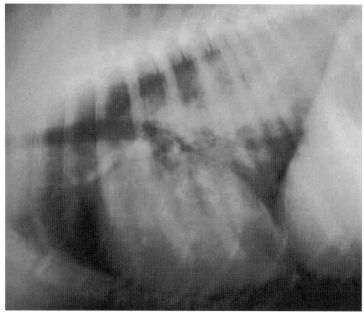

■ **Figure 51-2** Lateral thoracic radiograph of a dog with severe heartworm disease showing dilated pulmonary arteries, pulmonary thromboembolism, and right ventricular enlargement.

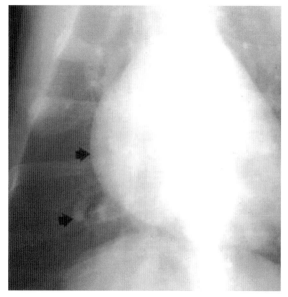

■ **Figure 51-3** Dorsoventral thoracic radiograph of a dog with severe heartworm disease showing right ventricular enlargement (*top arrow*) and enlarged truncated right caudal pulmonary artery (*lower arrow*).

- Diffuse, symmetrical, alveolar, and interstitial infiltrates—occasionally occur because of an allergic reaction to microfilaria
- Echocardiography—often unremarkable and therefore not a cost-effective test
- Echocardiogram—may show right ventricular dilation and wall hypertrophy; parallel linear echodensities produced by heartworms may be detected in the RV, RA, and PA (inconsistent finding in dogs)
- Angiography—of little practical clinical importance
- ECG—usually normal; may reflect RV hypertrophy in dogs with severe (Class III) infection; heart rhythm disturbances rarely seen but may include atrial fibrillation (most common) in severe infection

 # THERAPEUTICS

- Hospitalization—Some patients may need hospitalization during adulticide administration.
- Hospitalization—recommended for dogs experiencing thromboembolic complications
- Severe restriction of activity—required for 4–6 weeks after adulticide administration.
- Cage confinement—recommended for 3–4 weeks after adulticide administration for severe (Class III) disease.
- Cage confinement for 7 days—recommended for dogs experiencing pulmonary thromboembolic complications
- Class III disease—treat CHF until stable before administering adulticide; use diuretics, cage rest, and sodium restriction
- Stabilize pulmonary failure—with antithrombotic agents (e.g., aspirin or heparin) and anti-inflammatory doses of corticosteroid; monitor using clinical and radiographic parameters
- Dogs with vena cava syndrome—surgical removal of adult worms from right heart and PA via jugular vein by use of fluoroscopy and a long, flexible alligator forceps; highly effective for treating high worm burden when employed by an experienced operator
- Determine justification of adulticide treatment in older dogs—Outcome may be worse than not treating because benefit of treatment may not be realized in dog's lifetime.

Drugs of Choice

Treatment of Infected Dogs

- Melarsomine dihydrochloride (Immiticide; Merial)—low toxicity (hepatotoxicity); good efficacy (>90%) against both sexes of adult worms but has no activity on worms <4 months of age; adverse effects include pulmonary thromboembolism (usually 7–30 days after therapy), anorexia (13% incidence), injection site reaction (myositis—32% incidence but mild and lasts 1–2 days), lethargy or depression (15% incidence); causes elevations of hepatic enzymes

- Class I infection—two injections 24 hours apart are given into the epaxial muscles (first injection on one side, second injection on opposite side, using 22-gauge needles); apply pressure over the injection site during and after needle withdrawal; check antigen test 6 months later and, if positive, repeat treatment. This regimen kills about 90% of adult worms (may want to use the alternative dose schedule as below).
- Class II and Class III infections (after CHF stabilization)—use alternative dose schedule: first injection administered initially (40% kill rate); 1 month later, two injections 24 hours apart are recommended.
- Alternative dose schedule—spreads the adulticide killing effect and thromboembolism over 2 treatments; kills about 98% of adult worms.
- Alternative dose schedule—used by many veterinarians for treating Class I infections because of its increased adulticide killing effect and less thromboembolism
- Pretreat patients—a macrocyclic lactone preventative for 2–3 months prior to starting the course of melarsomine injections; will ensure that susceptible heartworm larvae will be killed (preventing reinfection) and allows juvenile adult worms to reach an age where they are susceptible to melarsomine.
- Pretreat patients – doxycycline (10 mg/kg, PO, q12h) for 4 weeks prior to starting melarsomine injections to kill any *Wolbachia* in adult heartworms; found to reduce pulmonary pathology associated with the death of the heartworms and may reduce any renal pathology also
- Exercise restriction—begin at the time of heartworm diagnosis, making it most stringent during the 4 weeks after the first melarsomine injection and continue it for 6 months after the last injection
- Microfilaricide administration—begin immediately after diagnosis (see above) and continue throughout treatment and for life:
  - Milbemycin (Interceptor; Novartis; 0.5 mg/kg) or ivermectin (multiple preparation, 50 mg/kg)—administered in the morning, and the patient observed for signs of microfilarial anaphylaxis (shock, vomiting, diarrhea, circulatory collapse) for the day and discharged in the evening
  - Likelihood of shock developing—highest in dogs with high microfilaremias
  - If shock occurs—administer high-dose glucocorticoids and shock doses of IV fluids; observe in hospital for 24 hours; excellent prognosis if treated quickly
  - Ivermectin—given as a prophylaxis (6 mg/kg, monthly); will eventually remove microfilaria after 8 months in most dogs
- Corticosteriods (prednisone, 0.5 mg/kg, PO, q12h for 7 days, then 0.5 mg/kg, PO, q24h for 7 days, then 0.5 mg/kg q48h for 7 to 14 days)—often started after the first injection of melarsomine to directly treat or decrease the development of pulmonary thromboembolism; does not affect the efficacy of melarsomine
- Perform an antigen test 4–6 months after adulticide treatment—if positive, repeat adulticide treatment.
- Some dogs with persistent adult infection—may not require retreatment; determined by age, severity of infection, degree of improvement since the first treatment, strength of the positive antigen test result, concomitant disease

Alternative therapies

- If Melarsomine is declined by the owner, rejected on other ground, or unavailable:
  - Prophylactic doses of ivermectin, moxidectin, and selamectin are effective in reducing the life span of juvenile and adult heartworms; may take a year or two to result in a removal of all worms; pulmonary pathology worsens over this time and is more severe than treating with melasomine; severely limit exercise during this time and examine the dog biyearly at least
  - Monthly prophylactic doses of ivermectin in association with periodic doses of doxycycline can result in about a 75% reduction of adult heartworm numbers over time.

Prophylaxis of Noninfected Dogs

- Heartworm prophylaxis—should be provided for all dogs at risk
- New patients starting on prophylaxis for the first time—a test to detect microfilaria may be indicated because some macrolide endectocides (milbemycin) may induce a shock syndrome within 24 hours of the first dose; antigen test before starting preventive treatment in such cases is indicated to rule out possible adult infection (if positive, consider adulticide treatment options but start prophylaxis treatment immediately as long as patient is microfilaremic negative).
- Ivermectin (Heartgard; Merial)—highly effective monthly preventive; retroactive efficacy as long as 4 months after infection when monthly administration is continued for 12 months; when combined with pyrantel pamoate (Heartgard Plus; Merial), also controls hookworm and roundworm infection; can be given safely to microfilaremic dogs, including so-called ivermectin-sensitive dogs
- Milbemycin oxime (Interceptor; Novartis)—highly effective monthly preventive; also controls hookworms, roundworms, and whipworms; the preventive dosage is microfilaricidal; acute reactions may occur when given to microfilaremic dogs
- Moxidectin (ProHeart tablets; Fort Dodge Animal Health)—a monthly preventive; can be given to microfilaremic dogs
- Moxidectin (ProHeart6 injectable; Fort Dodge Animal Health)—prophylactic effective for at least 6 months after injection; currently not available in the United States
- Selamectin (Revolution; Pfizer)—monthly topical preventive; also controls fleas, ear mites, sarcoptic mange, and some tick infestations
- Macrocide endectocide preventives (milbemycin oxime, ivermectin, selamactin, and moxidectin)—provide retroactive efficacy of 100% for 1 month and at least 75% for 2 months; ivermectin may provide up to 4 months of protection if continued for 12 months thereafter.
- Diethylcarbamazine citrate (Filaribits [Pfizer]; Nemacide [Boehringer Ingelheim])—daily administration (6.6 mg/kg) is required to ensure prophylaxis; cheaper than macrolides; need to continue dosing 2 months beyond the end of transmission season; if miss a few doses (which voids protection), administer one dose of a macrolide endectocide (ivermectin, milbemycin, etc.) at prophylaxis doses

- All of the prophylactic drugs can be administered safely to collies or collie-like breeds at the appropriate preventive dosages.

 ## COMMENTS

Precautions/Interactions

- Adulticide treatment—not indicated in patients with renal failure, hepatic failure, or nephrotic syndrome
- Standard adulticide therapy in dogs with severe infection—associated with high mortality due to subsequent pulmonary thromboembolism
- Prognosis in Class I—usually excellent
- Prognosis in Class III—guarded, with a higher risk of complications
- Old dogs—may not require treatment, because heartworm infection may not be the life-limiting factor
- Zoonosis—Heartworms represent no zoonotic potential.
- Adulticide treatment—should be delayed in pregnant animals
- Transplacental infection by microfilaria—can occur

Abbreviations

CBC, complete blood count; CHF, congestive heart failure; COPD, chronic obstructive pulmonary disease; ECG, electrocardiogram; PA, pulmonary artery; PCV, packed cell volume; PPP, prepatent period; RA, right atrium; RV, right ventricle.

Suggested Reading

American Heartworm Society. 2007. Current canine guidelines. Available at: http://www.heartworm society.org/veterinary-resources/canine-guidelines.html.

Helicobacter Infection

chapter **52**

DEFINITION/OVERVIEW

- A bacterial cause of inflammatory changes or glandular degeneration in the stomachs of cats and dogs

ETIOLOGY/PATHOPHYSIOLOGY

- *Helicobacter* spp. (specifically *H. felii, H. canis, H. bizzozeronii, H. salomonis, H. heilmannii, H. bilis, H. pametensis,* and *Flexispira rappini* in cats and dogs)—microaerophilic, gram-negative, urease-positive bacteria ranging from coccoid to curved to spiral
- *H. pylori*—most important species affecting humans, causing gastritis, peptic ulcers, and gastric neoplasia
- Experimentally—*H. pylori* causes gastritis, lymphoid follicle proliferation, and humoral immune responses in dogs and cats, but role in disease is currently unknown
- *Helicobacter* spp.—have been associated with the development of cholangiohepatitis in some cats

SIGNALMENT/HISTORY

- Infection with gastric *Helicobacter* spp.—appears to be acquired at a young age
- Most healthy cats and dogs harbor *Helicobacter* spp. in their stomachs.
- Asymptomatic *Helicobacter* infection—common
- Vomiting, anorexia, abdominal pain, weight loss, and/or borborygmis—seen in dogs and cats with gastric *Helicobacter* spp., but the signs may not be caused by *Helicobacter* infection
- Diarrhea in dogs—may be associated with *H. canis* infection, but a lot of normal dogs also have *H. canis* present
- Vomiting, weakness, and sudden death seen in one dog with hepatic *H. canis*.

CLINICAL FEATURES

- As well as the above historical signs—may have signs of dehydration from fluid and electrolyte loss (from vomiting or diarrhea)

 # DIFFERENTIAL DIAGNOSIS

- High *Helicobacter* spp. prevalence rates exist in dogs and cats—Exclusion of other causes of gastric disease and a positive test for *Helicobacter* infection are necessary before a diagnosis of GI disease due to *Helicobacter* spp. infection can be made.
- Identify other causes of vomiting, diarrhea, or liver disease—Because *Helicobacter* is ubiquitous, it requires a diagnosis by exclusion.

 # DIAGNOSTICS

- CBC and biochemical panel—nonspecific changes; reflect fluid and electrolyte abnormalities, secondary to vomiting and/or diarrhea, or hepatic disease
- Impression smears from the gastric mucosa obtained during endoscopy (stained with May-Gruüwald-Giemsa, Gram's, or Diff-Quick stains)—sensitive and easy test to perform (Fig. 52-1)

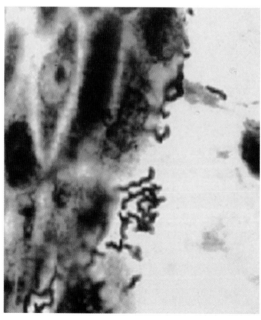

■ **Figure 52-1** *Helicobacter* organisms bordering the lining of the stomach mucosa in a dog (Warthin–Starry silver stain, 1400×).

- Rapid-urease test—requires gastric biopsy specimen; easy to perform in animals that undergo gastroduodenoscopy
- 13C-urea breath or blood test—shown to be reliable in identifying infected dogs
- Culture—requires special techniques and media; low success rate
- PCR of DNA extracted from biopsy specimens or from gastric juice—sensitive
- Serology (ELISA) measure of circulating IgG in serum—cannot distinguish among different HLOs

Diagnostic Feature

- **Endoscopy to obtain histopathology—enables definitive diagnosis of gastric *Helicobacter* infection; grossly, may see superficial nodules (suggest lymphoid follicle hyperplasia), diffuse gastric rugal thickening, mucosal flattening, punctate hemorrhages, and erosions**

THERAPEUTICS

- No unanimously accepted guidelines for treatment because pathogenicity remains unclear
- Currently no indication for treating asymptomatic animals
- Attempt eradication of gastric *Helicobacter* spp. in infected dogs and cats that have compatible clinical signs not attributable to other causes
- A triple therapy (combination of two antibiotics and one antisecretory drug for 2–3 weeks); effective in humans with *H. pylori* infection
- Triple therapy cure rates approach/exceed 90% in humans.
- Combination therapy in dogs and cats is less effective in eliminating *Helicobacter* infection than in humans.

Drugs of Choice

- Combination 1: metronidazole, amoxicillin, and famotidine—effectively eradicated *Helicobacter* infection in 6 of 8 dogs evaluated 3 days post-treatment; all dogs were recolonized by day 28 after completion of treatment.
- Combination 2: metronidazole, clarithromycin, ranitidine, and bismuth—effective in eradicating *H. heilmannii* in 11 of 11 cats by 10 days; 2 cats were reinfected 42 days post-treatment.
- Combination 3: amoxicillin, metronidazole, and omeprazole—transiently eradicated *H. pylori* in 6 cats; all were reinfected 6 weeks post-treatment.
- Combination 4: amoxicillin, metronidazole, and clarithromycin—100% effective in 12 chronically infected cats (Table 52-1)
- Recurrent infection after therapy—unclear whether due to reinfection or recrudescence of infection

TABLE 52-1 Drug Therapy Combinations for the Treatment of Helicobacteriosis in Dogs and Cats

Regimen (Species)	Drug	Dose (mg/kg)	Route	Interval (h)	Duration (days)
1 (Dogs)	Metronidazole	15	PO	12	14
	Amoxicillin	20	PO	12	14
	Famotidine	0.5	PO	12	14
2 (Cats)	Metronidazole	30[a]	PO	12	4
	Clarithromycin	30[a]	PO	12	4
	Ranitidine	20[a]	PO	12	4
	Bismuth	40[a]	PO	12	4
3 (Cats)	Metronidazole	10	PO	8	21
	Amoxicillin	20	PO	8	21
	Omeprazole	0.7	PO	24	21
4 (Cats)	Metronidazole	10	PO	12	14
	Amoxicillin	20	PO	12	14
	Clarithromycin	7.5	PO	12	14

[a]Total dose per cat.

Precautions/Interactions

- Avoid metronidazole and tetracycline in pregnant and young animals.
- High doses of metronidazole can cause neurologic toxicity.
- Avoid bismuth subsalicylate in cats.

COMMENTS

- Explain to clients—the difficulty of establishing a diagnosis, the high prevalence rates of infections with HLOs in normal dogs and cats, the potential for recurrence, and the zoonotic potential of the disease
- The zoonotic risk of the disease is likely very small.
- Serologic tests—not useful to confirm eradication of gastric HLOs; serum IgG titers may not decrease for up to 6 months after cleared infection
- 13C-urea breath and blood test—has been evaluated to monitor the eradication of HLOs in dogs and cats; shows promise for routine application
- If vomiting persists or recurs after cessation of combination therapy—may need to repeat endoscopic biopsy to determine whether the infection has been successfully eradicated

Abbreviations

CBC, complete blood count; DNA, deoxyribonucleic acid; ELISA, enzyme-linked immunosorbent assay; GI, gastrointestinal; HLO, *Helicobacter*-like organism; PCR, polymerase chain reaction; TNF, tumor necrosis factor.

Suggested Reading

Greiter-Wilke A, Scanziani E, Sokiati S, et al. Association of *Helicobacter* with cholangiohepatitis in cats. *J Vet Intern Med* 2006;20:822–827.

Neiger R, Simpson KW. Helicobacter infection in dogs and cats: facts and fiction. *J Vet Intern Med* 2000;14:125–133.

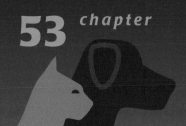

53 *chapter*

Hemotropic Mycoplasmosis

DEFINITION/OVERVIEW

- RBC destruction and anemia caused by parasite attachment to the external surface of RBCs and immune response by the host

ETIOLOGY/PATHOPHYSIOLOGY

- Rickettsial bacteria previously known as *Haemobartonella felis* (cats) and *Haemobartonella canis* (dogs)
- Three species infect cats:
  - *Mycoplasma haemofelis* for a large form of *H. felis*
  - *Mycoplasma haemominutum* for the small form of *H. felis*
  - *Mycoplasma turicensis* for a form not yet identified on RBCs but by PCR only
- One species infects dogs:
  - *Mycoplasma haemocanis* (previously *H. canis*).
- The large species of mycoplasmal organisms infecting cats—generally causes more severe disease than small species; other causes of hemolytic anemia should be considered in cats testing positive for *M. haemominutum* and *M. turicensis*.
- Cats—anemia more severe if FeLV infected
- Dogs—rarely show disease unless splenectomized or severe splenic pathology occurs in which case anemia can occur
- Anemia (usually due to extravascular hemolysis)—Mechanism may be due to direct damage by organisms to RBC surface or immune-mediated mechanisms.
- After recovery from acute anemia—Cats remain infected, but rarely will clinical manifestations of infection occur.
- Transmission—To date, no single vector has be definitely implicated in transmission; bites received and given during fighting between cats might explain why prevalence is higher in males; blood transfusion is a mode of transmission.

SIGNALMENT/HISTORY

- Worldwide distribtution
- Most common in adults (dogs and cats)
- More common in males (cats)
- No sex prevalence in dogs

CLINICAL FEATURES

Cats

- Variable disease severity—ranges from inapparent infection to marked depression and death
- Intermittent fever (50% of the time) during the acute phase
- Depression
- Weakness
- Anorexia
- Pale mucous membranes
- Splenomegaly
- Icterus—rare (Fig. 53-1)

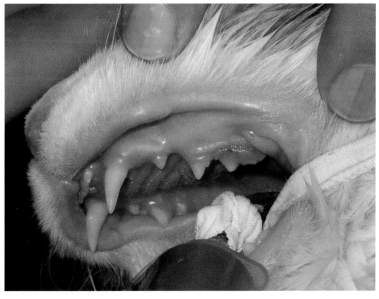

■ **Figure 53-1** Severe icterus in a cat infected with *M. haemofelis*.

Dogs

- Mild or inapparent signs—pale mucous membranes and listlessness
- In splenectomized dogs—signs more like in cats

 DIFFERENTIAL DIAGNOSIS

- Other causes of hemolytic anemia include IMHA, babesiosis (not in cats in the United States), cytauxzoonosis (cats only), Heinz body hemolytic anemia, microangiopathic hemolytic anemia, pyruvate kinase deficiency, phosphofructokinase deficiency (dogs only)
- Differentiated from IMHA—only by recognition of parasites in blood (stained blood film or PCR-based assays); both disorders may have a positive Coombs' test result
- *Babesia* and *Cytauxzoon* spp.—differ in morphology from these mycoplasmal organisms
- New Methylene Blue stain—used to identify Heinz bodies
- Enzyme assays or specialized DNA tests—used to diagnose pyruvate kinase and phosphofructokinase deficiencies

 DIAGNOSTICS

- CBC:
  - Anemia—usually with reticulocytosis if regenerative
  - Anemia—may appear poorly regenerative if a precipitous decrease in PCV has occurred early in the disease or if there are other concurrent disorders (e.g., FeLV or FIV infections in cats)
  - Autoagglutination—may be seen in feline blood samples after they cool to below body temperature
  - Variable total and differential leukocyte counts of little diagnostic assistance
  - Hemoglobinemia—rarely observed, so no hemoglobinuria reported
- Biochemical profile:
  - Hyperbilirubinemia—seen in some cases but seldom severe
  - Substantial bilirubinuria—seen in some dogs
  - Abnormalities related to anemic hypoxia—may be shown by clinical chemistry profiles, but profile can be normal
  - Hypoglycemia—possible in moribund cats (not specific to this disease)
  - Plasma protein concentrations—usually normal but may be increased
- Routine blood stains (e.g., Wright–Giemsa)—to identify organisms in blood films; examine before treatment is begun because treatment increases false-negative results
- Reticulocyte—Stains cannot be used because punctate reticulocytes in cats appear similar to the parasites.

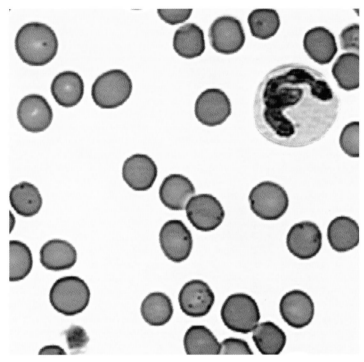

■ **Figure 53-2** Small blue-staining cocci with some ring forms typical of *M. haemominutum* in a cat (courtesy of Dr. Joanne Messick, Cornell University).

- Organisms must be differentiated from precipitated stain—Refractile drying or fixation artifacts, poorly staining Howell–Jolly bodies, and basophilic stippling can confuse diagnosis.
- Feline organisms—small blue-staining cocci, rings, or rods on RBCs (Figs. 53-2 and 53-3)

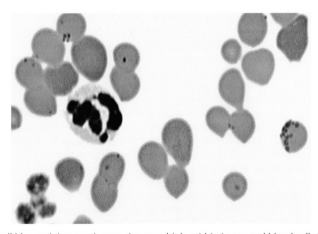

■ **Figure 53-3** Small blue-staining cocci, sometimes multiple within in one red blood cell, typical of *M. haemofelis* in a blood sample from a cat (courtesy of Dr. Joanne Messick, Cornell University).

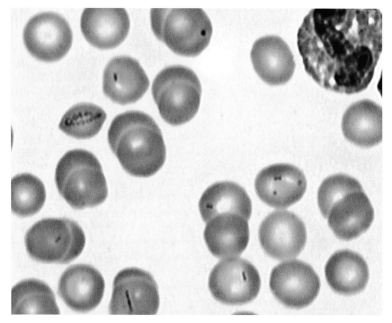

■ **Figure 53-4** Blue-staining cocci often in chains on the surface of dog red blood cells with *M. haemocanis* (courtesy of Dr. Joanne Messick, Cornell University).

- Canine organisms—commonly form chains of organisms that appear as filamentous structures on the surface of RBCs (Fig. 53-4)
- Parasitemia—cyclic, and thus organisms not always identifiable in blood (especially in cats)
- PCR-based assays—can detect parasites in blood below the number required to make a diagnosis from a stained blood film but may not consistently identify infection in asymptomatic carriers; assays widely available commercially
- Direct Coombs' test—may be positive

THERAPEUTICS

- Without therapy—Mortality with the larger form may reach 30% in cats.
- Outpatient treatment—unless severely anemic or moribund
- Blood transfusions—required when the anemia is considered life-threatening
- IV administration of glucose-containing fluid—recommended in moribund animals
- Drug therapy is only indicated in cats with clinical signs; treatment of PCR-positive but nonanemic asymptomatic cats is not indicated.
- *M. hemominutum* infections do not respond as well as *M. hemofelis* to doxycycline treatment.
- Antibiotic therapy can not be reliably used to clear infections from the blood from potential blood donors.

TABLE 53-1 Drug Therapy for Haemobartonellosis (Erythrocytic Mycoplasmal Infections) in Dogs and Cats

Drug	Dose (mg/kg)	Route	Interval (h)	Duration (weeks)
Doxycycline	5	PO, SC	12	3
Tetracycline	22	PO	8	3
Oxytetracycline	22	PO	8	3
Enrofloxacin	5–10	PO, IM	12	1–2
Prednisolone	1–2	PO	12	2[a]

[a]Gradually decrease dose as anemia improves; taper in 50% decrements every 2 weeks.

Drugs of Choice

- Doxycycline—primary drug of choice
- Tetracycline, or oxytetracycline—can also be used in the place of doxycycline
- Enrofloxacin—efficacious alternative for cats that do not tolerate tetracycline antibiotics; pradofloxacin is also an alternative
- Prednisolone—may be given to severely anemic animals (to treat immune-mediated destruction of RBCs); gradually decrease dosage as the PCV increases (Table 53-1)

Precautions/Interactions

- Tetracycline antibiotics—may produce fever or evidence of GI disease in cats; use a lower dosage or a different drug, or discontinue drug therapy altogether
- Doxycycline—may cause esophagitis and stricture in cats; give with food or a bolus of water orally after administration
- Enrofloxacin—has been associated with blindness in cats at doses >5 mg/kg; may cause arthropathy in young cats
- Chloramphenicol—may be used in dogs; can cause dose-dependent erythroid hypoplasia in cats

  COMMENTS

- Examine animal after 1 week of treatment—to confirm that PCV has risen
- Alert owner—Cats may remain carriers even after completion of treatment but seldom relapse with disease once PCV returns to normal.
- Prognosis usually excellent in cats—if treated early in disease
- Mycoplasma can survive up to a week in stored blood products; never use a positive cat as a blood donor even after drug treatment.
- Zoonotic potential – *M. haemofelis* has been detected by PCR in an immunodeficient human, so it has the potential to infect people.

Abbreviations

CBC, complete blood count; DNA, deoxyribonucleic acid; IMHA, immune-mediated hemolytic anemia; FeLV, feline leukemia virus; FIV, feline immunodeficiency virus; GI, gastrointestinal; PCR, polymerase chain reaction; PCV, packed cell volume; RBC, red blood cell.

Suggested Reading

Sykes JE. Feline hemotropic mycoplasmas. *J Vet Emerg Crit Care* 2010;20:62–69.

Sykes JE, Drazenovich NL, Ball LM, et al. Use of conventional and real-time polymerase chain reaction to determine the epidemiology of hemoplasma infections in anemic and nonanemic cats. *J Vet Intern Med* 2007;21:685–693.

Sykes JE, Terry JC, Lindsay LL, et al. Prevalences of various hemoplasma species among cats in the United States with possible hemoplasmosis. *J Am Vet Med Assoc* 2008;232:372–379.

Tasker S, Peters IR, Papasouliotis K, et al. Description of outcomes of experimental infection with feline haemoplasmas: copy numbers, haematology, Coombs' testing and blood glucose concentrations. *Vet Microbiol* 2009;139:323–332.

Hepatozoonosis

DEFINITION/OVERVIEW

- A systemic tick-borne protozoal infection of mammalian carnivores (foxes, coyotes, hyenas, and large cats, including lions, leopards, and cheetahs), including dogs, and very rarely cats
- Infection in dogs is mainly characterized by severe periosteal proliferation, but may affect multiple organ systems.

ETIOLOGY/PATHOPHYSIOLOGY

- *Hepatozoon americanum*—infects dogs in south cental and southeastern United States (Texas to Georgia) and seems to be moving northward
- Domestic cats—extremely rare (one case reported in Hawaii)
- Infection—ingestion of tick vector (*Amblyomma maculatum*); predation of prey harboring infected ticks or containing cystozoites of *H. americanum* in their tissues constitutes other modes of transmission
- Vertical transmission to puppies—can occur
- Complex pathogenesis—complicated by other factors affecting immune status
- Factors include—concurrent infections, such as with distemper, parvovirus, *Babesia*, *Ehrlichia*, and *Leishmania*
- Age at infection—an important determinant of clinical disease development
- If infected young—more chance of developing periosteal bone proliferation
- Experimental infections—develop bloody diarrhea 3 days postinfection (lasts 2–14 days), pyrexia (day 7 and lasting weeks), lymphadenopathy (by 3 weeks postinfection); leukocytosis with cachexia and ocular discharge present by 4 weeks postinfection
- Amyloid deposits—occur in multiple organs, with vasculitis and glomerulonephritis developing in fatal cases
- Humoral immunity—not protective and may even facilitate fatal immune complex disease

SIGNALMENT/HISTORY

- Young dogs—most severely affected mainly during warmer months (coinciding with rising and falling parasitemias)

 # CLINICAL FEATURES

Dogs

- Usually subclinical
- Clinically affected—chronic antibiotic-unresponsive fever and cachexia
- Anorexia
- Diarrhea
- Paraparesis
- Signs may vary between localities—Bloody diarrhea seems to be a feature of dogs infected in Texas.
- Generalized muscle atrophy and hyperesthesia—causes stiffness and reluctance to move
- Cervical and trunk rigidity—caused by periosteal pain
- Ocular abnormalities—Low tear production, focal retinal scarring, hyperpigmentation, papilledema, and uveitis have all been reported.
- Prolonged course of disease—with periods of apparent remission interspersed with periods of fever and pain
- Periods of remission—longer in surviving cases; shorter in fatal cases
- Cats—asymptomatic, with schizonts being found in tissues at necropsy

 # DIFFERENTIAL DIAGNOSIS

Dogs

- Few other causes of persistent antibiotic-resistant fever, cachexia, periosteal bone proliferation, with profound leukocytosis in dogs in southern and southwestern United States
- Other possible causes include leishmaniasis, chronic erhlichiosis, babesiosis, systemic mycotic infections, pyelonephritis (lumbar hyperesthesia), neoplasia, endocarditis, immune-mediated polyarthritis or polymyositis, diskospondylitis.

 # DIAGNOSTICS

- CBC—profound leukocytosis (sometimes as high as 200,000 cells/ml blood) with left shift; sometimes eosinophilia (up to 20%); mild normocytic, normochromic

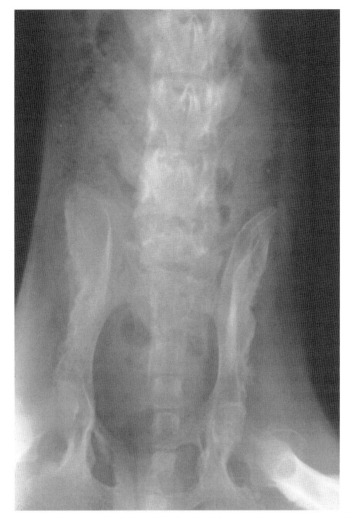

■ **Figure 54-1** Ventrodorsal radiograph of the pelvis of a dog infected with *H. americanum* showing periosteal bone proliferation over the ileum and vertebrae.

regenerative anemia; often a thrombocytosis (as opposed to thrombocytopenia, characteristic of *Erhlichia* infection)
■ Serum chemistry—hypoalbuminemia, hyperglobulinemia, increased SAP activity.
■ Profound hypoglycemia—probably artifact due to high neutrophil counts metabolizing glucose after sample collection
■ Elevated urine protein/creatine ratio—dogs with glomerulopathy
■ Radiology—periosteal bone proliferation, particularly at the attachment sites of muscles in all bones, with the usual exception of the head (Fig. 54-1)
■ Not all dogs develop bone proliferative lesion—more common in younger dogs (<1 year)

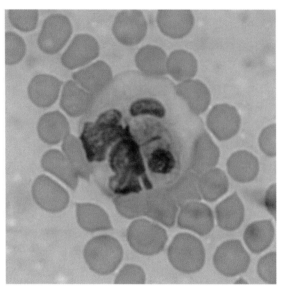

■ **Figure 54-2** Gamont of *H. americanum* in a neutrophil on a peripheral blood smear (Wright–Giemsa stain, 1000×).

Diagnostic Feature

- **Diagnosis—made by finding gamonts in neutrophils or monocytes in buffy coat blood smears (Giemsa stain best) (Fig. 54-2)**
- Gamonts—difficult to find in WBCs in North American strains
- Muscle biopsy—Muscle cysts are more consistently found than gamonts in WBCs in North American infections (Fig. 54-3).

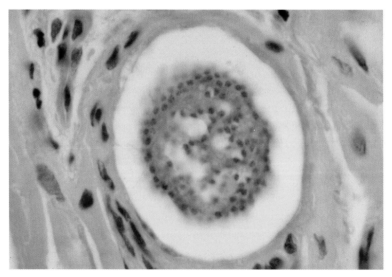

■ **Figure 54-3** *H. americanum* cyst in a muscle biopsy section from an infected dog (hematoxylin and eosin, 800×).

THERAPEUTICS

- Mostly palliative—complete recovery rare, with relapses occurring 3–6 months after treatment
- Symptomatic palliative treatment—nonsteroidal anti-inflammatory agents provide best relief
- Glucocorticoids—provide short-term temporary relief, but must be avoided over the long term
- Combinations of therapies—provide the best outcome

Drugs of Choice

Initial Therapy (Give All Drugs Together)

- TMS (Tribrissen; Schering-Plough)
- Clindamycin (Antirobe; Pharmacia and Upjohn)
- Pyrimethamine (Daraprim; Burroughs Welcome)

Long-Term Therapy

- Decoquinate (Deccox; Alpharma) (Table 54-1)
- Medicated feed additive for cattle
- Supplied as a 6% (each pound contains 27.2 g of decoquinate) feed medication mixed in corn meal, soybean oil, lecithin, and silicon dioxide

Precautions/Interactions

- TMS—may induce keratoconjunctivitis sicca, hepatotoxicity, immune-mediated polyarthritis, retinitis, glomerulonephritis, vasculitis, thrombocytopenia, erythema multiforme, toxic epidermal necrolysis, and other cutaneous drug eruptions
- Do not use pyrimethamine in pregnant animals—may cause teratogenesis

TABLE 54-1 **Drug Therapy for Hepatozoonosis in Dogs**				
Drug	Dose (mg/kg)	Route	Interval (h)	Duration (days)
Trimethoprim-sulfadiazine (Tribrissen)	15	PO	12	2[a]
Clindamycin (Antirobe)	10	PO	8	2[a]
Pyrimethamine (Daraprim)	0.25	PO	24	2[a]
Decoquinate (Deccox)	10–20	PO	12	33 months[b]

[a]Initial therapy.
[b]Long-term therapy; 1/4 oz. of feed additive will medicate 20–40 kg body weight of dog.

- TMS and pyrimethamine—may induce folate deficiency and augment myelo-suppression
- Folate deficiency—supplement with 5–15 mg/day, PO of folinic acid
- Clindamycin—GI signs with vomiting and diarrhea

COMMENTS

- Improvement—best monitored by clinical signs, not organisms in peripheral blood or on muscle biopsy
- Most cases—asymptomatic
- Cases with severe periosteal disease—Even symptomatic therapy may not be enough to improve an animal's quality of life.
- Avoid glucocorticoids if possible—often exacerbate clinical disease
- Humans—have been reported to be infected with *Hepatozoon* spp.
- Role of the infected dog as a source of infection to humans—probably insignificant

Abbreviations

CBC, complete blood count; GI, gastrointestinal; SAP, serum alkaline phosphatase; TMS, trimethroprim-sulfadiazine; WBCs, white blood cells.

Suggested Reading

Holman PJ, Snowden KF. Canine hepatozoon and babesiosis, and feline cytauxzoonosis. *Vet Clin North Am Small Anim Pract* 2009;39:1035–1053.

Johnson EM, Panciera RJ, Allen KE, et al. Alternate pathway of infection with *Hepatozoon americanum* and the epidemiologic importance of predation. *J Vet Intern Med* 2009;23:1315–1318.

Potter TM, Macintire DK. *Hepatozoon americanum*: an emerging disease in the southcentral/southern United States. *J Vet Emerg Crit Care* 2010;20:70–76.

chapter 55

Histoplasmosis

DEFINITION/OVERVIEW

- Systemic fungal infection resulting in mainly intestinal tract disease in the dog, and respiratory disease in the cat, but affecting multiple organs (including liver, spleen, bone marrow, bone, lung and lymph nodes) in both species

ETIOLOGY/PATHOPHYSIOLOGY

- *Histoplasma capsulatum*—mycelial form, which grows in bird manure or organically enriched soil produces infectious spores (microconidia)
- Microconidia—inhaled into terminal airways; spores germinate in lungs and develop into yeast form
- Yeast form—phagocytized by macrophages and distributed throughout the body
- Ingested organisms—may directly infect the intestinal tract, especially in dogs
- Immune response—determines whether disease will develop
- Affected animals—often develop transient asymptomatic infection

Dogs

- Main organs affected—intestinal tract, but also liver, lung, spleen, and lymph nodes
- Systems less frequently affected—bones, bone marrow, kidneys, adrenals, oral cavity, tongue, eyes, and testes

Cats

- Respiratory tract—mainly affected
- Also often affected—bone, bone marrow, liver, spleen, skin, and lymph nodes
- Systems less frequently affected—intestinal tract, eyes, kidneys, adrenals, and brain

SIGNALMENT/HISTORY

- Low prevalence of clinically relevant cases

- Endemic areas—Ohio, Missouri, Mississippi, Tennessee, St. Lawrence rive basins; also present in Texas, Oklahoma, southeastern United States, and occasionally the Great Lakes region

Dogs

- Most often—young dogs affected, but all ages
- Historically—weight loss, depression, and large-bowel diarrhea are most common
- Cough and dyspnea—often noted by owner
- Lameness, ocular and skin changes—noted less commonly by owner

Cats

- Usually <1 year of age, but also all ages
- Historically—more insidious onset of anorexia, weight loss, dyspnea, and cough
- Lameness, ocular discharge, diarrhea—noted less commonly by owner

 CLINICAL FEATURES

Dogs

- Emaciation
- Fever
- Generalized lymphadenopathy
- Hepatosplenomegaly
- Pale mucous membranes
- Easily elicited cough and harsh lung sounds
- Icterus, rarely

Cats

- Fever
- Increased respiratory effort
- Harsh lung sounds
- Pale mucous membranes
- Generalized lymphadenopathy
- Lameness
- Ocular signs

 DIFFERENTIAL DIAGNOSIS

Dogs

- Severe chronic diarrhea and weight loss—GI lymphoma; IBD (lymphocytic plasmacytic, eosinophilic), exocrine pancreatic insufficiency, and chronic parasitism (whipworms)

- Respiratory signs—a general differential diagnosis for respiratory signs and cough includes such categories as:
  - Cardiovascular (pulmonary edema; enlarged heart, especially the left atrium; left-sided heart failure; pulmonary emboli) and congenital (hypoplastic trachea)
  - Allergic (bronchial asthma, chronic bronchitis, eosinophilic pneumonia or granulomatosis, pulmonary infiltrate with eosinophilia)
  - Trauma (foreign body, irritating gases, collapsing trachea)
  - Neoplasia (not only of the respiratory tree but also associated structures such as ribs, lymph nodes, muscles)
  - Inflammatory (pharyngitis; tonsillitis; kennel cough from such agents as *Bordetella bronchoseptica*, parainfluenza virus, infectious laryngotracheitis virus, and mycoplasma; bacterial bronchopneumonia; chronic pulmonary fibrosis; pulmonary abscess or granuloma; COPD); other fungal agents (blastomycosis, cryptococcosis); pleural space diseases
  - Parasites (*Oslerus [Filaroides] osleri, Crenosoma vulpis, Capillaria aerophila, Filaroides milksi, Paragonimus kellicotti, Dirofilaria immitis*—heartworm disease)
  - Lymph node enlargement—similar to lymphosarcoma differentiated by lymph node aspirate cytology
- Chronic large-bowel disease with severe weight loss unresponsive to antibiotics and motility modifiers in young dogs from endemic regions suggests the diagnosis.

Cats

- Respiratory signs—differentiate from heart disease, feline asthma, parenchymal lung disease (pneumonia, parasitic lungworms, neoplasia, toxoplasmosis), and pleural disease (pyothorax, neoplasia)
- Lameness—differentiate from trauma, cat bite abscess, spinal lymphoma, and polyarthritis
- Ocular disease—lymphoma, toxoplasmosis, and FIP

DIAGNOSTICS

- CBC—usually moderate to severe nonregenerative anemia; usually normal leukocyte counts but can have leukocytosis (rarely leukopenia from bone marrow involvement); frequently see thrombocytopenia
- Peripheral blood smears—may find *Histoplasma* organisms in monocytes or neutrophils (Fig. 55-1) or bone marrow aspirate (Fig. 55-2)
- Biochemical panel—elevated hepatic enzymes (liver involvement), hypoalbuminemia (intestinal tract involvement), hyperglobulinemia
- AGID test—detects antibodies against *H. capsulatum*; supports diagnosis; positive result usually indicates active infection, although false-positive result can occur (suggests past infection); false-negative results are common
- Coombs' test—may be positive because antibodies to *H. capsulatum* may cross-react with RBCs

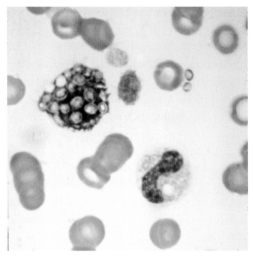

■ **Figure 55-1** Peripheral blood smear of a dog with systemic histoplasmosis, showing the organisms within a monocyte (may also be found in neutrophils and very rarely, eosinophils). Note the two extracellular organisms; these have been torn out of cells during the fixation procedure (Wright's stain, 1000×).

- Imaging:
  - Thoracic radiographs—diffuse interstitial-to-nodular pneumonia; enlarged tracheobronchial lymph nodes compressing the tracheal bifurcation (Fig. 55-3) in dogs (rare in cats)
  - Abdominal imaging—organomegaly (liver, spleen, lymph nodes)
  - Bones—predominantly osteolytic lesions, usually distal to elbows and stifles (especially cats)

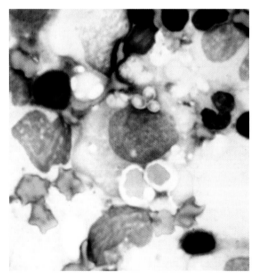

■ **Figure 55-2** *Histoplasma* organisms can be identified in mononuclear cells within bone marrow aspirates from dogs systemically affected by the fungus. Note also that the same cell containing the organisms has phagocytosed two red blood cells, a common occurrence (Wright's stain, 1000×).

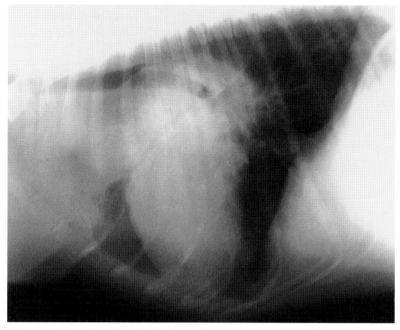

■ **Figure 55-3** Lateral thoracic radiograph of a dog with pulmonary histoplasmosis, showing diffuse interstitial and nodular lung infiltrates and markedly enlarged hilar lymph nodes.

Diagnostic Feature

- **Definitive diagnostic method of choice—identify organism on cytology, histopathology, or culture; obtain samples by rectal scraping (Fig. 55-4), lymph node aspirates, bone marrow aspirates, or lung aspirates; lung aspirates are best (tracheal wash relatively low yield)**
- Rectal scraping—with gloved fingernail of index finger, scrape the dorsal wall of the rectum; smear scraping on microscope slide, air dry, and stain (Wright–Giemsa)

 THERAPEUTICS

- Usually outpatient—if stable (use oral itraconazole)
- Inpatient—if administering intravenous amphotericin B (dogs with severe intestinal disease and malabsorption)
- Dogs receiving amphotericin B—monitor carefully for renal toxicity (examine urinary sediment for appearance of casts)
- Administer total parenteral nutrition—to reverse wasting until intestinal disease is resolved enough for adequate food absorption
- Oxygen therapy—may be required for dogs in respiratory distress

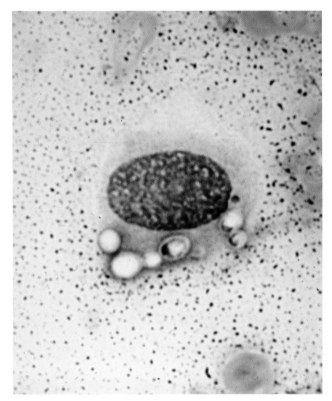

■ **Figure 55-4** Cytologic preparation of a rectal scraping from a dog with intestinal histoplasmosis, showing organisms within a macrophage (Wright's stain, 750×). This is the method of choice to definitively diagnose intestinal histoplasmosis in the dog.

Drugs of Choice

Itraconazole (Sporanox; Janssen)

- Drug of choice in animals with good intestinal absorption
- Less expensive than fluconazole
- Give with a fat-rich meal (canned dog food) for the first 3 days to achieve a therapeutic blood concentration as soon as possible.
- For cats, have drug compounded (by an appropriate pharmacy) or open the 100-mg capsules containing pellets and mix with palatable food.

Amphotericin B (Fungizone; E. R. Squibb)

- Check for nephrotoxicity by monitoring urine for appearance of casts; discontinue when they appear and maintain hydration.
- Use liposomal or lipid complex formulations to reduce nephrotoxicity; more expensive
- Use until patient begins to gain weight, and then switch to itraconazole.

TABLE 55-1 Drug Therapy for Histoplasmosis in Dogs and Cats

Drug	Dose (mg/kg)	Route	Interval (h)	Duration (months)
Itraconazole (Sporanox)	5–10	PO	12–24	3–6[a]
Amphotericin B (Fungizone)	0.25–0.5[b]	IV	48[c]	[d]
Fluconazole (Diflucan)	5	PO	12–24	3–6[a]

[a]Give with a fatty meal for a minimum of 3 months depending on response.
[b]Reconstituted in 5% dextrose (do not reconstitute in electrolyte solutions that precipitate the drug) and dilute to administer; if normal renal function, dilute in 60–120 ml 5% dextrose given over 15 minutes; if renal compromise, dilute in 0.5–1 liter 5% dextrose given over 3–4 hours to reduce further renal toxicity.
[c]Or 3 times a week.
[d]Administer until a total cumulative dose of 5–10 mg/kg in dogs and 4–5 mg/kg in cats is reached.

Fluconazole (Diflucan; Pfizer)

- Use in dogs that cannot receive amphotericin B.
- Penetrates all body cavities and tissues, including eye and CNS; use in cases with ocular and/or CNS involvement (Table 55-1)

Precautions/Interactions

- Renal failure—precludes the use of amphotericin B; may use less nephrotoxic formulations
- Steroids—use with caution; will allow proliferation of *H. capsulatum*; life-threatening respiratory distress due to infiltrative lung disease or hilar lymphadenopathy justifies the use of dexamethasone (dosage: 0.2 mg/kg, IV or IM, q24h, for 2–3 days) to decrease inflammation while the patient receives antifungal treatment
- Itraconazole and fluconazole—hepatic toxicity; temporarily discontinue if patient becomes anorexic or if serum ALT activity >300 U/L (check monthly); restart at half dose after appetite returns
- Itraconazole—not teratogenic at therapeutic doses but is at high doses in rats (no dog or cat studies, but one dog delivered normal litter when given drug half way through pregnancy)

COMMENTS

- Follow-up—obtain chest radiographs after 60 days of treatment, and stop treatment when infiltrates are clear or remaining lung lesions fail to improve (continue treatment for 1 month after there is no change observed on radiographs); monitor bone lesions by radiology; monitor ocular lesions
- Identify high-risk environments to inform owners of risk to them—no risk of spread from animals to humans (although veterinarians need to take care with needle sticks

such as for aspirate cytology or necropsies on infected animals, because cuts can become infected)

- Duration of treatment is usually 4 months—Warn owners of expense of drugs.
- Prognosis is good for stable patients without dyspnea when starting treatment—Prognosis worsens in debilitated, emaciated animals or those with severe lung involvement.
- Recovered dogs are probably immune—Recurrence is possible, requiring a second course of treatment.

Abbreviations

AGID, agar gel immunodiffusion; ALT, alanine aminotransferase; CBC, complete blood count; CNS, central nervous system; COPD, chronic obstructive pulmonary disease; FIP, feline infectious peritonitis; GI, gastrointestinal; IBD, inflammatory bowel disease; RBC, red blood cell.

Suggested Reading

Bromel C, Sykes JE. Histoplasmosis in dogs and cats. *Clin Tech Small Anim Pract* 2005;20:227–232.

Greene CE. Histoplasmosis. In: Greene CE, ed. *Infectious Diseases of the Dog and the Cat*. Philadelphia: WB Saunders, 2006:577–584.

Kerl ME. Update on canine and feline fungal disease. *Vet Clin North Am Small Anim Pract* 2003;33:721–747.

Schulman RL, McKiernan BC, Schaeffer DJ. Use of corticosteroids for treating dogs with airway obstruction secondary to hilar lymphadenopathy caused by chronic histoplasmosis: 16 cases (1979–1997). *J Am Vet Med Assoc* 1999;214:1345–1348.

chapter 56

Hookworms

DEFINITION/OVERVIEW

- Nematode parasites—Adults (and 4th-stage larvae) are voracious blood feeders while attached to the small intestinal tract of dogs and cats, causing blood loss anemia.

ETIOLOGY/PATHOPHYSIOLOGY

- *Ancylostoma tubaeforme*—cats
- *Ancylostoma caninum*—dogs
- *Ancylostoma braziliense* and *Uncinaria stenocephala*—cats and dogs
- *A. caninum*—most widely distributed; subtropical and temperate regions
- *A. braziliense*—tropical/subtropical; southern United States
- *A. tubaeforme* and *U. stenocephala*—temperate states
- Infection—ingestion of infective larvae or by skin penetration (except *A. tubaeforme* in cats)
- *A. braziliense*—also transmitted via colostrum to pups
- Adults and 4th-stage larvae—cause blood-loss anemia and enteritis by ingesting large quantities of blood
- Once detached—Parasite bite wounds and anticoagulants cause continual seepage of blood and serum in bowel lumen.
- Neonates—particularly susceptible to peracute and acute blood loss

SIGNALMENT/HISTORY

- Neonates and young puppies—acute disease
- Mature dogs and cats—chronic blood loss anemia

CLINICAL FEATURES

Dogs

- Peracute disease—as a result of transmammary infection

- Pups that are healthy in the first week of life—deteriorate rapidly in the second week, with severe anemia; soft, liquid, tarry, bloody feces; and sudden death before eggs appear in feces
- Acute disease—older puppies (and some mature dogs) exposed to large numbers of infective larvae
- Develop signs of anemia
- Weakness
- Tarry stools—even before eggs appear in feces
- Chronic (compensated) disease—usually asymptomatic but with anemia and eggs in feces
- Secondary disease—older dogs with other conditions (usually with severe weight loss) causing debilitation, resulting in profound anemia
- Other signs—dry cough from larval migration through lungs of pups (rare)
- Mild acanthosis
- Hyperkeratinization over site of larvae entry in skin; erythematous pruritic lesions; papules between toes on feet

Cats

- Usually asymptomatic—only rarely develop signs of anemia and loose, tarry stools

 DIFFERENTIAL DIAGNOSIS

- Other causes of loss of RBC mass, including:
  - Hemolysis—caused by toxins (zinc, acetaminophen, onion), immune-mediated hemolytic anemia, parasites (*Babesia, Haemobartonella* spp.), microangiopathic hemolysis (splenic torsion, vena caval syndrome), RBC cell disorders (pyruvate kinase deficiency), and drugs (propylthiouracil, gold salts)
  - Acute or chronic blood loss—bowel lumen (neoplasia, parasites, ulcers), from skin (external parasitism—fleas); chronic blood loss often results in iron-deficiency anemia

 DIAGNOSTICS

CBC

- Acute—regenerative anemia (regeneration may not be present in the very young because blood loss and death can occur before regeneration has time to occur)
- Chronic—iron-deficiency anemia (microcytic hypochromic nonregenerative anemia)
- Eosinophilia

Fecal Flotation

- Eggs in stools (Fig. 56-1); *A. caninum*—elongated ellipsoid (60 × 40 mm), thin-shelled (usually in eight-cell-stage); indistinguishable from *A. braziliensis*
- *A. caninum* egg is smaller than *U. stenocephala*—(70 mm long)

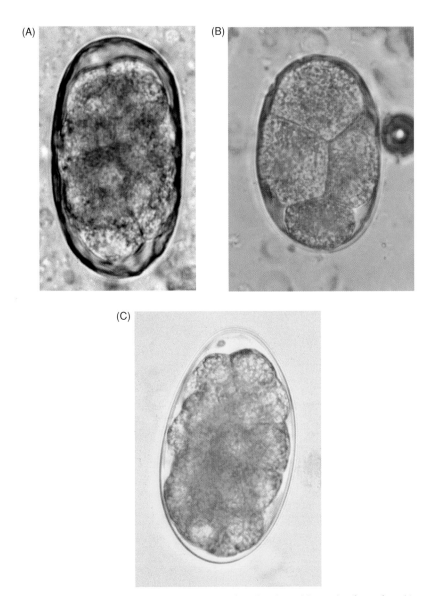

■ **Figure 56-1** The eggs of hookworms—(A) *A. caninum* found in dogs; (B) *A. tubaeforme* found in cats; and (C) *U. stenocephala* found in both dogs and cats.

THERAPEUTICS

- Pups in a heavily contaminated environment—treat at 2-week intervals to weaning
- Peracute—often too late, but administer anthelmintic first (pyrantel), then blood transfusion (in neonates, give intraosseous) and fluid support
- Alert owners—to the potential of sudden death
- Acute and chronic primary hookworm cases—respond rapidly to anthelmintics alone

- Animals with secondary disease—need supplementation (iron, vitamin, blood transfusion, high-protein diet), as well as regular anthelmintic therapy
- Hookworms constantly repopulate the bowel from larvae sequestered in tissues—can continue for months or even years
- Queen—treat with adulticide/larvicide anthelmintic prior to breeding and after littering; fenbendazole from day 40 of gestation to day 14 of lactation or ivermectin, 4–9 days prior to whelping, and again 10 days later—kills reactivated hookworm larvae before they reach the pups and should prevent pup loss
- Pups—begin biweekly anthelmintic treatment of pups at 2 weeks of age; continue until weaned, especially pups at high risk of infection from bitch or environment; treat monthly after weaned
- Kittens—begin anthelmintic treatment at 3–4 weeks of age; treat monthly thereafter
- Promptly remove and dispose of feces to prevent contamination of environment with larvae.
- Prevent hunting and scavenging—to prevent ingestion of potential transport hosts

Drugs of Choice

Adult Larvae Anthelmintic Activity

- Fenbendazole (Panacur Granules 22.2%; Intervet)
- Milbemycin oxime (Interceptor or Sentinel; Novartis)
- Cats—emodepside (3 mg/kg)/praziquantel (12 mg/kg) (Profender; Bayer); topical

Adulticide Activity

- Pyrantel (Nemex; Pfizer)
- Praziquantel/pyrantel/febantel (Drontal Plus; Bayer)
- Praziquantel/pyrantel (Drontal [Bayer, Shawnee Mission, KS]).
- Ivermectin and pyrantel (Heartguard Plus; Merial)
- Dichlorvos (Task Tabs; Boehringer Ingelheim) (Table 56-1)

Adulticide Activity

DOGS
- Adult larvae dewormer (fenbendazole)—during third trimester of pregnancy to kill migrating larvae in somatic tissue and adult worms
- Adult larvae dewormer—on daily or monthly basis for pups and mature dogs
- Treat pups biweekly until weaning—if at high risk

Adulticide Activity

CATS
- Adult larvae dewormer for queen—before breeding and after littering
- Start adulticide dewormer—by 4 weeks of age for kittens

TABLE 56-1 Drug Therapy for Hookworms in Dogs and Cats						
Drug	**Parasite Stage**	**Species**	**Dose (mg/kg)**	**Route**	**Interval (H)**	**Duration (Days)**
Fenbendazole (Panacur)	AL	D	50	PO	24	3
Milbemycin oxime (Interceptor)	AL	D	0.5	PO	Once	30[a]
Emodepside/prazequantel (Profender)	AL	C	3/12.5	Topical	Once	
Pyrantel pamoate (Nemex)	A	D	15	PO	Once	14[b]
	A	C	20–30	PO	Once	14[b]
Praziquantel/pyrantel/febantel (Drontal Plus)	A	D	[c]	PO	Once	14[b]
Praziquantel/pyrantel (Drontal)	A	C	[d]	PO	Once	14[b]
Ivermectin/pyrantel (Heartgard Plus)	A	D	[e]	PO	Once	30[a]
Dichlorvos (Task Tabs)	A	B	11	PO	Once	14[b]

[a]Repeat every month.
[b]Repeat in 14 days.
[c]Dose for praziquantel (5–12 mg/kg), pyrantel (5–12 mg/kg), and febantel (25–62 mg/kg).
[d]Dose for praziquantel (5 mg/kg) and pyrantel (20 mg/kg).
[e]Dose for ivermectin (0.006 mg/kg) and pyrantel (5 mg/kg).
AL, adults and larvae; A, adults; B, both cats and dogs; C, cats, D dogs.

Precautions/Interactions

- Do not give dichlorvos to animals with heartworm disease.
- Do not give dichlorvos concurrently with other organophosphates (e.g., insecticides).
- Pay particular attention to the manufacturers' recommendations regarding use of drugs in pregnant animals and in puppies and kittens <4 weeks of age.

 COMMENTS

- CLM ("creeping eruption")—*A. braziliense* most often causes these linear, tortuous, erythematous, pruritic eruptions on humans as a result of larval migration into the skin.
- VLM—*A. caninum* larvae; can migrate to GI tract causing abdominal pain and eosinophila without becoming patent
- Contaminated environments—*Ancylostom* (but not *Uncinaria* eggs) are destroyed by freezing, so a hard winter often stops clinical hookworm infections.
- Sodium borate (10 pounds/100 square feet) raked into ground destroys larvae (and vegetation as well).
- Paved areas—physically cleaned, then spray with 1% sodium hypochlorite (3 cups of bleach/gallon of water)
- Puppies with peracute or acute *A. conainum* infections often die in spite of treatment.

- Older dogs—expect full recovery.
- Adult dogs—Anthelmintic treatment of dogs with dormant larvae in their tissues can result in larval activation and repopulation of small intestine.

Abbreviations

CLM, cutaneous larval migrans; GI, gastrointestinal; RBC, red blood cell; VLM, visceral larva migrans

Suggested Reading

Bowman DD. *Georgis' Parasitology for Veterinarians*, 9th ed. St. Louis, MO: Elsevier Science, 2009:179–185.

Infectious Canine Hepatitis Virus Infection

chapter 57

DEFINITION/OVERVIEW

- Viral disease of dogs and other Canidae affecting mainly the liver but also eyes and endothelium

ETIOLOGY/PATHOPHYSIOLOGY

- CAV-1—serologically homogeneous but antigenically distinct from respiratory CAV-2
- Oronasal exposure—leads to viremia (4–8 days)
- Virus—shed in saliva and feces
- After viremia—virus initially dispersed to hepatic macrophages (Kupffer cells) and endothelium
- Replicates in Kupffer cells—damage to adjacent hepatocytes and massive viremia when released
- Adequate antibody response clears organs in 10–14 days—persists in renal tubules and may be shed in urine for 6–9 months
- Chronic hepatitis—follows infection in dogs with only partial neutralizing antibody response
- Cytotoxic ocular injury—anterior uveitis leading to classic "hepatitis blue eye"

SIGNALMENT/HISTORY

- No breed or sex predilections
- Most common in dogs <1 year of age

CLINICAL FEATURES

Peracute

- Fever
- CNS signs

- Vascular collapse
- DIC
- Death within hours

Acute

- Fever
- Anorexia
- Lethargy
- Vomiting
- Diarrhea
- Hepatomegaly
- Abdominal pain
- Abdominal effusion
- Vasculitis (petechia, bruising)
- DIC
- Lymphadenopathy—rarely
- Nonsuppurative encephalitis

Uncomplicated

- Lethargy
- Anorexia
- Transient fever
- Tonsillitis
- Vomiting
- Diarrhea
- Lymphadenopathy
- Hepatomegaly
- Abdominal pain
- Late—20% of cases develop anterior uveitis and corneal edema 4–6 days postinfection; recover within 21 days; may progress to glaucoma and corneal ulceration

DIFFERENTIAL DIAGNOSIS

- Other infectious hepatopathies—leptospirosis
- Granulomatous hepatitis
- Toxic hepatitis
- Fulminant infectious disease—e.g., parvovirus, canine distemper

DIAGNOSTICS

- CBC—schistocytes; leukopenia during acute viremia, followed by leukocytosis with reactive lymphocytosis and nucleated RBCs

- Biochemistry profile—hepatic enzyme activity high initially, begins declining within 14 days; low glucose and albumin reflect fulminant hepatic failure, vasculitis, and endotoxemia; low sodium and potassium levels reflect GI losses; hyperbilirubinemia
- Urinalysis—proteinuria reflects glomerular injury; granular casts reflect renal tubule damage; bilirubinuria
- Coagulation tests—reflect severity of liver injury and DIC
- Serologic test for antibodies to CAV-1—fourfold rise in IgM and IgG; vaccine-induced antibodies confuse interpretation
- Viral isolation—anterior segment of eye, kidney, tonsil, and urine
- Isolation difficult in parenchymal organs (especially liver)—unless first week of infection
- Abdominal radiography—normal or large liver; poor detail due to effusion
- Abdominal ultrasonography—may observe hepatomegaly, hypoechoic parenchyma (multifocal or diffuse pattern), and effusion

 THERAPEUTICS

- Usually inpatient—fluid therapy (balanced polyionic fluids; carefully monitor fluids to avoid overhydration in context of increased vascular permeability and hypoalbuminemia)
- In fulminant hepatic failure (acute/peracute presentation)—lactate may be contraindicated (inability to metabolize)
- Judicious potassium and magnesium supplementation—electrolyte depletion may augment hepatic encephalopathy (monitor serum electrolytes closely)
- Avoid neuroglycopenia—Supplement fluids with dextrose (2.5–5.0%) if patient becomes hypoglycemic.
- Blood component or synthetic colloids—for coagulopathy and low colloidal osmotic pressure
- Synthetic colloids—for low colloid oncotic pressure
- With overt DIC—fresh blood products and low-molecular-weight heparin (e.g., enoxaparin 100 U/kg [1 mg/kg] q24h)
- Nutritional support—frequent small meals as tolerated; optimize nitrogen intake to patient; inappropriate protein restriction may impair tissue repair and regeneration
- If oral feeding is not tolerated—provide partial parenteral nutrition (maximum of 5 days) or, preferably, total parenteral nutrition
- MLV using CAV-2 at 6–8 weeks of age—two boosters 3–4 weeks apart until 16 weeks of age; booster at 1 year; highly effective vaccine; boosters may not be needed
- MLV using CAV-1—produces life-long immunity with one dose, but the virus can localize in the kidneys to produce subclinical nephritis and persistent shedding, as well as a small percentage developing severe keratitis ("blue eye") and uveitis (Fig. 57-1) when given subcutaneously

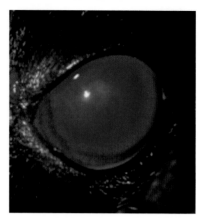

■ **Figure 57-1** Diffuse corneal edema and keratitis ("blue eye") after vaccination with canine adenovirus-1 modified live vaccine (courtesy of Dr. R. Riis, Cornell University).

- Maternal antibody—may protect some pups for first 8 weeks; depends on antibody concentration in bitch and on effective passive transfer
- Vaccination of pups with high levels of passively acquired antibodies—successful at 14–16 weeks of age

Drugs of Choice

- Prophylactic antimicrobials (for anticipated transmural migration of enteric flora and endotoxemia in the context of hepatic failure)—ticarcillin combined with metronidazole (at a reduced dose)
- Antiemetics—for vomiting; metoclopramide or ondansetron
- H_2-receptor antagonists—famotidine
- Gastric protectants—sucralfate for gastrointestinal bleeding
- Ursodeoxycholic acid—choleretic and hepatoprotectant; give indefinitely for chronic hepatitis
- Antioxidants—vitamin E and S-adenosylmethionine until hepatic enzymes and dog fully recovers; indefinitely with chronic hepatitis (Table 57-1)

Precautions/Interactions

- Consider severity of hepatic injury, protein depletion, and age when calculating dosages of drugs.

 COMMENTS

- Routinely monitor—fluid, electrolyte, acid–base, and coagulation status to adjust supportive measures; monitor for acute renal failure
- Prognosis: peracute—poor; death within hours
- Prognosis: acute—guarded to good

- Poor antibody response (titer 1:16 to 1:50)—chronic hepatitis may develop
- Good antibody response (titer >1:500 IgG)—complete recovery in 5–7 days possible
- Recovered patients—may develop chronic hepatic or renal disease

TABLE 57-1 Drugs Used in the Treatment of Infectious Canine Hepatitis Virus Infections

Drug	Dose (mg/kg)	Route	Interval (H)	Duration (Days)
Ticarcillin	33–50	PO	6–8	14
Metronidazole[a]	7.5	IV, PO	8–12	14
Metoclopramide	0.2–0.5	SC, PO	6–8	5[b]
Ondansetron	0.5–1	PO	12	5[b]
Famotidine	0.5	SC, IV, PO	12–24	7[b]
Sucralfate	0.25–1 g[c]	PO	8–12	7[b]
Ursodeoxycholic acid	10–15	PO	24	28[d]
Vitamin E	10 U/kg	PO	24	28[d]
S-Adenosylmethionine	20	PO	24	28[d]

[a]Use in combination with ticarcillin.
[b]Or for as long as needed to control vomiting.
[c]Total dose.
[d]Or indefinitely for chronic hepatitis.

Abbreviations

CAV, canine adenovirus; CBC, complete blood count; CNS, central nervous system; COPD, chronic obstructive pulmonary disease; DIC, disseminated intravascular coagulation; GI, gastrointestinal; MLV, modified live virus.

Suggested Reading

Decaro N, Martella V, Buonavoglia C. Canine adenoviruses and herpesvirus. *Vet Clin North Am Small Anim Pract* 2008;38:799–814.

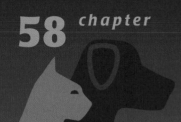

58 *chapter*

Infectious Canine Tracheobronchitis (Kennel Cough)

DEFINITION/OVERVIEW

- Any contagious respiratory disease of dogs that is manifested by acute onset of paroxysmal coughing

ETIOLOGY/PATHOPHYSIOLOGY

- Etiology—usually complex involving viral (canine distemper virus, CAV-2, CPI, CAV-1, canine reovirus types 1, 2, or 3, canine respiratory coronavirus, CIV, and canine herpes virus), bacterial (*Bordetella bronchiseptica* as a primary pathogen and other secondary pathogens, including *Pseudomonas* spp., *Escherichia coli*, *Klebsiella* spp., *Pasteurella* spp., and *Streptococcus* spp.), and mycoplasma
- CAV-2 and CPI—may damage respiratory epithelium to such an extent that invasion by bacteria and mycoplasma causes severe airway disease
- *B. bronchiseptica*—a gram-negative bacterium with an incubation period of about 6 days, replicates on cilia of respiratory epithelium; produces a number of toxins that impair phagocytosis and cause ciliastasis; produces strong local immunity but may persist in the respiratory tract for up to 3 months
- *Mycoplasma* spp.—endogenous to the nasopharynx, but not usually found in the lower respiratory tract; takes advantage of damaged mucosa (such as viral, or physical damage); infection leads to a purulent bronchitis

SIGNALMENT/HISTORY

- All ages susceptible—puppies 6 weeks to 6 months of age most severely affected
- Dogs with preexisting respiratory conditions—at higher risk for developing severe disease
- History of exposure—often in kennel/boarding situation with high-density housing, where rapid spread from seemingly healthy dogs to others can occur
- Signs—usually develop 4–7 days after exposure

- Historically—In uncomplicated cases, cough develops in otherwise healthy animal.
  - Dry and hacking, soft and dry, moist and hacking or paroxysmal coughing followed by gagging or expectoration of white foamy mucus often worse after exercise (clients often complain that dog is vomiting up white foam)
- Severe complicated cases:
  - Anorexia
  - Moist, productive cough
  - Lethargy
  - Dyspnea and exercise intolerance

 # CLINICAL FEATURES

- Uncomplicated—cough readily induced with tracheal pressure in an otherwise healthy animal; other physical examination findings, including lung sounds, usually normal; cough may be dry and hacking, soft and dry, moist and hacking or paroxysmal followed by gagging or expectoration of mucus; cough also induced by exercise, excitement, changes in air temperature or humidty
- Severe—low-grade fever with inappetance, tachypnea, dyspnea, cough, increased lung sounds, crackles, and wheezes (less frequently)
- Paroxysmal cough—easily elicited on tracheal palpation

 # DIFFERENTIAL DIAGNOSIS

- A general differential diagnosis for cough includes such categories as:
  - Cardiovascular (pulmonary edema; pleural effusions; enlarged heart, especially the left atrium; pulmonary emboli)
  - Allergic (bronchitis, eosinophilic pneumonia or granulomatosis, pulmonary infiltrate with eosinophilis)
  - Trauma (foreign body, irritating gases, collapsing trachea)
  - Neoplasia (not only of the respiratory tree but also associated structures such as ribs, lymph nodes, muscles)
  - Inflammatory (pharyngitis, tonsillitis, bacterial bronchopneumonia, chronic pulmonary fibrosis, pulmonary abscess or granuloma, chronic obstructive pulmonary disease)
  - Parasites (*Capillaria aerophila, Oslerus [Filaroides] osleri, Filaroides hirthi, Filaroides milksi, Paragonimus kellicotti, Dirofilaria immitis*—heartworm disease)
- Kennel cough—often a clinical diagnosis based on a history of sudden onset, recent exposure to likely pathogens (boarding), lack of recent vaccinations for the respiratory pathogens, lack of other clinical signs other than cough, and cough easily induced upon even slight tracheal palpation

DIAGNOSTICS

- CBC—usually normal; in severe cases, leukocytosis with neutrophilia and left shift
- Serum biochemical profile and urinalysis—normal
- Thoracic radiography—normal or mild bronchial pattern; in severe cases and those complicated by bronchopneumonia, interstitial and alveolar lung pattern found, often with a cranioventral distribution typical of bacterial pneumonia
- Transtracheal wash—perform only if resistant to initial therapy; to isolate organism by culture for antibacterial sensitivity studies; examine cytology for type of inflammation and other causes (parasitic)

THERAPEUTICS

- Strongly recommend—to treat uncomplicated cases as outpatients to prevent hospital contamination
- Hospitalize—only those with pneumonia that require IV fluid support
- Enforced rest—for at least 14–21 days (uncomplicated cases); 2 months in cases of pneumonia
- Owner should be aware of infectivity of dog to other dogs—should be encouraged to isolate the patient from other dogs (even up to months after recovery because *B. bronchiseptica* can be present in respiratory tract for months after infection)
- Dogs with uncomplicated disease—should respond to treatment in 10–14 days

Drugs of Choice

- Broad-spectrum antibiotics in uncomplicated cases—amoxicillin/clavulanic acid, doxycycline, or TMS
- Severe cases that are resistant to first-choice antibiotic therapies above—combination therapy of an aminoglycoside (gentamicin or amikacin) with a cephalosporin (cefazolin); may use enrofloxacin as alternative to gentamicin
- In severe cases (bronchopneumonia)—continue at least 2 weeks past radiographic resolution of signs
- Resistant bacteria (*B. bronchiseptica* and others)—important to culture and establish the bacterial sensitivity; may need to deliver antibiotics by nebulization (kanamycin 250 mg; gentamicin 50 mg; polymixin B 333,000 IU) for 3–5 days
- Cough suppressants—butorphanol (Torbutrol; Fort Dodge Animal Health) or hydrocodone bitartrate (Hycodan; DuPont Pharma) often effective in suppressing a dry, nonproductive cough
- Bronchodilators (theophylline or aminophylline)—offer little help but may relieve clinically apparent wheezing (Table 58-1)

TABLE 58-1 Drug Therapy for Canine Infectious Tracheobronchitis (Kennel Cough)				
Drug	Dose (mg/kg)	Route	Interval (h)	Duration (days)
Amocicillin-clavulanic acid	12.5–25	PO	12	10–14
Doxycycline	5	PO	12	10–14
Trimethoprim-sulfadiazine	15	PO, IV	12	10–14
Gentamicin[a]	6	IV, SC, IM	24	14
Amikacin[a]	6.5	IV, SC, IM	8	14
Cefazolin[b]	20–35	IV, IM	8	14–28
Enrofloxacin[c]	2.5–5	PO, IV, IM	12	14–28
Butorphanol	0.55	PO	8–12	[d]
Hydrocodone bitartrate	0.22	PO	6–8	[d]
Theophylline	10	PO	8	[d]
Aminophylline	10	PO, IM, IV	8	[d]

[a]Use in combination with a cephalosporin or penicillin; monitor for nephrotoxicity by examining urine for cast formation.
[b]Use in combination with an aminoglycoside.
[c]Use as an alternative to aminoglycosides.
[d]Use for extended periods to suppress cough.

- Vaccination—available for *B. bronchiseptica*, CIV, and CPI; intranasal vaccines generally considered to offer superior protection because they induce both local and systemic immunity, they are not affected by maternal antibody, and they protect against challenge more rapidly than parenteral vaccines; vaccinate puppies intranasally as early as 2–4 weeks of age, followed by revaccination annually; may vaccinate mature dogs with a one-dose intranasal vaccination; a single booster at least 5 days before exposure in dogs not vaccinated in the previous 6 months is recommended
- CIV vaccine—inactivated vaccine available (see chapter on CIV)
- Best protection is achieved when both intranasal and parenteral vaccines given together or sequentially.

Precautions/Interactions

- Do not use cough suppressants in patients with pneumonia or productive coughs.
- TMS—multiple adverse reactions, including:
  - KCS—monitor tear production weekly throughout treatment
  - Hepatotoxicity—anorexia, depression, icterus; monitor ALT—if prolonged therapy
  - Megaloblastic-folate acid deficiency anemia—especially in cats after several weeks; supplement with folinic acid (2.5 mg/kg/day)

- Immune-mediated polyarthritis, retinitis, glomerulonephritis, vasculitis, anemia, thrombocytopenia, urticaria, toxic epidermal necrolysis, erythema multiforme, and conjunctivitis—remove from drug
- Renal failure and interference with renal excretion of potassium—leading to hyperkalemia
- Salivation, diarrhea, and vomiting (cats)
- May interfere with thyroid hormone synthesis (dogs)—check T_3 and T_4 after 6 weeks
- TMS—Use with caution in neonates and pregnant patients.
- Fluoroquinolones—avoid use in pregnant, neonatal or growing animals (medium-sized dogs <8 months of age; large or giant breeds <12–18 months of age) because of cartilage lesions
- Fluoroquinolones and theophylline derivatives—used together may increase the plasma theophylline concentrations to toxic levels
- Intranasal vaccine—can induce a cough or nasal discharge 2–5 days postinoculation, whereas parenteral vaccination does not

 COMMENTS

- If infection is established in a kennel situation, evacuate the kennel for 1–2 weeks and disinfect with sodium hypochlorite (1:30 dilution), chlorhexidine, or benzalkonium.
- Uncomplicated cases should resolve within 10–14 days; if patient continues to cough beyond 14 days, question the diagnosis of uncomplicated disease.
- Dogs recovering from *B. bronchiseptica* infection are immune for at least 6 months.

Abbreviations

ALT, alanine aminotransferase; CAV, canine adenovirus; CBC, complete blood count; CIV, canine influenza virus; CPI, canine parainfluenza; KCS, keratoconjunctivitis sicca; TMS, trimethoprim-sulfadiazine.

Suggested Reading

Ellis JA, Krakowka GS, Dayton, et al. Effect of vaccination on experimental infection with *Bordetella bronchiseptica* in dogs. *J Am Vet Med Assoc* 2001;218:367–375.

Ford BB, Canine infectious tracheobronchitis. In: Greene CE, ed. *Infectious Diseases of the Dog and Cat*. Philadelphia: WB Saunders, 2006:54–61.

Radhakrishnan A, Drobatz KJ, Culp WT, et al. Community-acquired infectious pneumonia in puppies: 65 cases (1993-2002). *J Am Vet Med Assoc* 2007;230:1493–1497.

Kidney Worm (*Dioctophyma*)

chapter 59

DEFINITION/OVERVIEW

- A nematode parasite (the largest in existence), the adults of which are found in the abdominal cavity and renal pelvis of dogs (rarely infect cats)

ETIOLOGY/PATHOPHYSIOLOGY

- *Dioctyophyma renale*—mink are the definitive host (in which the adult worm is much smaller); occasionally found in dogs
- Female worm (can reach 1 meter in length)—lays brownish, thick-shelled eggs with bipolar plugs
- Eggs—passed in the urine; mature to larvated eggs (if enter water) over about a month
- Larvated eggs—infect earthworms to hatch L1 that develop to L3
- Dogs—become infected after ingesting paratenic hosts (intestines of fish or frogs) or earthworms containing the L3
- L3 larvae—migrate through the stomach wall, cross the peritoneal cavity to enter the liver, where they molt to L4
- L4 larvae—enter the peritoneal cavity, molt to adults before entering the renal capsule
- Adult worms—migrate to the renal pelvis (usually of the right kidney)
- Exact mechanism of how adult worms destroy the renal parenchyma—unknown
- Hydronephrosis and pyelonephritis may play a role in the pathogenesis.
- Histopathology—shows destruction of the renal tubules surrounded by chronic inflammation, with preservation of many glomeruli
- Worms in the peritoneal cavity—produce a serofibrinous to chronic fibrinous peritonitis
- Worms in close proximity to the liver—cause large erosions on the liver (and even severe hemorrhage from liver rupture)
- Eggs—often found within chronic granulomas within the peritoneal cavity
- The severity of renal disease—depends on the number of parasites in the kidney, the number of kidneys infected, duration of infection, and the presence of concomitant renal disease

SIGNALMENT/HISTORY

Dogs

- Exceptionally rare in the dog, given its relatively high prevalence in the wild
- Usually dogs have a history of ingesting earthworms or the raw viscera of fish.

Cats

- Last natural infection—reported in the 1930s

 CLINICAL FEATURES

- Most cases—asymptomatic
- Most infections—restricted to the abdominal cavity, producing a mild peritonitis
- Infections involving the kidneys—hematuria, right renomegaly, and UTI
- Renal failure—if both kidneys are infected (very rare)
- Renomegaly (especially right kidney)—on abdominal palpation

 DIFFERENTIAL DIAGNOSIS

- Other causes of hematuria with unilateral renomegaly:
  - Neoplasia (renal carcinoma, hemangiosarcoma)
  - Unilateral hydronephrosis
  - Trauma

 DIAGNOSTICS

- Urinalysis—large (68 × 44 mm) brown, thick-shelled eggs with bipolar plugs
- Urinalysis—occult blood, elevated protein, and RBCs and WBCs per high-power field too numerous to count, consistent with pyelonephritis or UTI
- Serum biochemistry profile—usually normal unless in renal failure (BUN and creatine, low urine specific gravity)
- Abdominal ultrasound—coiled parasite within the pelvis of the right kidney; mild fibrinous peritonitis
- Renal function tests—often show reduced function of the right kidney (if only one infected) and compensation of the left kidney

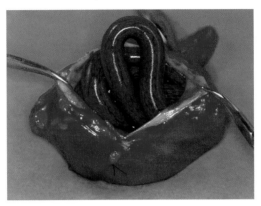

■ **Figure 59-1** A kidney removed surgically from a dog containing an adult *D. renale* worm (courtesy of Dr. Carl A. Osborne, University of Minnesota).

 ## THERAPEUTICS

- If no biochemical signs of renal insufficiency exist, and infection is confined to one kidney—surgically remove that kidney (Fig. 59-1)
- If both kidneys are infected, but renal function tests show good renal function—attempt to remove the worms from one renal pelvis by surgery
- Examine abdominal cavity thoroughly for the presence of adult worms at the time of surgery.

Drugs of Choice

- None identified

 ## COMMENTS

- Although *D. renale* has been reported in humans (exceptionally rare), they cannot become infected by ingesting eggs passed in the urine of dogs.
- Dogs should be prevented from ingesting raw fish (especially their viscera) or earthworms.

Abbreviations

BUN, blood urea nitrogen; RBCs, red blood cells; UTI, urinary tract infection; WBCs, white blood cells.

Suggested Reading

Ferreira VL, Medeiros FP, July JR, et al. Dioctophyma renale in a dog: clinical diagnosis and surgical treatment. *Vet Parasitol* 2010;168:151–155.

L-Form Bacterial Infections

DEFINITION/OVERVIEW

- Infections, usually at the site of entry (arthritis in dogs, bite wounds in cats), caused by bacteria that have lost their cell wall or that have a defective cell wall

ETIOLOGY/PATHOPHYSIOLOGY

- Soft pleomorphic spherical and osmotically fragile organisms
- Also called L-organisms, cell wall-deficient (CWD)-forms
- Differ from mycoplasma by lack of sterols in their membranes
- Grow and replicate by cell fission; yield daughter cells that vary in size, nucleic acid content, and amount of cytoplasm
- Formed as spontaneous variants of bacteria or when cell wall synthesis is inhibited or impaired by antibiotics, specific immunoglobulins, or lysosomal enzymes that degrade cell walls
- Includes both unstable (able to revert back to normal walled bacteria) L-forms with reversible loss of cell wall organization due to phenotypic variants of bacteria, and stable (unable o revert) L-forms with irreversible loss of cell wall due to genomic mutations
- Virtually all gram-positive or gram-negative bacteria are capable of forming L-forms.
- Formation stimulated by antibiotic use, resistance of host, suitability of in vivo site in host for developing infective foci, and relatively low to moderate virulence of infecting bacterium
- May revert to normal cell wall strain in a suitable host
- Usually no pathogenicity
- Can be isolated from humans, animals, and plants

SIGNALMENT/HISTORY

- Sporadic in cats and dogs
- Most common in free-roaming cats; all ages

CLINICAL FEATURES

Dogs

- Arthritis
- Fever
- Local lymphadenopathy

Cats

- Penetrating wounds (usually cat bites)
- Infected surgical sites
- Cellulitis
- Fever
- Arthritis
- Synovitis

 # DIFFERENTIAL DIAGNOSIS

Dogs

- Other causes of arthritis—immune-mediated disease; Lyme disease; mycoplasma; rickettsia; and fungal

Cats

- Other causes of suppurative skin infections—wounds infected with bacteria; mycobacterium; yeast; and fungi

 # DIAGNOSTICS

- CBC—neutrophilia with left shift; monocytosis; lymphocytosis; eosinophilia; occasionally, mild normocytic normochromic anemia (anemia of chronic disease)
- Cytologic examination of infected wound—nondiagnostic (suppurative inflammation)
- Joint fluid from infected joint—high neutrophil count
- Radiologic examination of joint—shows periarticular joint swelling (nonspecific)

Diagnostic Feature

- **Culture—difficult; requires special medium (Hayflick) on which colonies appear as "fried-eggs" on solid agar**
- Light microscopy—usually of no help
- Electron microscopy—used to differentiate from mycoplasma

THERAPEUTICS

- Gentle cleaning of the wound will degrade organisms.
- Allow open wounds to heal by secondary intention.

Drugs of Choice

- Variable antibiotic sensitivity
- Tetracycline (dosage: 22 mg/kg, PO, q8h for 10 days after signs disappear)

Precautions/Interactions

- Antibiotics that interfere with cell wall synthesis (β-lactam antibiotics)—not effective

COMMENTS

- Usually, once tetracyclines are begun and wound is appropriately drained (if necessary), fever will resolve in 24–48 hours.
- Public health significance of having an infected animal around humans—unknown

Abbreviation

CBC, complete blood count.

Suggested Reading

Allan EJ, Holschen C, Gumpert J. Bacterial L forms. *Adv Appl Microbiol* 2009;68:1–39.
Greene CE. Mycoplasmal, ureaplasmal, and L-form infections. In: Greene CE, ed. *Infectious Diseases of the Dog and Cat*. Philadelphia: WB Saunders, 2006:264–265.

Leishmaniasis

chapter 61

DEFINITION/OVERVIEW

- An uncommon protozoal infection of dogs affecting skin, liver, spleen, kidneys, eyes, and joints
- Cats—rarely (skin)

ETIOLOGY/PATHOPHYSIOLOGY

- Protozoan—genus *Leishmania*
- Acquisition—in the United States, dogs acquire infection in two different ways:
  - Overseas, usually from an infected vector—*Leishmania donovani infantum* (Mediterranean basin, Portugal, and Spain; sporadic cases in Switzerland, northern France, and the Netherlands); *L. donovani* complex or *Leishmania braziliensis* (endemic areas of South and Central America and southern Mexico)
  - Endemic—in the Foxhound population in North America (*L. donovani infantum*)
- Sandfly vector—transmit flagellated parasites into the skin of a host
- Vector unknown in North America—transfusion of blood products, direct contact with other dogs, or transplacentally are other methods of transmission that can occur in dogs
- Dogs—organism invariably spreads throughout the body to most organs
- Renal failure—most common cause of death in dogs
- Cats—organism often localizes in skin
- Incubation period—1 month to several years

SIGNALMENT/HISTORY

Dogs

- Virtually all develop visceral or systemic disease
- 90% also have cutaneous involvement
- No sex or breed predilection

Cats

- Cutaneous disease is rare
- No sex or breed predilection

CLINICAL FEATURES

Dogs

- Exercise intolerance
- Severe weight loss and anorexia
- Fever (33% of patients)
- Splenomegaly (33% of patients)
- Diarrhea
- Vomiting
- Epistaxis and melena (less common)
- Generalized lymphadenopathy
- Cutaneous lesions—hyperkeratosis most prominent finding, often bilaterally symmetrical over the head (Fig. 61-1); excessive epidermal scale with thickening, depigmentation, and chapping of the muzzle and foodpads; dry brittle hair coat with hair loss; intradermal nodules and ulcers may be seen (Fig. 61-2); abnormally long or brittle nails in some patients
- Signs of renal failure terminally—polyuria, polydipsia, vomiting
- Rare signs—neuralgia, polyarthritis, polymyositis, osteolytic lesions, and proliferative periostitis
- In utero transmission can occur.

Cats

- Cutaneous nodules—especially on the ears

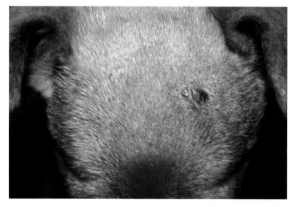

■ **Figure 61-1** Hyperkeratosis, excessive epidermal scale, nodule, and some alopecia over the head of a dog with leishmaniasis.

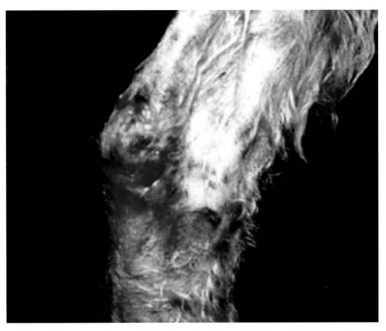

■ **Figure 61-2** Dermal ulcers over the hock of a dog with advanced leishmaniasis. Impression smear of such a lesion would easily demonstrate typical intracellular organisms.

DIFFERENTIAL DIAGNOSIS

- Visceral—mycoses (blastomycosis, histoplasmosis); SLE; metastatic neoplasia; distemper; and vasculitis
- Cutaneous—other causes of hyperkeratosis: primary idiopathic seborrhea and nutritional dermatoses (vitamin A responsive, zinc responsive); idiopathic nasodigital hyperkeratosis, lichenoid-psoriasiform dermatosis, mucocutaneous syndrome, pemphigus foliaceus, epidermal dysplasia, and Schnauzer comedo syndrome are rare and breed-specific
- Skin biopsy—hyperkeratotic and nodular lesions; existence of organisms confirms diagnosis of leishmaniasis
- Hyperglobulinemia—need to differentiate from chronic ehrlichiosis and multiple myeloma

DIAGNOSTICS

- Hyperproteinemia with hyperglobulinemia—100% of cases
- Hypoalbuminemia—95% of cases
- Proteinuria—85% of cases

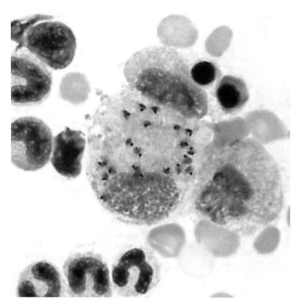

■ **Figure 61-3** Bone marrow aspirate showing typical intracellular organisms containing both a nucleus and kinedoplast typical of *Leishmania* (Wright–Geimsa stain, 1000×).

- High hepatic enzyme activity—55% of cases
- Thrombocytopenia—50% of cases
- Azotemia—45% of cases
- Leukopenia with lymphopenia—20% of cases
- Coombs', ANA, and lupus erythematosus cell tests—sometimes positive
- Serologic diagnosis by IFA or ELISA available—most tests give cross-reaction to *Trypanosoma cruzi* (closely related organism); differentiate based on clinical signs, history, and likelihood of exposure
- Culture of skin, spleen, bone marrow, or lymph node tissue—send to the CDC

Diagnostic Feature

- **Cytology is diagnostic method of choice (same samples as cultured)—identify typical intracellular organisms (Fig. 61-3)**

 THERAPEUTICS

- Outpatient
- Use multiple drugs (if able to obtain them)—induce initially with amphotericin B or sodium stibogluconate (if available) and keep on allopurinol for entire life (maintenance)
- Emaciated, chronically infected animals—consider euthanasia; prognosis very poor

TABLE 61-1 Drug Therapy for Leishmaniasis in Dogs

Drug	Dose (mg/kg)	Route	Interval (h)	Duration (months)
Sodium stibogluconate (Pentostam)	30–50	IV, SC	24	1
Allopurinol	7–10	PO	8	3–24[a]
Amphotericin B (Fungizone)	0.25–0.5[b]	IV	48[c]	[d]
Meglumine antimonite[e] (Glucantime)	100	IV, SC	24	1

[a]Or for rest of dog's life.
[b]Reconstituted in 5% dextrose (do not reconstitute in electrolyte solutions, which precipitate the drug) and dilute to administer; if normal renal function, dilute in 60–120 ml 5% dextrose given over 15 minutes; if renal compromise, dilute in 0.5–1 liter 5% dextrose given over 3–4 hours to reduce further renal toxicity.
[c]Or 3 times a week.
[d]Administer until a total cumulative dose of 5–10 mg/kg is reached.
[e]Not available in the United States.

- Diet—high-quality protein; special for renal insufficiency, if necessary
- Cats—single dermal nodule lesions are best surgically removed
- Vaccination—A canine vaccine is available in Europe and some areas of South America.

Drugs of Choice

- Sodium stibogluconate (Pentostam; available from the CDC); interferes with energy metabolism; expensive; excellent initial clinical response; relapses common months to years after stop treating
- Allopurinol—organism hydrolyzes the drug to an aberrant isomer of inosine, which becomes incorporated into RNA and interferes with protein synthesis; cheap and nontoxic; produces clinical cure, but relapses occur; best when used in combination with other drugs for long-term maintenance; probably does not prevent transmission in endemic regions
- Amphotericin B (Fungizone; BM Squibb)—poorly absorbed into bone, eyes, and body cavities; nephrotoxic; when combined with allopurinol, has improved efficacy
- Meglumine antimonite (Glucantime; Merial [not available in North America])—probably the most efficacious drug when combined with allopurinol (Table 61-1)

Precautions/Interactions

- Seriously ill dogs—start antimonial drugs at lower doses
- Renal insufficiency—treat before giving antimonial drugs; prognosis depends on renal function at the onset of treatment
- Sodium stibogluconate—pain at injection site; resistance has been identified in Europe due to underdosing of drug
- Amphotericin B—Nephrotoxicity needs to be monitored by examining renal sediment for casts; perivascular injection can cause severe phlebitis.

- Treatment efficacy—monitor by clinical improvement and identification of organisms in repeat biopsies
- Relapses—a few months to a year after therapy; recheck at least every 2 months after completion of treatment
- Relapses—identified by monitoring rise in blood globulins or reappearance of clinical signs in a dog previously in remission
- Prognosis for a cure—very guarded, even when using best treatment (meglumine with allopurinol)

 COMMENTS

- Leishmaniasis is a notifiable disease—Confirmed cases must be reported to the CDC.
- Advise client—Potential zoonotic transmission of organisms in lesions to humans is possible.
- Inform client—Organisms will never be eliminated, and relapses, requiring treatment, are inevitable.

Abbreviations

ANA, antinuclear antibody; CDC, Centers for Disease Control and Prevention; ELISA, enzyme-linked immunosorbent assay; IFA, immunofluorescence assay; RNA, ribonucleic acid; SLE, systemic lupus erythematosus.

Suggested Reading

Lemesre JL, Holzmuller P, Goncalves RB, et al. Long-lasting protection against canine visceral leishmaniasis using the LiESAp-MDP vaccine in endemic areas of France: double-blind randomised efficacy field trial. *Vaccine* 2007;25:4223–4234.

Petersen CA, Barr SC. Canine Leishmaniasis in North America: emergine or newly recognized? *Vet Clin North Am Small Anim Pract* 2009;39:1065–1074.

Schantz PM, Steurer FJ, Duprey ZH, et al. Autochthonous visceral leishmaniasis in dogs in North America. *J Am Vet Med Assoc* 2005;226:1316–1322.

Leptospirosis

DEFINITION/OVERVIEW

- A systemic bacterial infection of dogs (and very rarely, cats), causing mainly acute nephritis and hepatitis, vasculitis, and chronic carrier states

ETIOLOGY/PATHOPHYSIOLOGY

- Pathogenic members of the genus *Leptospira*—Main serovars causing disease in dogs include *L. pomona* and *L. grippotyphosa*, occasionally *L. autumnalis* and *L. bratislava*, and, rarely, *L. canicola* and *L. icterohaemorrhagiae*.
- Direct transmission—host-to-host contact via infected urine, postabortion discharge, infected fetus/discharge, and sexual contact (semen)
- Indirect transmission—exposure (via urine) to a contaminated environment (vegetation, soil, food, water, and bedding) under conditions in which *Leptospira* organisms can survive
- *Leptospira* spp.—penetrate intact or cut skin or mucous membranes; rapidly invade bloodstream (4–7 days); spread to all parts of the body (2–4 days)
- Invasion—leads to transient fever, leukocytosis, transitory anemia (hemolysis), mild hemoglobinuria, and albuminuria; capillary and endothelial cell damage (occasionally results in petechial hemorrhages); liver necrosis and jaundice; acute nephritis with leptospiruria (organism replicates readily in tubular epithelial cell)
- Vasculitis—may cause interstitial pneumonia, anterior uveitis, myocardial damage and meningitis (rare), and abortions
- Death—usually a result of interstitial nephritis, vascular damage, and renal failure; may result from acute septicemia or DIC
- Usually one or more serovars account for endemic disease in a geographic area—overall reported incidence probably falsely low because most infections are inapparent (undiagnosed)
- Distribution—worldwide, especially in warm, wet climates or seasons
- Standing water and neutral or slightly alkaline soil—promote presence in environment
- Most cases—occur during late summer/fall in northeastern United States

SIGNALMENT/HISTORY

- Dogs in rural habitat
- Young dogs without passive maternal antibody are more likely to exhibit severe disease.
- Old dogs with adequate antibody titer levels seldom exhibit clinical disease unless exposed to a serovar not in the vaccine.
- Dense animal population (kennels and urban settings) increases chances of urine exposure, exposure to rodents, and other wildlife (hunting dogs).
- Historically:
  - Peracute/acute—fever, sore muscles, stiffness, weakness, anorexia, depression, acute onset of vomiting, rapid dehydration, diarrhea (occasional bloody), occasionally icterus, cough with mild respiratory distress if respiratory component severe, and polyuria/polydipsia progressing to anuria
  - Chronic—usually no apparent illness; polyuria/polydipsia if chronic renal failure

 CLINICAL FEATURES

- Peracute/acute disease
  - Tachypnea
  - Tachycardia, sometimes with arrhythmias
  - Poor capillary perfusion
  - Hematemesis
  - Hematochezia
  - Melena
  - Epistaxis
  - Injected mucous membranes
  - Petechial and ecchymotic hemorrhages
  - Reluctance to move, stiff gait
  - Paraspinal hyperesthesia
  - Conjunctivitis, uveitis (Fig. 62-1), blepharospasm
  - Hematuria
  - Harsh respiratory sounds on auscultation
  - Mild lymphadenopathy (occasionally)

 DIFFERENTIAL DIAGNOSIS

Dogs

- Subacute/acute disease—any severe systemic disease involving mainly the liver or kidneys alone, or together: heartworm disease, immune-mediated hemolytic anemia,

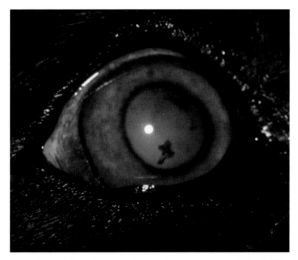

■ **Figure 62-1** Hyphema and uveitis in a dog with leptospirosis (courtesy of Dr. R. Riis, Cornell University).

bacteremia/septicemia (bite wound, prostatitis, endocarditis, dental disease), infectious canine hepatitis virus, CHV, hepatic neoplasia, lupus, RMSF, ehrlichiosis, toxoplasmosis, acute nephritis, renal neoplasia, and renal calculi, trauma
■ Reproductive failure—brucellosis, distemper, and herpes

Cats

■ Much more rare; consider other causes of acute systemic hepatic and nephritic disease: haemobartonellosis, bacteremia/septicemia, FIV- and FeLV-associated diseases, cholangitis, toxoplasmosis, FIP, hepatic neoplasia, autoimmune disease (e.g., SLE), renal calculi, renal neoplasia, trauma, drugs (acetaminophen)

 DIAGNOSTICS

■ CBC—signs of dehydration (PCV and total plasma solids elevated), leukocytosis with left shift, thrombocytopenia
■ Serum biochemistry profile—Elevated BUN, creatine, and hepatic enzymes are main changes.
■ Other changes—due to dehydration or renal failure (electrolyte changes include hyponatremia, hypochloremia, hyperkalemia, hyperphosphatemia, hypoalbuminemia)
■ Urinalysis—proteinuria, isosthenuria usually, and casts
■ Chronic carrier states—may only see isosthenuria, with few granular casts in urine
■ Serologic examination—MAT; test in acute stage and 3–4 weeks later (convalescent serum); in unvaccinated patients, titers may be low initially (1:100 to 1:200), then rise during convalescents (1:800 to 1:1600 or higher); several serovars usually show elevated titer but make serovar diagnosis based on highest titer

- MAT titers in vaccinated dogs—vaccination causes elevation of MAT titer in most cases but usually only to serovars vaccinated against (no cross-reactivity); do get MAT titer elevations to *L. autumnalis* after vaccination with subunit vaccines against *L. grippotyphosa* and *L. pomona* (Fort Dodge Animal Health)
- Dogs vaccinated with whole cell bacteria—usually develop higher MAT titers (up to 1:800) than subunit vaccines (negative to 1:400)
- MAT titers induced by vaccination—usually only last up to 4 months
- MAT titers induced by infection—usually last >12 months
- Dark field microscopy of urine—often inconclusive because it is difficult to read and requires fresh urine
- FA test of urine—more conclusive because leptospires do not need to be viable; submit urine to laboratory on ice by overnight courier; pretreatment with furosemide (2 mg/kg, SC) 15 minutes before urine collection will increase success rate
- PCR on urine—offered by some commercial laboratories; shown in 1 of 8 dogs to detect organisms in urine before development of serologic titer; needs more work in experimentally infected dogs before being well validated
- Culture—usually unrewarding

 THERAPEUTICS

- Tissue diagnosis (kidney biopsy)—FA, immunohistochemistry, Warthin–Starry silver stain, and PCR are all effective.
- Inpatient for acute severe disease—extent of supportive therapy depends on severity; renal failure requires closely monitored diuresis, attention to DIC development; care must be taken not to overhydrate, because vasculitis of respiratory endothelium can lead to pulmonary edema during diuresis
- Vaccines—bacterin and subunit vaccines available against *L. canicola* and *L. icterohaemorrhagiae*, and subunit vaccine available against *L. pomona, L. grippotyphosa*; most claim year efficacy except those subunit vaccines covering *L. pomona* and *L. grippotyphosa* (protect for 2–21$^1/_2$ weeks after booster); no cross-protection outside of the serovars used in vaccine serogroup); revaccination at least yearly; vaccinate dogs at risk (hunter, show dogs, dogs with access to water/ponds) every 4–6 months, especially in endemic areas; does not protect against carrier state; associated with a high incidence of anaphylaxis (particularly bacterin vaccines) after booster doses occurring within 1 hour of booster

Drugs of Choice

- Doxycycline (Vibramycin; Pfizer)—use alone to clear leptospiremia and leptospiruria, as well as carrier state
- If doxycycline to be used, unnecessary to use penicillin

TABLE 62-1 Drug Therapy for Leptospirosis in Dogs				
Drug	Dose (mg/kg)	Route	Interval (h)	Duration (weeks)
Doxycycline	5	PO, IV	12	2
Penicillin G	25,000–40,000 U/kg	IM, SC, IV	12	2
Ampicillin	22	PO, SC, IV	6–8	2
Amoxicillin	22	PO	8–12	2

- Penicillin compounds—may be used during acute leptospiremic phase if unable to administer doxycycline (Table 62-1)
- Streptomycin—will clear organisms from kidneys but difficult to obtain and may potentiate renal insufficiency

Precautions/Interactions

- If vomiting, use injectable doxycycline.

 COMMENTS

- Inform client of zoonotic potential from contaminated urine of affected dogs and their environment.
- Kennels—strict sanitation to avoid contact with infected urine; control rodents; monitor and remove carrier dogs until treated; isolate affected animals during treatment; disinfect premises, using iodine-based disinfectant or stabilized bleach solutions
- Activity—limit access to marshy/muddy areas, ponds, low-lying areas with stagnant surface water, heavily irrigated pastures, and wildlife
- Chronic active hepatitis and chronic interstitial nephritis—can occur as chronic disease

Abbreviations

BUN, blood urea nitrogen; CBC, complete blood count; CHV, canine herpes virus; DIC, disseminated intravascular coagulation; FA, fluorescent antibody; FeLV, feline leukemia virus; FIP, feline infectious peritonitis; FIV, feline immunodeficiency virus; MAT, microagglutination titer; PCR, polymerase chain reaction; PCV, packed cell volume; RMSF, Rocky Mountain spotted fever; SLE, systemic lupus erythematosus.

Suggested Reading

Adlera B, de la Peña Moctezuma A. Leptospira and leptospirosis. *Vet Microbiol* 2010;140:287–296.
Alton GD, Berke O, Reid-Smith R, et al. Increase in seroprevalence of canine leptospirosis and its risk factors, Ontario 1998–2006. *Can J Vet Res* 2009;73:167–175.

Goldstein RE. Canine Leptospirosis. *Vet Clin North Am Small Anim Pract* 2010;40:1091–1101.

Goldstein RE, Lin RC, Langston CE, et al. Influence of infecting serogroup on clinical features of leptospirosis in dogs. *J Vet Intern Med* 2006;20:489–494.

Greene CE, Sykes JE, Brown CA, et al. In: Greene CE, ed. *Infectious Diseases of the Dog and Cat.* Philadelphia: WB Saunders, 2006:402–417.

Moore GE, Guptill LF, Glickman NW, et al. Canine leptospirosis, United States, 2002–2004. *Emerg Infect Dis* 2006;12:501–503.

Sykes JE, Hartmann K, Lunn KF, et al. 2010 ACVIM small animal concensus statement on leptospirosis diagnosis, epidemiology, treatment, and prevention. *J Vet Intern Med* 2011;153:1–13.

Liver Fluke Infection

chapter **63**

DEFINITION/OVERVIEW

- A parasitic (trematode) infection of cats in Florida, Hawaii, and many other tropical parts of the world

ETIOLOGY/PATHOPHYSIOLOGY

- *Platynosomum concinnum*—acquired from ingestion of an infected intermediate host (usually lizards or frogs)
- Endemic areas—15–85% of cats infected
- Adults parasites—reside in the bile ducts and gallbladder of infected cats
- Embryonated eggs—passed in cat feces to be ingested by first intermediate host (land snails)
- Sporocysts emerge from eggs within the snail—ingested by second intermediate host (anole lizards, skinks, geckos, frogs, toads), which are then ingested by cats
- Cats—Cercariae are released in upper digestive tract before migrating to bile ducts.
- Cercariae mature to adults in bile ducts—shed eggs
- PPP = 8 weeks
- Adult parasites—if they cause disease, produce intrahepatic bile duct obstruction and hepatic necrosis

SIGNALMENT/HISTORY

- Typical patient—Feral cat, 6–24 months old, with access to local fauna

CLINICAL FEATURES

- Depend on severity of infection
- Most affected cats show no clinical signs.

- Affected cats may show:
  - Jaundice
  - Emaciation
  - Anorexia
  - Mucoid diarrhea
  - Hepatomegaly—abdominal distention
  - Polycystic liver disease
  - Vomiting
  - Malaise

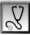

DIFFERENTIAL DIAGNOSIS

- Cholangiohepatitis, hepatic lipidosis, bile duct carcinoma, hepatic lymphoma, pancreatitis, and any disorder causing major bile duct occlusion
- Differentiated by examination of cytologic specimens from hepatic or bile aspirates.

DIAGNOSTICS

- CBC—usually eosinophilia beginning 3 weeks after infection; persists for months
- Serum biochemistry profile—elevated hepatic enzyme activities (especially ALT and AST; ALP may be normal or only slightly elevated) and bilirubinemia (markedly high in advanced severe disease)
- Urinalysis—bilirubinuria
- Fasting/postprandial bile acid—increased (not necessary to perform if bilirubinemia present)

Diagnostic Feature

- **Definitive diagnostic test—identification of *P. concinnum* eggs (Fig. 63-1) using sedimentation (formalin-ether or sodium acetate most reliable; demonstrates eight times more eggs than direct fecal examination)**
- Fecal eggs—detected in only 25% of cats
- Patients with few parasites (1–5 flukes)—may shed only 2–10 eggs/gram of feces that may not be found on fecal testing, making serial examinations necessary
- Abdominal radiographic examination—nonspecific mild hepatomegaly
- Abdominal ultrasonography—differentiates biliary obstruction from hepatocellular disease; shows one or more of the following:
  - Biliary obstruction—dilated gallbladder, common bile duct (>2 mm), and intrahepatic ducts

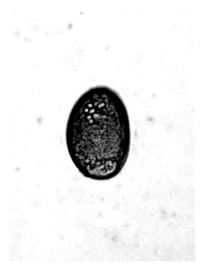

■ **Figure 63-1** *P. concinnum* eggs in the feces of a cat infected with the liver fluke (sodium acetate sedimentation, 400×).

- Gallbladder—sediment with flukes (oval hypoechoic structures with an echoic center), mildly thick gallbladder wall with a double-layered appearance (cholecystitis)
- Overall hypoechoic hepatic parenchyma—with prominent hyperechoic portal areas (ducts) associated with cholangiohepatitis
- May reveal polycystic liver disease
- Cholecystocentesis—reveals fluke eggs
- Histopathology of biopsied liver tissue—usually definitive

THERAPEUTICS

- Outpatient versus inpatient—depends on severity of illness
- Inpatient—balanced polyionic solution with potassium supplementation
- Nutritional support—important to avoid development of hepatic lipidosis:
  - Feed—high-protein canned food
  - Ensure—cat is taking in food
  - If anorectic—use feeding tube (nasogastric initially, place esophageal or PEG once condition is stable)
  - Cats with severe clinical signs—partial parenteral nutrition (not >5 days) or total parenteral nutrition may be necessary
  - Hepatic encephalopathy—rare, but may develop, necessitating protein restriction
- B vitamin supplementation—important for anorectic and ill cats on fluid therapy (2 ml of B-soluble vitamins/liter fluids)

TABLE 63-1 Drug Therapy for Liver Flukes in Cats

Drug	Dose (mg/kg)	Route	Interval (h)	Duration (days)
Praziquantel (Doncit)	20	SC	24	3–5
Prednisolone	2	PO	24	2–4[a]
Ursodeoxycholic acid	10–15	PO	24	6[b]
Amoxicillin/clavulanic acid	10–20	PO	12	2
Vitamin E	10 U	PO	24	6[b]
S-Adenosylmethionine	20	PO	24	4[c]
Metoclopramide	0.2–0.5	PO, SC, IV	6–8[d]	1[b]

[a]Then taper in 50% decrements every 2 weeks.
[b]Or until clinical signs have resolved.
[c]Until hepatic enzymes normalize.
[d]Or by constant rate infusion.

Drugs of Choice

- Praziquantel (Droncit injectable, 56.8 mg/ml solution; Bayer)—Eggs may pass in feces for up to 2 months after treatment.
- Prednisolone—initial dose for cats showing eosinophilia to decrease eosinophilic infiltration around bile ducts in liver
- Ursodeoxycholic acid—unless there is biliary obstruction
- Broad-spectrum antibiotic (amoxicillin/clavulanic acid)—protect from retrograde biliary tree infection with enteric organisms introduced by parasite; growth permissively encouraged by parasite death in tissues
- Antioxidant therapy (vitamin E and S-adenosylmethionine)—suggested by necrotic inflammatory tissue injury
- Antiemetics (metoclopramice)—for vomiting (Table 63-1)

Precautions/Interactions

- Watch for signs of biliary tree obstruction—from dying adult parasites after starting praziquantel
- Avoid ursodeoxycholic acid—in cats with biliary obstruction

 COMMENTS

- Restrict outdoor access
- Praziquantel prophylaxis—every 3 months, especially for outdoor cats in endemic, tropical climates
- Uncomplicated recovery in most patients treated

- However, can lead to severe fatal liver disease including polycystic and severe choliastatic disease if undiagnosed and left untreated.
- Zoonosis—no records of it infecting humans

Abbreviations

ALP, alkaline phosphatase; ALT, alanine aminotransferase; AST, aspartate aminotransferase; CBC, complete blood count; PEG, percutaneous endoscopic gastrostomy; PPP, prepatent period.

Suggested Reading

Bowman DD, Hendrix CM, Lindsay DS, et al. *Platynosomum concinnum.* In: Bowmann DD, ed. *Feline Clinical Parasitology.* Ames, IA: Iowa State University Press, 2002:148–150.

Haney DR, Christiansen JS, Toll J. Severe cholestatic liver disease secondary to liver fluke (*Platynosomum concinnum*) infection in three cats. *J Am Anim Hosp Assoc* 2006;42:234–237.

Xavier FG, Morato GS, Righi DA, et al. Cystic liver disease related to high *Platynosomum fastosum* infection in a domestic cat. *J Feline Med Surg* 2007;9:51–55.

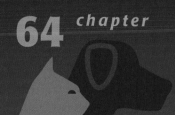

64

Lung Fluke Infection (*Paragonimus*)

DEFINITION/OVERVIEW

- Trematode parasite found in pulmonary cysts in dogs and cats and other mammals, including humans and mink

ETIOLOGY/PATHOPHYSIOLOGY

- *Paragonimus kellicotti*—female lays eggs in subpleural cysts that communicate directly with a bronchiole
- Eggs—swept up the airways, swallowed, and passed in feces
- Life cycle—requires two intermediate hosts; the first is an aquatic snail; the second is a crayfish
- Dogs and cats—become infected when they eat an infected crayfish
- Most common—north central and southeastern United States
- PPP = 4–5 weeks

SIGNALMENT/HISTORY

- No sex, breed, or age predisposition
- Hosts must have eaten a crayfish at some stage.

CLINICAL FEATURES

- Usually clinically inapparent
- Chronic cough unresponsive to antibiotics or other therapies.
- Hemoptysis, occasionally
- Pneumothorax, rarely

DIFFERENTIAL DIAGNOSIS

Dogs

- A general differential diagnosis for cough includes categories such as:
  - Cardiovascular (pulmonary edema; enlarged heart, especially the left atrium; left-sided heart failure; pulmonary emboli)
  - Allergic (bronchial asthma, eosinophilic pneumonia or granulomatosis, pulmonary infiltrate with eosinophilia)
  - Trauma (foreign body, irritating gases, collapsing trachea, hypoplastic trachea)
  - Neoplasia (not only of the respiratory tree but also associated structures such as ribs, lymph nodes, muscles)
  - Inflammatory (pharyngitis; tonsillitis; kennel cough from such agents as *Bordetella bronchiseptica*, parainfluenza virus, infectious laryngotracheitis virus, and mycoplasma; bacterial bronchopneumonia; aspiration pneumonia; fungal pneumonia; chronic pulmonary fibrosis; pulmonary abscess or granuloma; chronic obstructive pulmonary disease)
  - Parasites (*Oslerus* [*Filaroides*] *osleri*, *Crenosoma vulpis*, *Filaroides hirthi*, *Filaroides milksi*, *Dirofilaria immitis*—heartworm disease)

Cats

- Principally—allergy (feline asthma), other parasites (*Aelurostrongylus abstrusus*, *Capillariasis* spp., feline heartworm disease), and cardiac disease
- Consider—trauma (diaphragmatic hernia), pleural disease (pyothorax, chylothorax), neoplasia, and inflammatory diseases

 DIAGNOSTICS

Diagnostic Feature

- **Large, single, operculated eggs present in a fecal sample or occasionally in phlegm from the animal (Fig. 64-1)**
- Fecal sedimentation—best method for identifying eggs
- Centrifugal flotation (sucrose technique with specific gravity of 1.275 or ZSCT with specific gravity of 1.18)—successful but low sensitivity if egg numbers in fecal sample are low
- Thoracic radiographs may reveal multiloculated cysts in dogs and interstitial nodules in cats, usually within the caudodorsal lung fields (Fig. 64-2); pneumothorax may be present.

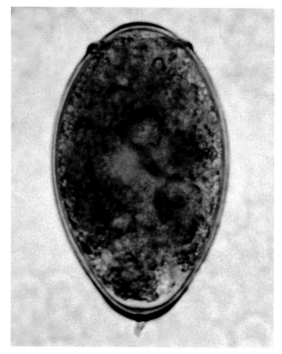

■ **Figure 64-1** Single operculated egg of *P. kellicotti* from the feces of an infected dog.

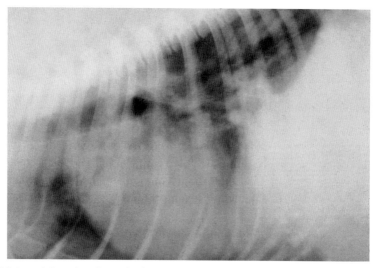

■ **Figure 64-2** Lateral thoracic radiograph of a dog with *P. kellicotti* infestation. Note the "coin" lesion in the dorsoventral lung fields typical of paragonimiasis.

TABLE 64-1 Drug Therapy for *P. kellicotti* in Dogs and Cats				
Drug	Dose (mg/kg)	Route	Interval (h)	Duration (days)
Praziquantel (Droncit)	25	PO	8	3
Fenbendazole (Panacur)	50	PO	24	10

THERAPEUTICS

- Pneumothorax—usually mild, requiring little treatment; excellent prognosis
- Tension pneumothorax—if present, institute continuous external drainage, which is usually successful; prognosis fair
- After 72 hours, if there is still constant flow of air into the pleural space, prognosis becomes very guarded and a thoracotomy may be the only hope of identifying and removing the lesion.

Drugs of Choice

- Praziquantel (Droncit; Bayer); preferred treatment
- Fenbendazole (Panacur; Intervet) (Table 64-1)

Precautions/Interactions

- Praziquantel—do not use in puppies under 4 weeks of age or kittens under 6 weeks of age

COMMENTS

- Praziquantel—results in resolution of radiographic lesions within 8 weeks
- Asymptomatic cases in which typical radiographic lesions have been found incidentally and eggs found on fecal examination—should be treated, because pneumothorax can occur at a later date
- If lung biopsies are performed during thoracotomy, a large adult fluke may be extracted from the affected lung tissue (Fig. 64-3).

Abbreviations

PPP, prepatent period; ZSCT, zinc sulfate concentration technique.

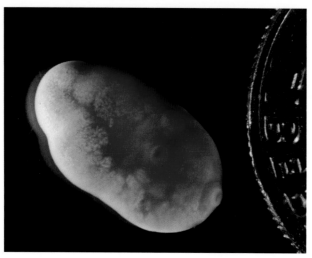

■ **Figure 64-3** Adult *P. kellicotti* removed from a lung lesion during thoracotomy.

Suggested Reading

Bowman DD. Helminths. In: *Georgi's Parasitolgy for Veterinarians*, 9ᵗʰ ed. St. Louis, MO; Elsevier-Saunders, 2009:115–239.

Conboy G. Helminth parasites of the canine and feline respiratory tract. *Vet Clin Small Anim Pract* 2009;39:1109–1126.

Lyme Borreliosis

chapter 65

DEFINITION/OVERVIEW

- A common bacterial tick-transmitted zoonotic diseases of dogs (rarely cats) causing recurrent arthritis with lameness and occasionally glomerulonephritis, cardiac, and neurologic disease

ETIOLOGY/PATHOPHYSIOLOGY

- *Borrelia burgdorferi* sensu lato group—a spirochete
- Acquisition—Dogs acquire infection from an infected tick bite by hard ticks (*Ixodes*) (Fig. 65-1).
- Produces a generalized infection—predominantly of connective tissues, joint capsules, muscle, and lymph nodes
- Incubation period in experimental dogs—2 to 5 months
- Persistent *B. burgdorferi*—found in skin, muscle, connective tissues, joints, and lymph nodes
- Rarely—found in body fluids (blood, CSF, and synovial fluid)
- Pathologic changes—with few exceptions, restricted to joints, local lymph nodes, skin at the tick bite site
- In specific cases—pathology of the glomeruli of the kidney
- Infection—only after tick (nymphal stage in spring or adult female in fall) is partially engorged; 24–48 hours after the initial infestation
- *Ixodes* ticks have a 2-year life cycle; larvae hatch in spring and become infected by feeding on white-footed mice (*Peromyscus leucopus*), which are persistently infected.
- Larvae molt into nymphs in the spring of the following year—stay infected or become infected by feeding on mice
- Nymphs molt into adults in late fall of the second year—Females engorge after mating on deer or other mammals, fall off, and hide under leaves until the following spring, when they each lay about 2000 eggs.
- Male ticks tend to stay on the deer.
- Seropositivity of dogs—varies greatly (5–80%) depending on tick exposure
- Seropositivity of dogs—Only about 5% of seropositive dogs in endemic areas ever develop clinical disease.

353

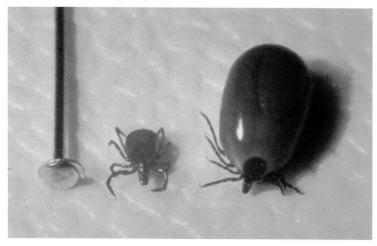

■ **Figure 65-1** An unengorged and engorged adult *Ixodes* tick next to a pin shows the small size of these ticks.

- Distribution—worldwide
- United States—90% of cases occur in the midatlantic to New England coastal states, northeastern states, and upper Midwestern states
- Certain dog breeds are reported to develop severe renal failure (Bernese Mountain dogs).

 SIGNALMENT/HISTORY

- Young dogs—appear more susceptible than older dogs
- Historically—exposure to ticks; running in rural habitat

 CLINICAL FEATURES

- Recurrent acute arthritis with lameness—characteristic
- Lameness—lasts for only 3–4 days; responds well to antibiotic treatment
- Acute lameness—one or more joints may be swollen, warm, and painful on palpation
- Affected dogs—may walk stiffly, with an arched back; sensitive to touch
- Arthritis—may be accompanied by fever, anorexia, and depression
- Superficial cervical and/or popliteal lymph nodes—may be swollen (Fig. 65-2)
- Cardiac—reported but rare; includes complete heart block
- Neurologic complications—rare
- Kidneys—reported glomerulonephritis with immune complex deposition in the glomeruli leading to fatal renal disease; viable *Borrelia* organisms are not present in the kidney

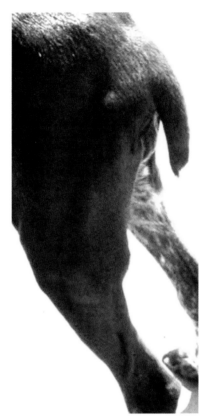

■ **Figure 65-2** Swollen popliteal lymph node and a swollen stifle joint are typical of an acute arthritis seen in dogs infected with Lyme disease.

- Patients may present with renal failure due to advanced glomerulonephritis—vomiting, diarrhea, anorexia, weight loss, polyuria/polydipsia, peripheral edema, or ascites
- Erythema migrans—observed at site of *Borrelia* inoculation in man; not seen in dogs

 DIFFERENTIAL DIAGNOSIS

- Differentiate from other nonerosive inflammatory arthritides—infectious (RMSF, anaplasmosis, ehrlichiosis, histoplasma, *Cryptococcus* infection, blastomycosis, leishmaniasis, *Streptococcus* or *Staphylococcus* infection), immune-mediated diseases (idiopathic, lupus erythematosus), non–immune-mediated diseases (hemarthrosis), specific breed diseases (Akita arthritis, Shar Pei fever)
- Cytology and culture of the joint fluid, serologic assays, and immune testing (ANA, lupus erythematosus preparations, although low sensitivity)—to rule out other disorders

DIAGNOSTICS

- Diagnosis—usually based on compatible clinical signs, response to antibiotic therapy, exclusion of other diagnoses, appropriate laboratory data, and history of exposure to an epidemiologic environment that provides an opportunity for infection
- CBC and serum biochemistry profile—unremarkable in dogs with arthritis only
- Dogs with protein-losing glomerulonephritis—uremia, proteinuria, hypercholesterolemia, hyperphosphatemia, and hypoalbuminemia usually occur
- Cytologic specimens from affected joints—acutely affected joints will have an increased volume of joint fluid, which will often be bloody (Fig. 65-3); on smear, markedly increased WBC (usually <75,000/µl; mainly neutrophils) counts (Fig. 65-4)
- Serologic examination ELISA—positive titer indicates previous exposure or vaccination
- Western blot—used to differentiate between those with a positive vaccine titer and exposed dogs (cross-reactions with antibody responses to *Leptospira* spp. minimal)
- Canine Snap 3Dx and 4Dx Diagnostic Tests (IDEXX Laboratories)—in-house snap tests for antibodies against Lyme disease, *E. canis*, and heartworm antigen; measures antibody to the C6 *B. burgdorferi* protein; convenient test and eliminates antibody responses to Lyme vaccines; however, 10% false-positive reactions were recently found with this test in field samples; C6-specific antibodies normally drop or may

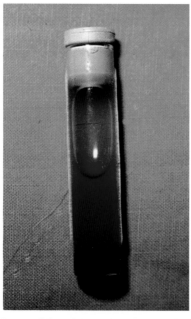

■ **Figure 65-3** An EDTA blood tube containing a joint aspirate from a stifle joint of a dog with Lyme disease arthritis. Note the increased volume and bloody color of the fluid.

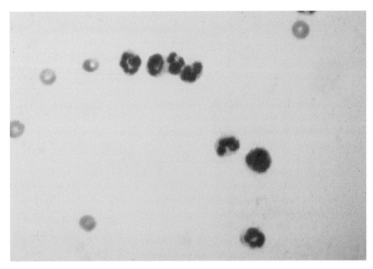

■ **Figure 65-4** Cytology of joint fluid from a dog with Lyme arthritis showing an increased neutrophil count (Wright's stain, 400×).

even disappear ∼4–6 months after antibiotic therapy; low to moderate pretherapy levels do not drop dramatically.
- PCR from skin biopsy specimens—*B. burgdorferi* frequently isolated or demonstrated; time-consuming, unreliable, and expensive (not practical); blood samples from infected dogs are typically negative on PCR

 THERAPEUTICS

- Vaccine—All vaccines currently available depend predominately on the effect of antibodies against the spirochetes' outer surface protein A (OspA). These antibodies prevent the spirochetes' migration within the feeding tick from the gut into the salivary glands.
- Commercially available vaccines—contain nonadjuvanted recombinant OspA or OspA and numerous antigens (e.g., OspC) in adjuvans (bacterins) produced from inactivated cultured *Bb* organisms; protection rate improves over time due to booster immunizations that induce higher and longer lasting vaccine antibody titers
- Cage rest while lameness occurs—use pain medication or NSAIDs

Drugs of Choice

- Doxycycline or amoxicillin are the drugs of choice; doxycycline is preferred when this is a coinfection with *Anaplasma phagocytophilum* (Table 65-1).
- Other drugs that are effective—include azithromycin, penicillin G, and chloramphenicol

TABLE 65-1 Drug Therapy for Lyme Disease in Dogs				
Drug	Dose (mg/kg)	Route	Interval (h)	Duration (weeks)
Doxycycline	10	PO	12	4
Amoxicillin	20	PO	8–12	4

- Antibiotics do not eliminate persistent infection—significantly improve clinical signs and pathology

Precautions/Interactions

- Doxycycline should not be used in very young pups—can cause teeth staining

 COMMENTS

- Inform client—may need to use antibiotic therapy to control arthritic reoccurrences because antibiotics are rarely totally curative
- Acute arthritis—If no response within 3 days of starting antibiotics, reconsider diagnosis.
- Prevent tick engorgement—use repellents containing DEET or permethrin; tick collars; groom dogs daily
- Controlling tick population in the environment—restricted to small areas; limited results from reducing deer and/or rodent population
- Disease may be recurrent, with intervals of weeks to months—should respond again to antibiotic treatment
- The nonresponsive chronic arthritis seen in humans—not known in dogs
- *B. burgdorferi* in the saliva or urine of affected dogs—not transmissible to humans; humans exposed to the same environment as infected dogs are at risk of infection.
- Dogs not a source of infected ticks to humans—Once a tick starts feeding on a dog, it feeds to repletion and does not change hosts.
- No convincing evidence that *B. burgdorferi* infection is transmitted in utero in dogs—pregnant animals tolerate antibiotic treatment (do not use tetracyclines); maternal C6-specific antibodies can be passed from dams to puppies.

Abbreviations

ANA, antinuclear antibody; CBC, complete blood count; CSF, cerebrospinal fluid; ELISA, enzyme-linked immunosorbent assay; NSAIDs, nonsteroidal anti-inflammatory drugs; PCR, polymerase chain reaction; RMSF, Rocky Mountain spotted fever; WBC, white blood cell.

Suggested Reading

Greene CE, Straubinger RK. Borreliosis. In: Greene CE, ed. *Infectious Diseases of the Dog and Cat.* Philadelphia: WB Saunders, 2006:417–435.

Krupka I, Straubinger RK. Lyme borreliosis in dogs and cats: background, diagnosis, treatment and prevention of infection with Borrelia burgdorferi sensu stricto. *Vet Clin North Am Small Anim Pract* 2010;40:1103–1119.

Littman MP, Goldstein RE, Labato MA, et al. ACVIM small animal consensus statement on Lyme disease in dogs: diagnosis, treatment, and prevention. *J Vet Intern Med* 2006;20:422–434.

Töpfer KH, Straubinger RK. Characterization of the humoral immune response in dogs after vaccination against the Lyme borreliosis agent. A study with five commercial vaccines using two different vaccination schedules. i 2007;25:314–326.

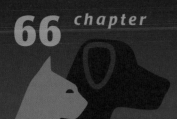

Mycobacterial Infections

DEFINITION/OVERVIEW

- Rare systemic and/or cutaneous bacterial infections of dogs and cats causing a myriad of clinical entities and syndromes depending on the organism species, how the organism enters the body, and the immune function of the host

ETIOLOGY/PATHOPHYSIOLOGY

- Mycobacteria—gram-positive, acid-fast bacteria (genus: *Mycobacterium*)
- Obligate or sporadic pathogens producing a wide range of syndromes in dogs and cats including those described in the following sections

Tuberculosis

- *Mycobacterium tuberculosis* (humans), *Mycobacterium bovis* (cattle and some wild mammals), and *Mycobacterium microti* (voles)
- Dogs and cats—exposed to infected primary hosts sporadically infected
- Dogs and cats—rare in developed countries
- Disseminated or multiorgan disease—caused by obligate parasitic organism

Leprosy

- *Mycobacterium lepraemurium* (from rodents) and two unnamed leprosy organisms

Cats

- Syndrome 1—affects young cats with localized nodular disease affecting limbs, with sparse to moderate numbers of acid-fast bacilli present in lesions (*M. lepraemurium*)
- Syndrome 2—affects old cats with generalized skin lesions with large numbers of acid-fast bacilli in lesions (unnamed species with affinity to *Mycobacterium malmoense*)

Dogs

- Canine leproid granuloma syndrome caused by unnamed and uncultured *Mycobacterium* spp. identified by DNA sequencing

Systemic or Noncutaneous Infection with Nontuberculosis Mycobacteria

- *M. chelonae-abscessus*, *M. avium* complex, *M. fortuitum*, *M. genavense*, *M. kansasii*, *M. smegmatis*, *M. thermoresistibile*, and *M. xenopi*
- Sporadic infections in dogs and cats
- Some patients with concurrent or immunosuppressing disease or the result of traumatic tissue introduction of saprophytic organism
- Syndromes include pleuritis, localized or disseminated granulomas, disseminated disease, neuritis, bronchopneumonia.

Cutaneous/Subcutaneous Infections Due to Rapidly Growing Mycobacteria (Mycobacterial Panniculitis

- Saprophytic mycobacteria *M. fortuitum*, *M. chelonae-abcessus*, *M. smegmatis*, *M. phlei*, and *M. thermoresistibile*

 SIGNALMENT/HISTORY

Tuberculosis

- Cats and dogs of any age
- Bassett hounds and Siamese cats reported as most susceptible—evidence unclear (possible statistical aberration)

Feline Leprosy

- Adult free-roaming cats and kittens
- Kittens and young adult cats in syndrome 1
- Older cats (average age 9 years) in syndrome 2

Canine Leproid Granuloma

- Reported cases—mainly in mostly short-haired, outdoor-housed, large-breed dogs, especially boxers, and German shepherd dogs

Systemic Nontuberculous Mycobacteriosis

- Sporadic diseas—can affect dogs and cats of any age

Mycobacterial Panniculitis

- Adult cats and dogs

   CLINICAL FEATURES

Tuberculosis

- Correlated with the route of exposure
- Major sites of involvement—oropharyngeal lymph nodes, cutaneous and subcutaneous tissues of the head and extremities, pulmonary system, GI system
- Dogs—respiratory, especially coughing; dyspnea uncommon
- Cats—from contaminated milk: weight loss, chronic diarrhea and thickened intestines; from predation: cutaneous nodules, ulcers, and draining tracts
- Virtually all dogs and many cats—pharyngeal and cervical lymphadenopathy; retching, ptyalism, or tonsillar abscess; lymph nodes are visible or palpably firm, fixed, tender; may ulcerate and drain
- Signs—fever, depression, partial anorexia, and weight loss
- Hypertrophic osteopathy—may occur
- Disseminated disease—body cavity effusion, visceral masses, bone or joint lesions, dermal and subcutaneous masses and ulcers, lymphadenopathy and/or abscesses, CNS signs, sudden death

Feline Leprosy

- Syndrome 1—initial localized nodules on limbs; progress rapidly, may ulcerate; aggressive clinical course; recurrence after surgical excision; widespread lesions develop in several weeks
- Syndrome 2—initial localized or generalized skin nodules that do not ulcerate, slowly progressive over months to years

Canine Leproid Granuloma

- One or more well-circumscribed painless nodules (2 mm to 5 cm) in dermis or subcutis; often on head or ear, but may be anywhere on the body; only very large lesions ulcerate (Fig. 66-1)
- No systemic signs of illness

Systemic Nontuberculous Mycobacteriosis

- Pulmonary and systemic infections with atypical mycobacteriosis are reported rarely in dogs—signs are as for TB
- With *M. avium* infection—disease is most often disseminated

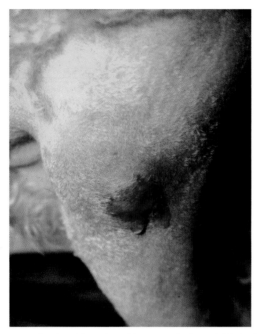

■ **Figure 66-1** This well-circumscribed, painless dermal lump on the lateral thigh of this dog was caused by *M. phlei.*

Mycobacterial Panniculitis

- Cutaneous traumatic lesion that fails to heal with appropriate therapy
- Spreads locally in the subcutaneous tissue (panniculitis)
- Original lesion enlarges, forming a deep ulcer that drains greasy hemorrhagic exudate
- Surrounding tissue becomes firm
- Satellite pinpoint ulcerations open and drain (Fig. 66-2)

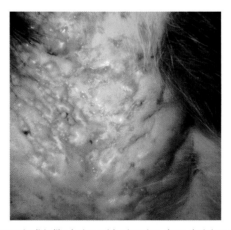

■ **Figure 66-2** A large, firm panniculitis-like lesion with pinpoint, deep draining ulcers covering the ventrum of a cat, caused by
M. smegmatis.

- Wound dehiscence at surgery sites
- Systemic signs uncommon

 ## DIFFERENTIAL DIAGNOSIS

Tuberculosis

- Systemic mycoses, neoplasia (lymphoma), disseminated mast cell tumor, systemic histiocytosis, plague, nocardiosis, and other myobacterial infections

Feline Leprosy

- Plague, L-form bacterial infections, *Rhodococcus equi* infection, chronic bite wound abscess, neoplasia, mycetoma, dermatophyte pseudomycetoma, and other mycobacterial infections (especially cutaneous tuberculosis)
- If acid-fast organisms are identified on cytology/biopsy—consider tuberculosis or cutaneous nocardiosis, both of which can be fastidious and slow growing in culture, leading to the suspicion of an unculturable leprosy organism

Atypical Mycobacteriosis

- Foreign body, bacterial abscess, L-form bacteria, feline leprosy, cutaneous tuberculosis, *R. equi* infection, nocardiosis, sterile nodular panniculitis, deep pyoderma and cellulites, leishmaniasis, mast cell tumor, and sweat gland neoplasia

 ## DIAGNOSTICS

- CBC—Nonregenerative normocytic normochromic anemia is common.
- Intradermal skin test with BCG—may produce false-positive results
- Radiographs—thoracic, abdominal, or skeletal lesions suggest granulomatous infectious disease
- No pathognomonic radiographic lesions for mycobacteriosis—pulmonary tuberculosis may become calcified or cavitated

Diagnostic Feature

- **Definitive diagnosis—made on biopsy and culture results**
- Ensure—biopsy uncontaminated by surface bacteria and incorporates the center of the granulomatous focus
- Aspirate cytologic specimens—from lesions, transtracheal wash, rectal cytology, enlarged lymph nodes, or smears from affected tissue to detect acid-fast bacilli can be effective
- Culture—submit heat-fixed smears and tissue; special media and techniques are required; isolate identification can take several weeks

THERAPEUTICS

- Feline leprosy—cured by surgical excision of lesions
- Subcutaneous atypical mycobacteriosis—may be aided by debulking surgery
- Benefit of surgery in conjunction with aggressive medical treatment—undefined

Tuberculosis

Primary

- Always—use double- or triple-drug oral therapy
- Never—attempt single-drug therapy of any organism
- Current recommendation—fluoroquinolone (e.g., enrofloxacin) combined with clarithromycin and rifampin for 6–9 months; enrofloxacin, orbifloxacin, ciprofloxacin
- Rifampin (Rifadin; Marion Merrell Dow)—reduce dosage in hepatic dysfunction or biliary obstruction; may cause hepatotoxicity, dermatologic signs in some cats (erythema, pruritus, dyspnea due to anaphylaxis
- Clarithromycin (Biaxin; Abbott Laboratories)—Side effects include GI tract upsets, anorexia, diarrhea, but usually less likely to occur than with erythromycin.

Alternatives

- Isoniazid and rifampin combination—mainly used in past; little known about their use in cats; one recent report of treatment in a cat with isoniazid, rifampin, and dihydrostreptomycin for 3 months noted weight loss but eventual cure
- Isoniazid (Laniazid; Novartis)—Side effects include vomiting, hepatoxicity, and vitamin B_6 deficiency causing tonic/clonic seizures in dogs.
- Ethambutol (Myambutol; Lederle)—reduce dose by extending dosing interval in renal insufficiency
- Pyrazinamide—instead of ethambutol
- Dihydrostreptomycin—not available currently for small animal use

Feline Leprosy

- Dapsone (Dapsone; Jacobus Pharmaceuticals)—reduced dosage in renal failure; may cause skin eruptions, vomiting, diarrhea, CNS signs, and myelotoxicity
- Clofazimine (Lamprene; Novartis)—not to be used in pregnant animals; avoid in pre-existing GI tract disease
- Rifampin

Atypical Mycobacteriosis

- Chemotherapy—may use in vitro sensitivity testing to choose drug
- Antibiotics—macrolides, sulfonamides, tetracyclines, aminoglycosides and fluoroquinolones generally effective

TABLE 66-1 Drug Therapy for Mycobacterial Infections in Cats and Dogs

Syndrome	Drug	Dose (mg/kg)	Route	Interval (h)	Duration (months)
Tuberculosis	Fluoroquinolone[a]	5–15	PO	24	6–9
	Clarithromycin	5–10	PO	24	6–9
	Rifampin	10–20	PO	24[b]	6–9
Feline leprosy	Dapsone[c]	1[d]	PO	12	1
	Clofazimine	2–8	PO	24	1[e]
	Rifampin	10–20	PO	24[b]	6
Atypical mycobacteriosis	Gentamicin	2	SC, IM	8–12	1[f]
	Kanamycin	5	SC, IM	12	1[f]
	Amikacin	5–10	SC, IM	8–12	1[f]
	Doxycycline	5–10	PO, IV	12	1–2
	TMS	15–30[g]	PO	12	1–2
	Enrofloxacin	5–15	PO	12–24	1–4
M. avium	Clofazimine	2–8	PO	24	1–2[e]
M. fortuitum subcutaneous disease	Enrofloxacin 2.27% topical[h]	1 ml[i]	Topical	12	2–6

[a]Enroflaxacin, orbifloxacin, or ciprofloxacin; use in combination with clarithromycin and rifampin.
[b]Or divided q12h to a maximal daily dose of 600 mg.
[c]Use in combination with clofazamine and rifampin.
[d]Up to a total dose of 50 mg/cat.
[e]After first month, every 3–4 days for 1–2 months.
[f]Four weeks is maximal treatment period (usually only 2 weeks needed); monitor for renal toxicity by examining urine for casts; combine with other nonaminoglycoside drugs.
[g]Use lower dose for cats (10–15 mg/kg).
[h]Topical solution in 90% DMSO at a 1:1 v/v ratio.
[i]Up to a total systemic dose of 5 mg/kg (each milliliter of solution contains approximately 12 mg).
TMS, trimethoprime-sulfadiazine.

- Fluoroquinolone combined with clarithromycin—good empirical treatment; use same dosages as for tuberculosis; treat for 2–6 months; relapses during course of or after completion of treatment common
- *M. avium*—clofazimine
- Subcutaneous disease (*M. fortuitum*)—topical treatment with a 1:1 solution of 2.27% enrofloxacin in 90% DMSO has been used successfully in cats; applied 1 ml, q12h, for a total systemic dosage of 5 mg/kg; continue treatment for 2–6 months; relapses after stop treatment are common (Table 66-1)

Precautions/Interactions

- Traditional antituberculosis drugs—be alert for any adverse reactions; experience limited, especially in cats
- Isoniazid—liver toxicity, seizures, neuritis, and drug eruption in humans

- Ethambutol—optic neuritis in humans
- Pyrazinamide—liver toxicity in humans
- Rifampin—anorexia, vomiting, and liver toxicity
- Dapsone—hemolytic anemia, other immune-mediated blood abnormalities, and liver toxicity
- Clofazimine—orange discoloration of fat, diarrhea and/or weight loss, and hepatic enzyme elevation
- Dihydrostreptomycin—hearing loss and renal toxicity
- Antituberculosis and antileprosy drugs—examine at least monthly; monitor for anorexia and weight loss

 COMMENTS

- Monitor—hepatic enzymes monthly
- Instruct clients—to report cutaneous lesions immediately
- Clinicians aware of a human tuberculosis case in a household with dogs or cats—should counsel owners about the risk to the pets in the household
- Tuberculosis—guarded prognosis, but currently undefined because experience of modern drug use is limited
- Feline leprosy—fair prognosis, especially if lesions are amenable to surgical removal
- Prognosis in subcutaneous atypical mycobacteriosis—good for survival but guarded for resolution; relapse after cessation of long-term antibiotic therapy occurs in >40% of cats treated with single-agent therapy
- Prognosis in pulmonary and disseminated atypical mycobacteriosis—guarded, but may be improved with modern agents and double-drug treatment
- Zoonosis—potentially
  - Tuberculosis—Affected pets pose a zoonotic threat to owners; public health authorities should be notified of any antemortum or postmortem diagnosis (required by law in some states); do not attempt treatment without concurrence of public health authorities.
  - *M. tuberculosis*—greatest potential for zoonosis, especially with draining cutaneous lesions
  - Disease transmission between pets and humans—very rarely recorded; in recent outbreaks of tuberculosis in cats, no transmission to humans was reported

Abbreviations

BCG, bacillus Calmette-Guérin; CBC, complete blood count; CNS, central nervous system; DMSO, dimethylsulfoxide; DNA, deoxyribonucleic acid; GI, gastrointestinal; TB, tuberculosis.

Suggested Reading

Courtin F, Huerre M, Fyfe J, et al. A case of feline leprosy caused by *Mycobacterium lepraemurium* originating from the island of Kythira (Greece): diagnosis and treatment. *J Feline Med Surg* 2007;9:238–241.

Greene CE. Mycobacterial infections. In: Greene CE, ed. *Infectious Diseases of the Dog and Cat*. Philadelphia: WB Saunders, 2006:462–488.

Moriello KA. Clinical snapshot. Feline leprosy. *Compend Contin Educ Vet* 2007;29:256–261.

Microsporidiosis

chapter 67

DEFINITION/OVERVIEW

- Uncommon protozoal disease (formally named Encephalitozoonosis) of dogs and cats with a wide host range (including humans, rabbits, mice, foxes) in the United States
- Causes lung, heart, kidney, and brain involvement

ETIOLOGY/PATHOPHYSIOLOGY

- *Encephalitozoon cuniculi* (and other species)—obligate intracellular protozoan (phylum Microspora)
- Mature spores—possess a polar filament and extrusion apparatus that distinguishes microsporidia from other protozoa
- Infection—ingestion or inhalation of spores from urine or feces shed by infected host
- Inoculation—transplacental and traumatic inoculation reported
- Once internalized—spores invade host cells, multiply by schizogony, rupture cells to invade others or are shed in urine or feces
- Localized infections—occur in kidney, liver, and brain of cats
- Natural infections—rare in cats and dogs (no prevalence data reported)
- Kennels of dogs—whole kennel can be infected at once

SIGNALMENT/HISTORY

- No sex or breed predilection
- Young animals (kittens) show more signs than older cats.

CLINICAL FEATURES

Neonates

- Signs—develop a few weeks postpartum
- Growth—stunted

- Unthriftiness—progresses to renal failure
- Neurologic abnormalities—possible

Adults

- Can include similar signs as neonates but usually not as severe
- Aggressive behavior
- Seizures
- Blindness

 ## DIFFERENTIAL DIAGNOSIS

- Other infectious diseases causing neurologic signs—rabies, distemper, toxoplasmosis, *Neospora* infections, FeLV, cuterebriasis, systemic mycoses, GME, toxins (lead), hepatic encephalopathy

 ## DIAGNOSTICS

- CBC—mild normocytic, normochromic anemia, lymphocytosis, monocytosis
- Biochemistry profile—elevated serum ALT and ALP
- Serologic examination—IFA on CSF or blood (commercially available)
- IFA serum titer >1:20 considered positive—suggests previous exposure and not necessarily active infection
- IFA—send refrigerated serum or CSF to Texas Veterinary Medical Diagnostic Laboratory
- Detect spores in urine, feces, or tissues—using Gram's or Ziehl–Neelson stains to identify organisms in renal epithelial cells
- Modified trichrome stains—excellent for tissue spores (stain bright pink with pink band and clear posterior vacuole; Fig. 67-1)

Diagnostic Feature

- **Electronmicroscopy—still considered the definitive diagnostic technique of choice**

 ## THERAPEUTICS

- None reported to be effective
- Euthanasia is indicated when severe neurologic signs develop.

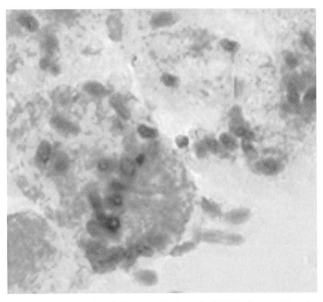

■ **Figure 67-1** Kidney aspirate from a dog infected with *E. cuniculi*. Note the bright pink organisms (modified trichrome stain, 1000×).

TABLE 67-1 **Suggested Drug Therapy for Encephalitozoonosis in Dogs and Cats**				
Drug	Dose (mg/kg)	Route	Interval (h)	Duration (days)
Fenbendazole (Panacur)	50	PO	24	14[a]
Albendazole (Valbazen)	50	PO	8	7[b]

[a]Proposed by consulting editor. A dose of 20 mg/kg, PO, q24h for 7 days treats rabbits, or medicated in feed for 4 weeks prevents infection in rabbits.
[b]This dose is effective in mice and humans; may cause myelosuppression in dogs and cats—monitor CBC.

Drugs of Choice

- Albendazole (Valbazen; Pfizer)
- Fenbendazole (Panacur; Intervet) (Table 67-1)

Precautions/Interactions

- Albendazole—reported to cause myelosuppression in cats and dogs

COMMENTS

- Currently—No effective drugs have been described in dogs and cats

- Fenbendazole—although not reported for the treatment of *E. cuniculi* infections in cats and dogs, would probably be worth trying
- Zoonosis—especially a risk to immunosuppressed humans
- Sanitation—70% ethanol

Abbreviations

ALP, alkaline phosphatase; ALT, alanine aminotransferase; CBC, complete blood count; CSF, cerebrospinal fluid; FeLV, feline leukemia virus; GME, granulomatous meningoencephalitis; IFA, indirect fluorescent antibody.

Suggested Reading

Didier PJ, Snowden K, Alvarez X, et al. Microsporidiosis. In: Greene CE, ed. *Infectious Diseases of the Dog and Cat*. Philadelphia: WB Saunders, 2006:711–716.

Snowden KF, Lewis BC, Hoffman J, et al. *Encephalitozoon cuniculi* infection in dogs: a case series. *J Am Anim Hosp Assoc* 2009;45:225–231.

Suter C, Muller–Doblies UU, Hatt JM, et al. Prevention and treatment of *Encephalitozoon cuniculi* infection in rabbits with fenbendazole. *Vet Rec* 2001;148:478–480.

Mycoplasmosis

chapter 68

DEFINITION/OVERVIEW

- A variety of systemic illnesses (respiratory, urogenital, gastrointestinal, ophthalmic, and musculoskeletal) in dogs and cats caused by a small group of prokaryotic organisms

ETIOLOGY/PATHOPHYSIOLOGY

- Fastidious, facultative anaerobic gram-negative rods—forming the smallest (0.2–0.3 mm) and simplest prokaryotic cells capable of self-replication (by binary fission)
- Lack a cell wall—makes them sensitive to lysis by osmotic shock, detergents, and alcohols
- Ubiquitous in nature as parasites, commensals, or saprophytes in animals, plants, and insects—many are pathogens of humans, animals, plants, and insects
- Often part of resident flora—commensals on mucous membranes of upper respiratory, digestive, and genital tracts
- Pathogenicity and role in disease—often controversial and poorly understood
- Frequent inhabitants of mucosal membranes—*Mycoplasma gateae* or *Mycoplasma felis* found in oral cavity or urogenital tract of 70–80% of healthy cats
- Rate of isolation in diseased dogs—much higher than in normal dogs (e.g., lung, uterus, prepuce)
- *Mycoplasma* spp.—show considerable host specificity
- Require—direct contact with host cell to obtain nutrients
- Induces primarily a humoral immune response—induces a fibrinous exudate, which protects organism from antibodies and antimicrobial drugs and contributes to chronicity of infection
- Secondary bacterial invaders—common

SIGNALMENT/HISTORY

- Commensals—occasionally cause systemic infection associated with immunodeficiency, immunosuppression, or cancer
- Impaired resistance of the host—may allow organisms to cross the mucosal barrier and disseminate
- Predisposing factors—stresses such as reproductive problems associated with overcrowded housing or local tissue injury (from urinary tract neoplasms or urinary calculi)
- Historical findings—reflect organ system involved

 ## CLINICAL FEATURES

Dogs

- Respiratory (often associated with fever, malaise):
  - Pneumonia
  - Upper respiratory tract infection
- Urogenital—urinary and genital tract infections:
  - Balanoposthitis
  - Urethritis
  - Prostatitis
  - Cystitis
  - Nephritis
  - Vaginitis
  - Endometritis
- Reproductive:
  - Infertility
  - Early embryonic death
  - Abortion
  - Stillbirths or weak newborns
  - Neonatal mortality
- Musculoskeletal—arthritis
- Gastrointestinal—colitis

Cats

- Ophthalmic—conjunctivitis
- Respiratory—pneumonia, uppper respiratory tract infection
- Musculoskeletal—chronic fibrinopurulent polyarthritis and tenosynovitis
- Urogenital—urinary tract infections
- Reproductive—abortions and fetal deaths
- Skin—chronic cutaneous abscesses

DIFFERENTIAL DIAGNOSIS

- Canine and feline upper respiratory tract infection—viruses (parainfluenza virus, canine distemper, herpes virus, feline calcivirus, reovirus); *Chlamydia psittaci*; bacteria (*Bordetella bronchiseptica*, staphylococci, streptococci, and coliforms)
- Canine and feline UTI—bacteria (staphylococci, streptococci, coliforms), fungi (*Candida* spp.), and parasites
- Canine infertility, early embryonic death, abortion, stillbirths or weak newborns, and neonatal mortality—bacteria (*Brucella, Salmonella* spp., *Campylobacter* spp., *Escherichia coli*, streptococcus), viruses (CHV, canine distemper, CAV), *Toxoplasma gondii*, and endocrinopathies (progesterone deficiency, hypothyroidism)
- Canine prostatitis—bacteria (*E. coli, Brucella canis*) and fungi (*Blastomyces dermatitidis, Cryptococcus neoformans*)
- Canine and feline arthritis—immune-mediated; bacteria (staphylococci, streptococci, coliforms, anaerobes), bacterial L-forms, rickettsia (*Ehrlichia* spp.), *Borrelia burgdorferi*; fungi (*Coccidioides* spp., *Cryptococcus neoformans, Blastomyces dermatitidis*), protozoa (*Leishmania* spp.), viruses (FCV)
- Feline conjunctivitis—FHV, FCV, feline reovirus, *Chlamydia psittaci*, and bacteria

DIAGNOSTICS

- CBC—mild anemia, neutrophilic leukocytosis (polyarthritis, pneumonia)
- Serum biochemical profile—hypoalbuminemia, hyperglobulinemia (polyarthritis)
- Urinalysis—proteinuria resulting from immune-complex glomerulonephritis
- Radiographic examination of arthritic joints—no radiographic changes
- Serologic assays are available in some diagnostic laboratories—Value of serology is controversial given that commensal organisms also produce a titer.
- PCR—becoming more available through some commercial diagnostic laboratories

Diagnostic Feature

- **Diagnostic challenge is to distinguish between commensal organisms and those causing pathology.**
- Organisms are difficult to demonstrate in and from tissues—extremely pleomorphic, in smears (e.g., conjunctival scrapings) seen as coccobacilli, coccal forms, ring forms, spirals, and filaments; stain poorly (gram-negative), preferred staining method is by Giemsa or other Romanowsky stains
- Scanning electron microscopy—demonstrates organism
- Definitive diagnosis based on isolation and identification or detection of the *Mycoplasma* organisms in tissues by a fluorescent antibody procedure—submit cotton swabs placed in Hayflicks broth medium or use commercially available swabs

(cool specimens and ship on ice if to arrive at lab in less than 24 hours; if longer, freeze samples and ship on dry ice)
- Culture—requires special medium (check that laboratory can perform culture before sending samples)

 ## THERAPEUTICS

Drugs of Choice

- Doxycycline—treat for extended periods (6 weeks)
- Tetracyclines
- Chloramphenicol
- Alternative drugs—gentamicin, kanamycin, spectinomycin, spiramycin, tylosin, erythromycin, nitrofurans, and fluoroquinolones (Table 68-1)
- Topical antibiotic—conjunctivitis
- Resistant—to sulfonamides and β-lactams that inhibit peptidoglycan synthesis because organisms lack a cell wall
- No standardized procedure for in vitro antimicrobial susceptibility tests

Precautions/Interactions

- Improper use of topical steroid ointments with conjunctivitis—may prolong infection and predispose to corneal ulceration
- Tetracycline and chloramphenicol should not be used in pregnant animals—use erythromycin instead
- Chloramphenicol—may cause myelosuppression (reversible if stop drug); warn owners to only handle the drug while wearing gloves because it can cause fatal, irreversible idiosyncratic pancytopenia in some humans.
- Doxycycline—may cause esophagitis and esophageal stricture in some cats
- Doxycycline—contraindicated in pregnant or lactating bitches
- Tetracyclines—may cause dental discoloration in young animals; do not give to animals with renal failure

TABLE 68-1 Drug Therapy for *Mycoplasma* Infections in Cats and Dogs				
Drug	Dose (mg/kg)	Route	Interval (h)	Duration (weeks)
Doxycycline	5	PO, IV	12	4–6
Tetracycline	22	PO	8	4–6
Chloramphenicol	50	PO, IV, IM, SC	8–12	4–6
Erythromycin	10–20	PO	8–12	4–6
Enrofloxacin	5	PO	12–24	4–6

COMMENTS

- Organisms readily killed by drying, sunshine, or any chemical disinfectant.
- Not generally considered zoonotic
- Suppurative mycoplasmal tenosynovitis has been reported in a veterinarian following a scratch from a cat being treated for colitis.

Abbreviations

CAV, canine adenovirus; CBC, complete blood count; CHV, canine herpes virus; FCV, feline calcivirus; FHV, feline herpes virus; PCR, polymerase chain reaction; UTI, urinary tract infection.

Suggested Reading

Chalker VJ. Canine mycoplasmas. *Res Vet Sci* 2005;79:1–8.

Greene CE. Mycoplasmal, ureaplasmal, and L-form infections. In: Greene CE, ed. *Infectious Diseases of the Dog and Cat*. Philadelphia: WB Saunders, 2006:260–265.

Sasaki Y. Mycoplasma. In: Chan VL, Sherman PM, Bourke B, eds. *Bacterial Genomes and Infectious Diseases*. Totowa, NJ: Humana Press, 2006:175–190.

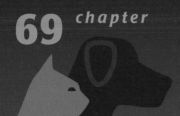

Nasal Capillariasis
(*Eucoleus*)

DEFINITION/OVERVIEW

- Nematode found in mucosa of nasal passages and sinuses of dogs
- Usually asymptomatic but can cause chronic sneezing and nasal discharge
- Often misidentified as *Eucoleus* (=*Capillaria*) *aerophilus* because eggs are nearly identical

ETIOLOGY/PATHOPHYSIOLOGY

- *Eucoleus boehmi*—capillarid parasite
- Life cycle—unknown but thought to be either direct or through earthworm paratenic hosts
- Adults (long; up to 4 cm, and thin) embed in epithelial lining of the nasal turbinates, frontal, and paranasal sinuses.
- Parasite produces—local inflammation and an allergic rhinitis
- PPP = 1 month

SIGNALMENT/HISTORY

- Few case reports but most described in young dogs

CLINICAL FEATURES

- Most cases are asymptomatic
- Chronic sneezing
- Mucopurulent nasal discharge (occasionally bloody)
- Epistaxis
- Face rubbing

DIFFERENTIAL DIAGNOSIS

- Signs of sneezing with nasal discharge—other parasitic infections (*Pneumonyssoides caninum* and *Linguatula serrata*), other infections (bacterial, fungal such as aspergillosis), allergic rhinitis, nasal foreign body, dental disease, and neoplasia
- Sneezing—more characteristic of parasitic infection or acute foreign body than neoplasia, which presents more often with nasal obstruction or discharge
- Reverse sneezing—not usually accompanied by nasal discharge

DIAGNOSTICS

Diagnostic Feature

- **Bi-operculate eggs in feces need to be differentiated from those of *Eucoleus* (=*Capillaria*) *aerophilus*, *Pearsonema* (=*Capillaria*) *plica* (eggs usually in urine but can be passed in feces if ingested by dog or urine contaminates feces), or *Trichuris vulpis* (Fig. 69-1).**
- Eggs—if in nasal discharges, will only be E. *boehmi*, unless dog has E. *aerophilus* and has coughed up lower airway discharges through the nose
- Nasal wash—diagnostic if contains bi-operculate eggs

THERAPEUTICS

- Ivermectin and fenbendazole are effective in alleviating clinical signs, but relapses may occur, so follow-up treatment may be necessary after a month of initial presentation.

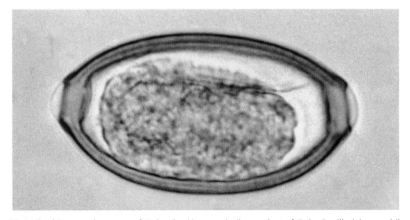

■ **Figure 69-1** The bi-operculate egg of *E. boehmi* is very similar to that of *E.* (=*Capillaria*) *aerophilus*, which resides in the lungs. Both eggs can be found in the feces of infected dogs and differ only in that the surface of *E. boehmi* eggs are covered in small pits similar to a thimble, whereas the eggs of *E. aerophilus* are not.

TABLE 69-1 Drug Therapy for Nasal Capillariasis (*E. boehmi*) in Dogs

Drug	Dose (mg/kg)	Route	Interval (h)	Repeat Interval (months)
Ivermectin	0.2	PO, SC	Once	1
Milbemycine oxime	2	PO	Once	1
Fenbendazole	50	PO	10–14	1

Drugs of Choice

- Neither drug is registered for the treatment of *E. boehmi* in the dog
- Ivermectin or milbemycin oxime
- Fenbendazole (Table 69-1)

Precautions/Interactions

- Ensure—dog does not have microfilaremia before administering ivermectin
- Ivermectin-sensitive collie and collie-cross—dogs may show neurologic signs with this dose of ivermectin

COMMENTS

- The life cycle of *E. boehmi* is unknown; however, it is reasonable to expect it to be similar to *Capillaria* and therefore implement similar control methods used for urinary capillariasis.
- Dogs should be maintained away from soil, on wire-bottomed enclosures or impervious pavements or at least sand devoid of vegetation (where earthworms, the probably intermediate host, are unlikely to survive).
- Direct sunshine effectively kills eggs.
- Treatment failures using fenbendazole and ivermectin have been reported—close follow-up is necessary.

Abbreviation

PPP, prepatent period.

Suggested Reading

Conboy G. Helminth parasites of the canine and feline respiratory tract. *Vet Clin Small Anim* 2009;39:1109–1126.

chapter 70

Nasal Mites (Pneumonyssoides)

DEFINITION/OVERVIEW

- Arthropod found in the nasal cavity and sinuses of dogs, leading to sneezing, chronic nasal discharge, and epistaxis

ETIOLOGY/PATHOPHYSIOLOGY

- *Pneumonyssoides caninum*—mite
- Transmission—direct contact with an infested animal
- The mite causes inflammation of the nasal mucosa (especially the olfactory area), possibly leading to a loss of sense of smell by the host.

SIGNALMENT/HISTORY

- Although not common in North America, the prevalence can be high in some northern European countries (20% in Sweden, 7% in Norway).
- No sex, breed, or age distribution, although dogs >3 years of age are more likely to be infested.
- Most clinically apparent infestations require large numbers (>50) of mites, whereas small numbers (<20) often cause no clinical signs.

CLINICAL FEATURES

- Sneezing—often reverse sneezing
- Epistaxis
- Chronic nasal discharge
- Signs of nasal irritation are pawing face, rubbing face against objects and the ground.
- May see mites on the outside of the nose (Fig. 70-1)
- One study suggests that nasal mite infestation predisposes large-breed dogs to gastric dilatation-volvulus because excessive aerophagia can occur during reverse sneezing.

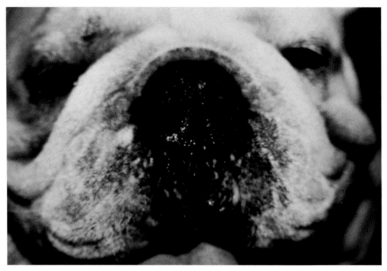

■ **Figure 70-1** Nose of an English bulldog covered in small white dots, which are the mites of *P. caninum*.

 ## DIFFERENTIAL DIAGNOSIS

- Sneezing with nasal discharge need to be differentiated from:
  - Other parasitic infestations, including *Linguatula serrata* and *Eucoleus boehmi*
  - Nasal foreign body
  - Neoplasia
  - Allergic rhinitis
- Sneezing is more characteristic of parasitic infection or acute foreign body rather than neoplasia (which presents more often with nasal obstruction or discharge).
- Reverse sneezing is not usually accompanied by nasal discharge.

 ## DIAGNOSTICS

- Large (pin head sized) white mites visible to the naked eye—can be detected by rhinoscopy (or otoscope inserted into the nares), or in nasal flushings
- Microscopy—Mites have uncomplicated leg tips unadorned by suckers or hooks (Fig. 70-2).
- Rhinoscopy—Mites scurry away from the bright light of the scope.

Diagnostic Feature

- **Mites dislike isoflurothane gas, so they will often appear at entrance of nares in anesthetized patient.**
- Mild eosinophilia may be present.

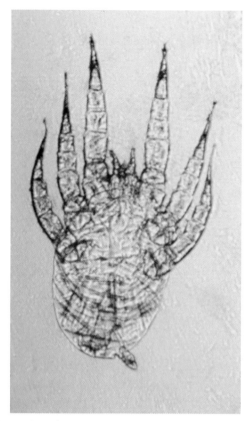

■ **Figure 70-2** The *P. caninum* mite is characterized by its large size and long legs without hooks or suckers.

Drugs of Choice

- Ivermectin (Ivermec; Merial)
- Milbemycin oxime (Interceptor; Novartis) (Table 70-1)
- Selamectin (Revolution; Pfizer Animal Health)—reported to be effective experimentally and in clinical cases
- All 3 drugs should provide prompt improvement of clinical signs.
- None of the drugs are registered for this use in dogs.

TABLE 70-1 **Drug Therapy for *P. caninum* in Dogs**				
Drug	Dose (mg/kg)	Route	Interval (weeks)	Duration (weeks)
Ivermectin (Ivermec)	0.2	PO, SC	1	3
Milbemycin oxime (Interceptor)	0.5–1	PO	1	3
Selamectin (Revolution)	6–24	Topical	2	6

Precautions/Interactions

- Ensure that patients do not have microfilaremia before administering ivermectin.
- Ivermectin-sensitive collie or collie-cross dogs may show neurologic signs with this dose of ivermectin.

 COMMENTS

- Treat all in contact animals.
- It is unlikely that mites survive in the environment for long.
- Keep dogs away from foxes, which can carry mites.

Suggested Reading

Gunnarsson LK, Moller LC, Einarsson AM, et al. Clinical efficacy of milbemycin oxime in the treatment of nasal mite infection in dogs. *J Am Anim Hosp Assoc* 1999;35:81–84.

Gunnarsson L, Zakrisson G, Christensson D, et al. Efficacy of selamectin in the treatment of nasal mite (*Pneumonyssoides caninum*) infection in dogs. *Am Anim Hosp Assoc* 2004;40:400–404.

Wills SJ, Arrese M, Torrance A, et al. *Pneumonyssoides* species infestation in two Pekingese dogs in the UK. *J Small Anim Pract* 2008;49:107–109.

chapter 71

Neosporosis

DEFINITION/OVERVIEW

- A protozoal (coccidian) disease causing tissue damage (by necrosis mainly of nerve tissue and muscle) from cyst rupture and tachyzoite invasion in dogs

ETIOLOGY/PATHOPHYSIOLOGY

- *Neospora caninum*—Tachyzoites and tissue cysts resemble *Toxoplasma gondii* under light microscopy.
- Dogs (and coyotes)—definitive host; excrete oocysts in feces
- Oocysts sporulate to become infective after 24 hours—infective to other dogs and intermediate hosts, including cattle, goats, horses, sheep, and cats (experimentally)
- Of little clinical significance in intermediate hosts—except cattle, in which abortion and stillbirths can cause a loss of production in some herds
- Transmission—transplacental, resulting in congenital infection
- Transmission—ingestion of sporulated oocysts passed in feces of dogs or coyotes or tissue cysts in tissues of intermediate hosts (e.g., dogs ingesting infected bovine fetal membranes)

SIGNALMENT/HISTORY

- Natural infections occur in dogs, with hunting/farm dogs over-represented.
- Serologic prevalence in farm dogs—usually >30%
- Puppies (<6 months of age)—over-represented
- Cats—no natural cases have been reported in cats.

CLINICAL FEATURES

- Similar to those of toxoplasmosis, except neurologic and muscular abnormalities predominate and are often more severe
- Young dogs (<6 months of age):
  - Ascending paralysis is common.
  - Distinguished from other forms of paralysis by gradual muscle atrophy
  - Stiffness of pelvic limbs; affected more than thoracic limbs
  - Progresses to rigid contracture of limbs
  - Lower motor neuron paralysis (Fig. 71-1)
  - Cervical weakness and dysphagia gradually develop, leading to death.
  - Cerebellar atrophy with associated ataxia is reported, although rare (Fig. 71-2).
- Older dogs:
  - Usually display CNS involvement (seizures, tremors)
  - Polymyositis and myocarditis reported
  - Like toxoplasmosis, virtually any organ can be affected.
  - Head tremors
  - Postural deficits from cerebellar disease
  - Horner's syndrome also reported.
- Generalized ulcerative and pyogranulomatous dermatitis reported in dogs on immunosuppressive therapy (mainly for SLE or lymphosarcoma)—large numbers of tachyzoites present in dermal lesions

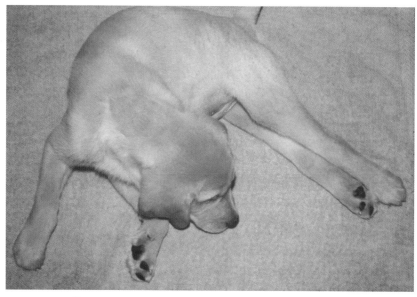

■ **Figure 71-1** Puppy affected with clinical neosporosis, showing pelvic limb muscle contracture forcing the limbs into rigid extension (courtesy of Dr. A. Delahunta, Cornell University).

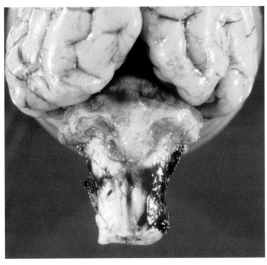

■ **Figure 71-2** Cerebellar atrophy can occur in young dogs from *N. caninum* infection (courtesy of Dr. A. Delahunta, Cornell University).

DIFFERENTIAL DIAGNOSIS

- Young dogs—other causes of peripheral multifocal neurologic signs, infectious diseases (toxoplasmosis, distemper), progressive polyradiculoneuritis, botulism, tick bite paralysis
- Other causes of diffuse lower motor neuron muscular diseases—are rare in young dogs
- Older dogs with CNS disease—other infectious diseases (fungal, rabies, pseudorabies), toxicity (lead, organophosphate, carbamate, chlorinated hydrocarbon, strychnine), nonsuppurative encephalitis, meningitis, GME, and metabolic disease (hypoglycemia, hepatic encephalopathy), and neoplasia

DIAGNOSTICS

- CBC, biochemical panel, urinalysis findings—nonspecific, depending on organ systems involved
- CK and AST activities—with muscle involvement
- CSF—usually a slight increase in protein concentration and nucleated cell counts (usually mononuclear but neutrophils can be seen); some cases have higher numbers of eosinophils
- Serologic testing (IFA)—CSF or serum; antibodies do not cross-react with *T. gondii* (ELISA available for testing cattle)

TABLE 71-1 Drug Therapy for Neosporosis

Drug	Dose (mg/kg)	Route	Interval (h)	Duration (weeks)
Clindamycin	12.5–25	PO, IM	12	4[a]
Trimethoprim-sulfadiazine	15–20	PO	12	4[a]
Pyrimethamine[b]	1	PO	24	4

[a]Continue at least until 2 weeks after signs have plateaued.
[b]Use in combination with trimethoprim-sulfadiazine.

- PCR—described but not yet commercially available; differentiate *N. caninum* from *T. gondii* in CSF; another differentiates *N. caninum* from *Hammondia* cysts in fecal samples

THERAPEUTICS

- Once muscle contracture or ascending paralysis has occurred—Prognosis for clinical improvement is poor.
- Progression of clinical signs—may be arrested by treatment

Drugs of Choice

- Clindamycin—continue for at least 2 weeks after clinical signs cleared or plateaued
- TMS and pyrimethamine—may also be used (Table 71-1)

Precautions/Interactions

- Reduce dose of clindamycin in renal failure, hepatic dysfunction, or biliary obstruction from any cause.
- May cause GI signs (vomiting, diarrhea, anorexia), and transient diarrhea—Temporarily discontinue dosing until signs stop, then reinstitute at half the dose, working up to full dose.

COMMENTS

- No zoonotic potential identified.
- Serologically test littermates and dam, along with any cattle if patient is from a farm.
- Prevent contamination of cattle feed with dog feces—Prevent dog from eating bovine fetal membranes.

- Only way to prevent transmission cycle between dogs and cattle—remove dogs from the farm
- Feeding raw meet to dogs increases risk of infection.

Abbreviations

AST, aspartate aminotransferase; CBC, complete blood count; CK, creatine kinase; CNS, central nervous system; CSF, cerebrospinal fluid; ELISA, enzyme-linked immunosorbent assay; GI, gastrointestinal; GME, granulomatous meningoencephalitis; IFA, immunofluorescent antibody; PCR, polymerase chain reaction; SLE, systemic lupus erythematosus; TMS, trimethoprim-sulfadiazine.

Suggested Reading

Dubey JP, Lindsay DS, Lappin MR. Toxoplasmosis and other intestinal coccidial infections in cats and dogs. *Vet Clin Small Anim Pract* 2009;39:1009–1034.

Dubey JP, Vianna MC, Kwok OC, et al. Neosporosis in Beagle dogs: clinical signs, diagnosis, treatment, isolation and genetic characterization of *Neospora caninum*. *Vet Parasitol* 2007;149:158–166.

Reichel MP, Ellis JT, Dubey JP. Neosporosis and hammondiosis in dogs. *J Small Anim Pract* 2007;48:308–312.

Windsor RC, Sturges BK, Vernau KM, et al. Cerebrospinal fluid eosinophilia in dogs. *J Vet Intern Med* 2009;23:275–281.

Nocardiosis

DEFINITION/OVERVIEW

- An uncommon bacterial infection of dogs and cats usually presenting as pyothorax, nonhealing cutaneous wounds, or systemic infection (although rarely)

ETIOLOGY/PATHOPHYSIOLOGY

- *Nocardia asteroides* (dogs and cats); *Nocardia brasiliensis* (cats only); *Nocardia nova* (common in Australia; now in the United States); *Proactinomyces* spp. (rare)
- *Nocardia*—a soil saprophyte that enters the body through contamination of wounds or by respiratory inhalation
- Compromised immune system—enhances likelihood of infection

SIGNALMENT/HISTORY

- Dogs and cats—of any breed
- Often animal is immunosuppressed—under treatment for neoplasia or immune-mediated disease

CLINICAL FEATURES

- Depend on the site of infection

Pleural

- Pyothorax; pneumonia or pyothorax in the cat
- Dyspnea
- Emaciation
- Fever

Cutaneous

- Chronic, nonhealing wounds
- Fistulous tracts, which may result in local lymphadenopathy

- Draining lymph nodes
- Osteomyelitis
- Specific eitiologies include—actinomycosis, atypical mycobacteriosis, leprosy, sporotrichosis, bite-wound abscess; foreign body draining tracts

Disseminated

- Most common in young dogs, usually originating in the respiratory tract
- Lethargy
- Fever, often cyclic
- Weight loss
- CNS may be affected, with diffuse neurologic signs
- Pleural and abdominal effusion may also occur
- Specifically for pleural disease—bacterial pyothorax, neoplasia, chronic diaphragmatic hernia
- Specifically for disseminated disease—systemic funal infection, FIP, plague

 DIFFERENTIAL DIAGNOSIS

Cutaneous

- Actinomycosis, atypical mycobacteriosis, leprosy, fungal, wound abscesses, foreign bodies draining tracts.

Pleural

- Bacterial pyothorax, thoracic neoplasia, chronic diaphragmatic hernia.

Disseminated

- Systemic fungal infection, FIP.

 DIAGNOSTICS

- CBC—neutrophilic leukocytosis, nonregenerative anemia (of chronic disease)
- Biochemical panel—usually normal; hypergammaglobulinemia in long-standing infections
- Radiographs—pleural or abdominal effusion, pleuropneumonia, or osteomyelitis
- Cytology—pleural fluid, abscess discharge, or abdominal fluid
- Stain with Romanowsky, Gram's, or modified acid-fast stains—reveals gram-positive, beaded, branching filamentous rods or cocci; sulfur granules (microaggregates) are infrequent in effusions; usually not able to differentiate from *Actinomyces* spp. (Fig. 72-1)
- Culture (definitive)—pleural fluid, abscess discharge, aspirated material from affected organ; grows under aerobic conditions on Sabouraud's medium

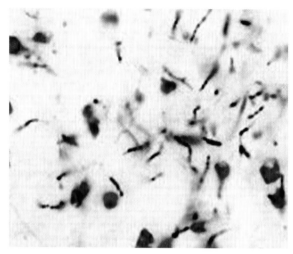

■ **Figure 72-1** Impression smear of a chronic fistulous tract on the thorax of a cat containing aggregates of branching filamentous gram-positive rods of *N. asteroides* (Gram's stain, 450×).

 # THERAPEUTICS

- Remove pleural effusion—usually by placing closed thorocostomy tube—through which to irrigate pleural cavity with warmed saline and remove any subsequent fluid accumulation
- Supportive care—IV fluid therapy, with or without nutritional support
- Antibiotic therapy
- Remove thorocostomy tube when fluid becomes noninfected and minimal in volume.
- Fistulous tracts and abscesses—surgically drain and debride; long-term antibiotic therapy

Drugs of Choice

- Antibiotics based on culture and sensitivity testing
- While awaiting culture and sensitivity results, good first-choice drugs include sulfonamides (sulfadiazine or trimethoprim-sulfadiazine combination).
- Other effective drugs include gentamicin, amikacin, doxycycline, tetracycline hydrochloride, minocycline, and erythromycin alone or combined with ampicillin or amoxicillin (Table 72-1).
- Can use amoxicillin in combination with an aminoglycoside
- Average treatment period is 6 weeks or for at least 2 weeks past the apparent remission of the disease.

Precautions/Interactions

- Tetracyclines may cause fever (especially cats); adjust dose (except doxycycline) in animals with renal insufficiency.

TABLE 72-1 Drug Therapy for Nocardiosis				
Drug	Dose (mg/kg)	Route	Interval (h)	Duration (days)
Sulfadiazine	100[a]	IV, PO	12	42
Trimethoprim-sulfadiazine	15	PO	12	42
Gentamicin[b]	2–4	IM, SC	8	10[c]
Amikacin[b]	6.5	IV, IM, SC	8	10[c]
Doxycycline	5	PO, IV	12	42
Tetracycline hydrochloride	15–20	PO	8	42
Minocycline	5–12.5	PO	12	42
Erythromycin	10–20	PO	8	42
Ampicillin	20–40	PO	8	42
Amoxicillin	6–20	PO	8–12	42

[a]As initial loading dose, then reduce to 50 mg/kg.
[b]Use in combination with ampicillin or amoxicillin; monitor for renal toxicity.
[c]Or for short period if clinical response occurring.

- Do not give aminoglycosides in poorly hydrated animals; monitor for renal tubular damage by monitoring urine sediment for the appearance of hyaline casts.
- Long-term use of sulfa drugs can cause polyarthritis, KCS, and blood dyscraisias; prevent by supplementing with folate administration (1 mg, PO, q24h)

 COMMENTS

- Even after apparent clinical remission, the patient should be monitored carefully for the development of fever, weight loss, neurologic signs, dyspnea, and lameness during the first year postinfection because of the possibility of bone and CNS involvement.

Abbreviations

CBC, complete blood count; CNS, central nervous system; FIP, feline infectious peritonitis; KCS, keratoconjunctivitis sicca.

Suggested Reading

Edwards DF. Nocardiosis. In: Greene CE, ed. *Infectious Diseases of the Dog and Cat*. Philadelphia: WB Saunders, 2006:456–461.

Malik R, Krockenberger MB, O'Brien CR, et al. *Nocardia* infections in cats: a retrospective multi-institutional study of 17 cases. *Aust Vet J* 2006;84:235–245.

Sivacolundhu, RK, O'Hara AJ, Read, RA. Thoracic actinomycosis (arcanobacteriosis) or nocardiosis causing thoracic pyogranuloma formation in three dogs. *Aust Vet J* 2001;79:398–402.

Thomovsky E, Kerl ME. Actinomycosis and nocardiosis. *Compend Contin Educ* 2008;10:4–10.

Ollulanus Infection

DEFINITION/OVERVIEW

- A trichostrongyloid nematode—Adult worms are found in the stomach wall of cats, causing chronic gastritis resulting in anorexia, vomiting, and weight loss.

ETIOLOGY/PATHOPHYSIOLOGY

- *Ollulanus tricuspis*—Adults (only up to 1 mm in length) coil into the gastric mucosa, causing superficial erosions.
- Over time, gastric erosions can become severe, with marked inflammation, accumulation of lymphoid aggregates, and fibrous changes in the mucosa and submucosa.
- Eggs—hatch within female worms; larvae develop to infective L3 larvae
- L3 larvae—passed into the stomach contents and vomited; infective to other cats
- Adult male and female worms passed in the vomitus—can infect other cats
- Distribution—throughout North America, Australia, New Zealand, Europe, Argentina, and Chile
- Germany—up to 40% of free-roaming cats may be infected

SIGNALMENT/HISTORY

- Colony cats—predisposed, probably because they have close access to other cats' vomitus
- Stray cats living in urban areas heavily populated with cats—high incidence of infection
- Captive cheetahs, lions, tigers, cougars—susceptible to infection
- Reported to occur in one cat with gastric adenocarcinoma

CLINICAL FEATURES

- Chronic vomiting
- Anorexia

- Weight loss
- Death from chronic gastritis

 DIFFERENTIAL DIAGNOSIS

- Other causes of vomiting including:
  - Dietary
  - Toxins—lead, ethylene glycol
  - Metabolic—diabetes mellitus, renal disease, hepatic disease, acidosis, heat stroke, hypoadrenocorticism, and hyperthyroidism
  - Gastric abnormalities—IBD, neoplasia, obstruction, atrophic gastritis, ulcers, dilatation/volvulus, and parasitic, such as *Physaloptera*
  - Gastroesophageal junction disorders—hiatal hernia
  - Small-intestine disorders—IBD disease, neoplasia, fungal, viral, obstruction, and paralytic ileus
  - Large-intestine disorders—colitis, obstipation, and IBD
  - Abdominal disorders—pancreatitis, gastrinoma, peritonitis, steatitis, pyometra, diaphragmatic hernia, and neoplasia
  - Neurologic disorders—psychogenic, motion sickness, vestibular lesions, head trauma, and brain neoplasia
  - Miscellaneous—heartworm disease and heart disease

 DIAGNOSTICS

- Larvae (or eggs)—seldom found in feces, because they are digested within the GI tract
- Vomitus—examine for L3 larvae
- Vomiting can be induced in the cat using xylazine (0.5 mg/kg IV or 1 mg/kg IM)—successful in about 70% of cases
- View worms through an endoscope (Fig. 73-1)—difficult due to size of worms
- Gastric lavage—using saline collection followed by centrifugation to precipitate L3 larvae or use Baermann's technique
- Histopathologic examination—Gastric biopsy specimen occasionally shows parasites.

 THERAPEUTICS

- Few treatments have been reported for this parasite.
- Fenbendazole, oxfendazole, and pyrantel pamoate have all been used but probably are ineffective.
- Although cats may improve clinically, parasites are not removed from stomach.

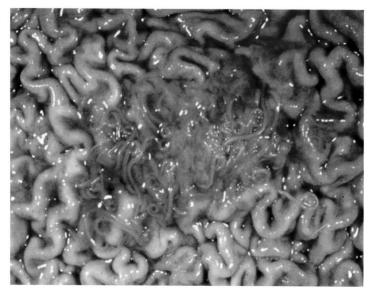

■ **Figure 73-1** Adult *O. tricuspis* worms in the stomach of a cat at necropsy examination.

Drugs of Choice

■ Tetramizole (give as a 2.5% formulation at 5 mg/kg, PO, once)—effective
■ Availability—Tetramizole is available in virtually every country but the United States.

Precautions/Interactions

■ Tetramizole at this dose should not cause any side effects in cats.

 COMMENTS

■ This author and others have successfully used tetramizole to treat *Ollulanus* infection in cats.

Abbreviations

GI, gastrointestinal; IBD, inflammatory bowel disease.

Suggested Reading

Bowman DD, Hendrix CM, Lindsay DS, et al. Ollulanus tricuspis. In: Bowman DD, ed. *Feline Clinical Parasitology*, Ames, IA: Iowa State University Press, 2002:262–265.

Cecchi R, Wills SJ, Dean R, et al. Demonstration of *Ollulanus tricuspis* in the stomach of domestic cats by biopsy. *J Comp Pathol* 2006;134:374–377.

Dennis MM, Bennett N, Ehrhart EJ. Gastric adenocarcinoma and chronic gastritis in two related Persian cats. *Vet Pathol* 2006;43:358–362.

chapter 74

Physaloptera Infection

DEFINITION/OVERVIEW

- A spirurid nematode—Adults and larvae are found attached to the gastric mucosa of cats (causing vomiting) and dogs (usually asymptomatic) with no larval migration.

ETIOLOGY/PATHOPHYSIOLOGY

- *Physaloptera* (*P. praeputialis* is cat-specific)
- Adults (3–5 cm long)—attach by their anterior end to the gastric mucosa of their vertebrate host
- Adults—pass ovoid eggs (50 × 35 mm) containing a fully formed larvae into the feces
- L1 larvae—infect intermediate hosts (beetles, crickets, and cockroaches)
- Intermediate hosts—eaten by paratenic hosts (lizards, hedgehog)
- Cats and dogs—become infected by eating paratenic hosts
- Distribution—worldwide
- PPP = 4–5 months

SIGNALMENT/HISTORY

- Cats usually have access to outdoors frequented by wildlife (raccoons, foxes, coyotes, bobcats, cougar, skunks) infected with *Physaloptera*.
- No age, sex, or breed predilection

CLINICAL FEATURES

Dogs

- Usually asymptomatic
- Can cause intermittent vomiting, anorexia, and slight weight loss

Cats

- Often asymptomatic
- Chronic vomiting
- Vomiting may continue for months
- Vomiting occasionally coupled with melena
- Vomitus can contain adult worms

 DIFFERENTIAL DIAGNOSIS

Cats

- Other causes of vomiting, including:
  - Dietary
  - Toxins—lead, ethylene glycol
  - Metabolic—diabetes mellitus, renal disease, hepatic disease, acidosis, heat stroke, hypoadrenocorticism, and hyperthyroidism
  - Gastric abnormalities—IBD, neoplasia, obstruction, atrophic gastritis, ulcers, dilatation/volvulus, and parasitic, such as *Ollunanus*
  - Gastroesophageal junction disorders—hiatal hernia
  - Small-intestine disorders—IBD, neoplasia, fungal, viral, obstruction, and paralytic ileus
  - Large-intestine disorders—colitis, obstipation, and IBD
  - Abdominal disorders—pancreatitis, gastrinoma, peritonitis, steatitis, pyometra, diaphragmatic hernia, and neoplasia
  - Neurologic disorders—psychogenic, motion sickness, vestibular lesions, head trauma, and brain neoplasia
  - Miscellaneous—heartworm disease and heart disease

 DIAGNOSTICS

- CBC—mild blood-loss anemia (in cats with melena); eosinophilia reported
- Vomitus—may contain adult parasites
- Eggs—containing larvae present in fecal flotation (Fig. 74-1)
- Flotation—may require sodium dichromate or magnesium sulfate flotation to identify eggs
- Endoscopy—reveals adult worms lying over the stomach wall (Fig. 74-2)

 THERAPEUTICS

- Cats and dogs rarely require any additional therapeutics other than an anthelmintic to remove the parasites.

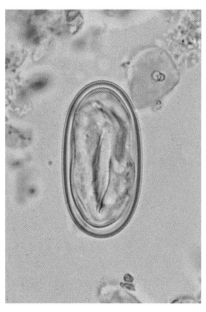

■ **Figure 74-1** *P. praeputialis* eggs in a fecal flotation.

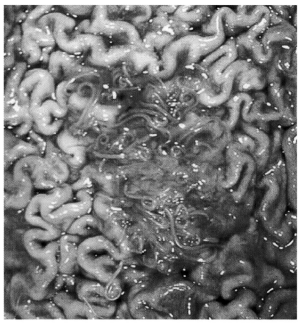

■ **Figure 74-2** Adult *P. praeputialis* worms in the stomach of a cat at necropsy examination (courtesy of Dr. J. King, Cornell University).

TABLE 74-1 Drug Treatment for *Physaloptera* Infection

Drug	Species	Dose (mg/kg)	Route	Interval (h)	Repeat (weeks)
Pyrantel pomoate (Strongid T)	B	5	PO	Once	3
Ivermectin (Ivomec 1% injectable)	B	0.2	SC, PO	Once	2
Fenbendazole (Panacur)	D	50	PO	24	3–5[a]

[a]Repeat if signs pesist.
B, both dogs and cats.

Drugs of Choice

- Pyrantel pomoate
- Ivermectin
- Fenbedazole (Table 74-1)
- Medications to reduce gastritis—famotadine (0.5 mg/kg, PO, q24h), sucralfate (0.25–1 g, PO, q8h)

Precautions/Interactions

- Ivermectin at this dose is not labeled for use in cats or dogs.
- No anthelmintic is specifically labeled for use against *Physaloptera.*

 # COMMENTS

- Both pyrantel and ivermectin will stop clinical signs and egg shedding in 5–8 days post-treatment.
- Recheck—2 weeks after finishing anthelmintic treatment; if eggs are still present on fecal exam or signs persist, repeat anthelmintics.
- Try to prevent pets from roaming; prompt disposal of feces will prevent infection of intermediate hosts.

Abbreviations

CBC, complete blood count; IBD, inflammatory bowel disease; PPP, prepatent period.

Suggested Reading

Campbell KL, Graham JC. *Physaloptera* infection in dogs and cats. *Comp Cont Vet Pract* 1999;21:299–314.

Theisen SK, LeGrange SN, Johnson SE, et al. *Pysaloptera* infection in 18 dogs with intermittent vomiting. *J Am Anim Hosp Assoc* 1998;34:74–78.

chapter 75

Plague

DEFINITION/OVERVIEW

- A systemic bacterial infection mainly of cats (dogs resistant)
- After skin inoculation, organisms rapidly migrate via lymphatics to regional lymph nodes to produce severe necrotic lymphadenopathy (buboes).
- Buboes—may rupture to the skin surface or cause septicemia.

ETIOLOGY/PATHOPHYSIOLOGY

- *Yersinia pestis*—a bipolar gram-negative staining rod found worldwide in wild rodents, squirrels, prairie dogs, rabbits, bobcats, and coyotes
- Most U.S. cases—New Mexico, Arizona, California, Colorado, Idaho, Nevada, Oregon, Texas, Utah, Washington, Wyoming, and Hawaii; movement of animals may result in occurrence in nonendemic areas.
- Common—May to October
- Infection—vector (fleas) transmit organism in bite
- After infection—organisms migrate from skin lymphatics to regional lymph nodes, multiply in phagocytic cells
- After infection—disease characterized by fever, painful lymphadenopathy (buboes), and intermittent bacteremia; lymph nodes may rupture
- Septicemia—can develop with or without lymph node involvement
- *Y. pestis* is a potential bioterrorist agent; occurrence of a cluster of pneumonia cases in companion animals may indicate animals as sentinels and the risk of human disease.

SIGNALMENT/HISTORY

- Cats—no sex, age, or breed predisposition
- Dogs—naturally resistant
- Outdoor (hunting) cats—increased risk
- Cats heavily infected with fleas or living near heavy rodent infestations—increased risk

CLINICAL FEATURES

Dogs

- Mild febrile signs with depression

Cats

Bubonic Plague

- Most common form
- Signs—develop 2–7 days after flea bite or after eating infected rodent
- Buboes—mainly develop on the head and neck
- Buboes—marked lymphadenopathy with hemorrhage, necrosis, and cellulitis
- If survives long enough—lymph nodes abscess, rupture, and drain through skin
- Signs of systemic illness—fever, depression, vomiting, diarrhea, dehydration, enlarged tonsils, anorexia, ocular discharge, weight loss, ataxia, coma, and oral ulcers

Systemic Plague

- Rare—usually rapidly fatal
- Septicemia—without lymphadenopathy or abscess formation
- Cats—unique in that they can develop bubonic pneumonia; high risk for zoonotic spread to people

 # DIFFERENTIAL DIAGNOSIS

Cats

- Lymphadenopathy:
  - Cat bite abscess formation
  - Foreign body migration
  - *Cuterebra* migration
- Systemic illness:
  - Tularemia
  - Cytauxzoonosis
  - Other acute bacterial causes of septicemia

 # DIAGNOSTICS

- CBC—leukocytosis with left shift and marked toxic changes in neutrophils
- Thrombocytopenia—if DIC occurs late in disease

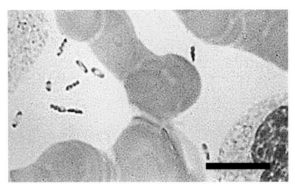

■ **Figure 75-1** *Y. pestis* organisms, the etiologic agent of the plague, in the blood of a patient with plague septicemia (Wright–Giemsa stain, bar = 10 mm).

- Biochemical profile—elevated hepatic enzyme activity and hyperbilirubinemia
- Occasionally—organisms visible on a peripheral blood smear (Fig. 75-1).
- Serology examination—performed by CDC and reference laboratories
- Serologic examination—Passive hemagglutination titers appear ~8 days postinfection; fourfold increase in titer between acute and convalescent serum samples.
- High titer—persists beyond a year in infected animals

Diagnostic Feature

- **Culture—definitive technique on peripheral blood, affected lymph node or abscess aspirate, or tissue biopsy before treatment**
- Fluorescent antibody test—on same samples used in culture will often give a quicker result

THERAPEUTICS

- High mortality—if not treated early and aggressively
- IV fluids and aggressive treatment of DIC—can save patient
- Important to treat fleas quickly to prevent personal exposure—use imidacloprid (Advantage; Bayer) for rapid flea kill
- Cats with pneumonic form—should be euthanatized to reduce extreme zoonotic potential

Drugs of Choice

- Tetracyclines (oxytetracycline, tetracycline, chlortetracycline)—25 mg/kg, PO, q8h for 10 days or parenterally 7.5 mg/kg, q12h
- Doxycycline—effectiveness not established but probably effective
- Chloramphenicol, gentamicin, TMS can be used if tetracyclines are contraindicated.

Precautions/Interactions

- Tetracyclines—may cause yellow staining of young animal's teeth
- Tetracyclines—may produce GI upsets
- Tetracyclines—use at reduced dose in animals with renal insufficiency

 COMMENTS

- Control exposure of pet to wildlife in endemic areas and treat with monthly flea preventatives.
- Pay particular attention—to controlling rodents near housing in endemic areas
- Pneumonic form is invariably fatal in cats—Euthanasia is often advised to decrease zoonotic risk and because prognosis is so poor.
- Bioterrism—Coordination with public health officials may be necessary.

Abbreviations

CBC, complete blood count; CDC, Centers for Disease Control and Prevention; DIC, disseminated intravascular coagulation; GI, gastrointestinal; TMS, trimethoprim- sulfa-diazine.

Suggested Reading

Gage KL, Dennis DT, Orloski KA, et al. Cases of cat-associated human plague in the Western US, 1997–1998. *Clin Infect Dis* 2000;30:893–900.

Gould LH, Pape J, Ettestad P, et al. Dog-associated risk factors for human plague. *Zoonoses Public Health* 2008;55:448–454.

Pneumocystosis

DEFINITION/OVERVIEW

- An atypical fungal disease of dogs (asymptomatic in cats) characterized by respiratory difficulty from parenchymal lung disease progressing over 1–4 weeks

ETIOLOGY/PATHOPHYSIOLOGY

- *Pneumocystis carinii (jirovecii)*—saprophytic atypical fungus whose life cycle is completed in the alveolar spaces
- Infection usually confined to the respiratory tract—but has been reported to disseminate throughout body
- Transmission (by respiratory route)—occurs in susceptible hosts within a species (i.e., transmission does not appear to occur from dogs to humans or cats)

SIGNALMENT/HISTORY

- Most reported cases have occurred in dachshunds <12 months of age.
- Shetland sheepdogs, Cavalier King Charles spaniels, a beagle, and a Yorkshire terrier—also reported with the disease
- Reduced immunity—may predispose to severe disease
- Cats—can be infected but do not show clinical signs

CLINICAL FEATURES

- Exercise intolerance (often primary complaint)
- Cough
- Mild fevers

- Gradual weight loss
- May progress to cachexia, respiratory distress, and cyanosis with severe infections
- Increased lung sounds on thoracic auscultation
- Vomiting and diarrhea occasionally noted

 DIFFERENTIAL DIAGNOSIS

- Cardiovascular (pulmonary edema; enlarged heart, especially the left atrium; pulmonary emboli)
- Allergic (bronchial asthma, eosinophilic pneumonia or granulomatosis, pulmonary infiltrate with eosinophils)
- Trauma (foreign body, irritating gases, collapsing trachea, diaphragmatic hernia)
- Neoplasia (not only of the respiratory tree but also associated structures such as ribs, lymph nodes, muscles); unlikely in young animals
- Inflammatory (pharyngitis; tonsillitis; kennel cough from such agents as *Bordetella bronchiseptica*, parainfluenza virus, infectious laryngotracheitis virus, and *Mycoplasma* spp.; bacterial bronchopneumonia; chronic pulmonary fibrosis; pulmonary abscess or granuloma; chronic obstructive pulmonary disease)
- Parasites (*Oslerus* [*Filaroides*] *osleri*, *Crenosoma vulpis*, *Filaroides hirthi*, *Filaroides milksi*, *Paragonimus kellicotti*, *Dirofilaria immitis*—heartworm disease in the dog)
- Other infectious agents—systemic mycoses (blastomycosis, histoplasmosis, and cryptococcosis), toxoplasmosis, and bacterial pneumonias

 DIAGNOSTICS

- CBC, serum biochemical profile, urinalysis—changes nonspecific
- Usually see leukocytosis—with neutrophilia and left shift, eosinophilia, and monocytosis
- PCV—may be elevated due to chronic hypoxia
- Arterial blood gas—reflects hypoxemia with ventilation–perfusion mismatch
- Thoracic radiography—changes not specific for pneumocystosis; diffuse interstitial pattern with peribronchial infiltrates progressing to alveolar pattern; middle lung lobes more severely affected than cranioventral lobes; cor pulmonale may be present in severe long-standing infections
- Serologic assays—unreliable
- Diagnosis made by visualizing organism on a transtracheal wash, BAL, or lung aspirate cytologic examination (Fig. 76-1)
- Immunohistochemistry on lung biopsy or aspirate cytologic examination—definitive diagnosis

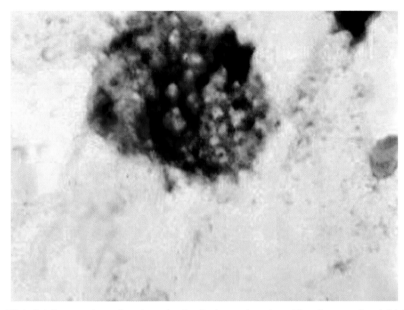

■ **Figure 76-1** Cytology specimen from bronchoalveolar lavage in a dog with pulmonary *P. carinii* infection. Note the small intracellular organisms within the mononuclear cell (Wright–Giemsa stain, 2000×).

 # THERAPEUTICS

- Inpatient—oxygen support for hypoxemic patients
- Nutrition—may need to institute enteral nutrition in cachexic patients
- Fluid therapy—may be needed while antimicrobial therapy is initiated
- Cage rest or restricted exercise

Drugs of Choice

- TMS—first-choice drug
- Pentamidine isethionate (Pentam 300 injection; LyphoMed)
- Carbutamide (Table 76-1)
- Caspofungin—β-glucan synthatase inhibitor prevents cysts developing (glucan is a major component of cyst wall); to date, no reports of use in dogs

TABLE 76-1 **Drug Therapy for Pneumocystosis**				
Drug	Dose (mg/kg)	Route	Interval (h)	Duration (weeks)
Trimethoprim-sulfonamide	15	PO	6	3
Pentamidine isethionate	4	IM	24	2
Carbutamide	50	IM	12	3

Precautions/Interactions

- Pentamidine isethionate—potentiates renal insufficiency and hepatic dysfunction, hypoglycemia, hypotension, hypocalcemia, urticaria, hematologic disorders, and localized pain at injection site

 COMMENTS

- Keep infected dogs away from other dogs, especially immunocompromised animals in an ICU.
- There is zoonotic potential reported.
- Human patients with HIV infection should be instructed to avoid contact with animals with pneumocystosis.

Abbreviations

BAL, bronchoalveloar lavage; CBC, complete blood count; HIV, human immunodeficiency virus; ICU, intensive care unit; PCV, packed cell volume; TMS, trimethoprim-sulfadiazine.

Suggested Reading

Lobetti RG. Common variable immunodeficiency in miniature dachshunds affected with *Pneumocystis caninii*. 2000:12;39–45.

Maddison JE, Page SW, Church DB. *Small Animal Clinical Pharmacology*, 2nd ed. Edinburgh: Saunders Elsevier, 2008:196.

Watson PJ, Wotton P, Eastwood J, et al. Immunoglobulin deficiency in Cavalier King Charles Spaniels with *Pneumocystis* pneumonia. *J Vet Intern Med* 2006;20:523–527.

Pox Virus Infection

chapter 77

DEFINITION/OVERVIEW

- Rare orthopoxvirus that affects cats and causes a papular, crusted, and ulcerative dermatitis

ETIOLOGY/PATHOPHYSIOLOGY

- Member of the genus *Orthopoxvirus*, family Poxviridae
- Enveloped DNA virus, resistant to drying (viable for years) but readily inactivated by most disinfectants
- Geographically limited to Eurasia
- Relatively common (10% infection prevalence in western Europe)

SIGNALMENT/HISTORY

- Cats—domestic and exotic
- No age, sex, or breed predisposition
- Reservoir host—wild rodents (voles, mice, gerbils, ground squirrels)
- Infection thought to be acquired during hunting—most common in young adults and active hunters, often from rural environment
- Lesions—often develop at the site of a bite wound (presumably inflicted by the prey animal carrying the virus)
- Most cases occur in autumn—when small wild mammals are at maximum population and most active
- Severe cutaneous and systemic signs with poor prognosis—frequently associated with immunosuppression (iatrogenic or coinfection with FeLV or FIV)
- Cat-to-cat transmission—rare; causes only subclinical infection
- Skin lesions—multiple, circular; dominant feature; usually develop on head, neck, or forelimbs
- Primary lesions—crusted papules, plaques, nodules, crateriform ulcers, or areas of cellulitis or abscesses

- Secondary lesions—erythematous nodules that ulcerate and crust; often widespread; develop after 1–3 weeks
- Pruritus—variable
- Systemic—20% of cases; anorexia, lethargy, pyrexia, vomiting, diarrhea, oculonasal discharge, conjunctivitis, and pneumonia

 # DIFFERENTIAL DIAGNOSIS

- Bacterial and fungal infections
- Eosinophilic granuloma complex
- Neoplasia—particularly mast cell tumor; lymphosarcoma
- Miliary dermatitis

 # DIAGNOSTICS

- Serologic testing—demonstrate rising titers; hemagglutination inhibition, virus neutralizing, complement fixation, or ELISA; titers may remain high for months or years
- Virus isolation from scab material—definitive diagnosis; 90% positive
- EM of extracts of scab, biopsy, or exudate—rapid presumptive diagnosis; 70% positive
- Skin biopsy—characteristic histologic changes of epidermal hyperplasia and hypertrophy; multilocular vesicle and ulceration; large eosinophilic intracytoplasmic inclusion bodies
- PCR—Assay is not readily commercially available as yet.

 # THERAPEUTICS

- No specific treatment
- Supportive (antibiotics, fluids) when necessary
- Elizabethan collar—to prevent self-induced damage
- Antibiotics—prevent secondary infections
- Immunosuppressive agents (e.g., glucocorticoids and megestrol acetate)—absolutely contraindicated because they can induce fatal systemic disease

 # COMMENTS

- Natural reservoir host is possibly small rodents; cats infected incidentally
- Vaccines—none available; vaccinia virus may be considered for valuable zoo collections, but its effects in nondomestic cats have not been investigated
- Most cats recover spontaneously in 1–2 months.

- Healing may be delayed by secondary bacterial skin infection.
- Prognosis is poor, with severe respiratory or pulmonary involvement.
- Rare human pox virus infections have been linked to contact with infected cats with skin lesions; use basic hygiene precautions (disposable gloves) when handling infected cats.
- Healthy humans—Infection usually mild and transient but can be severe and even life-threatening in immunocompromised individuals.
- May cause painful skin lesions and severe systemic illness, particularly in the very young or elderly, people with a pre-existing skin condition, and the immunodeficient

Abbreviations

DNA, deoxyribonucleic acid; ELISA, enzyme-linked immunosorbent assay; EM, electron microscopy; FeLV, feline leukemia virus; FIV, feline immuno deficiency virus; PCR, polymerase chain reaction.

Suggested Reading

Godfrey DR, Blundell CJ, Essbauer S, et al. Unusual presentations of cowpox infection in cats. *J Small Anim Pract* 2004;45:202–205.
Schulze C, Alex M, Schirrmeier H, et al. Generalized fatal cowpox virus infection in a cat with transmission to a human contact case. *Zoonoses Public Health* 2007;54:31–37.

Protothecosis

DEFINITION/OVERVIEW

- Blue–green algae infection causing either localized infection (cats) of the skin and GI, or systemic disseminated infection (dogs)

ETIOLOGY/PATHOPHYSIOLOGY

- *Prototheca wickerhamii* (usually cats) and *Prototheca zopfi* (usually dogs)—single-celled achlorophyllous blue–green algae
- Algae live on raw and treated sewage—survive as contaminants of soil, water, and food
- Occasionally isolated—from the feces of healthy individuals

SIGNALMENT/HISTORY

- Dogs and cats—rare
- Dogs—medium to large breeds, middle-aged females mostly affected
- Depressed cell immunity may predispose dogs to infection—no known predisposing factors for cats
- North American infections—confined to southeastern states

CLINICAL FEATURES

Dogs

- Mainly affected by the GI form of the disease
- Depends on the organ system involved; kidney, liver, heart, intestine, brain and eyes are most common sites for dissemination
- Signs can include:
    - Intermittent and chronic bloody diarrhea
    - Chronic weight loss

- Blindness, with posterior segment disease with retinal granulomas and/or detached retinas
- Neurologic signs
- Cutaneous lesions, with ragged ulcers and crusts usually on extremities and mucosal surfaces

Cats

- Chronic cutaneous or mucous membrane ulceration, with few if any systemic signs
- Cutaneous lesions, usually localized, extend deep into the subcutaneous tissues (usually on limbs and/or face) and consist of granulomatous inflammation in which there are a large number of organisms

 DIFFERENTIAL DIAGNOSIS

- Systemic—systemic mycoses (histoplasmosis, blastomycosis)
- Cutaneous—systemic or cutaneous mycoses; mycobacteriosis

 DIAGNOSTICS

- CBC, biochemical profile, and urinalysis—usually normal but may reflect organ damage in systemic disease (normal in the cat)
- CSF tap—pleocytosis with mononuclear cells reported; elevated protein; may see organisms in CSF if CNS infected

Diagnostic Feature

- **Cytology—most definitive diagnostic test to identify organism in skin lesions or organ aspirates (rectal or colonic mucosa, anterior chamber aspirations, or CSF); Wright–Giemsa best stain (Fig. 78-1)**
- Histopathologic examination—identify organism in biopsy of skin lesions (special stains: Gomori methenamine silver GMS), periodic acid–Schiff)
- Culture—grows on Sabouraud's dextrose agar at 25–37°C in 2–7 days

 THERAPEUTICS

- Dogs—require antimicrobials if systemically affected
- Cutaneous lesions (mainly cats)—excision is treatment of choice followed by systemic antifungal agents

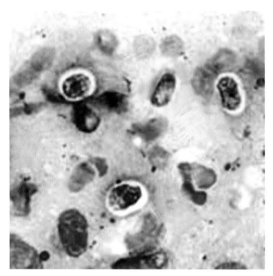

■ **Figure 78-1** Cytologic specimen of a rectal scraping from a dog with protothecosis. Organisms are identified by the halo and a thin cell wall and are of varying size (Wright's stain, 1000×).

Drugs of Choice

- Amphotericin B—use for localized disease after surgical excision; lipid formulations are also effective and produce fewer side effects
- Tetracyclines given concurrently with amphotericin B—may provide a synergistic effect; more effective for ocular disease
- Oral antifungal agents such as ketoconazole, fluconazole, and itraconazole—may be used in conjunction with amphotericin B or as sole agent in non–life-threatening cases (Table 78-1)

		Dose		Interval	Duration
TABLE 78-1 Drug Therapy for Protothecosis					
Drug	**Species**	**(mg/kg)**	**Route**	**(h)**	**(weeks)**
Amphotericin B	D	0.25–0.5	IV	3 times weekly	a
	C	0.25	IV	3 times weekly	b
Tetracycline	B	22	PO	8	c
Ketoconazole	B	10–15	PO	12–24	6
Itraconazole	B	5–10	PO	12	6
Fluconazole	B	2.5–5	PO	12	6

[a]Until total cumulative dose of 8 mg/kg or renal toxicity occurs.
[b]Until total cumulative dose of 4 mg/kg.
[c]Continue for as long as amphotericin B is administered.
D, dogs; C, cats; B, both dogs and cats.

Precautions/Interactions

- Amphotericin B—may cause toxic nephritis; monitor by examining urine for appearance of hyaline casts
- Amphotericin B—may also cause severe phlebitis
- Ketoconazole (and to a lesser extent itraconazole and fluconazole)—may induce hepatic enzymes and cause hepatotoxicity; monitor periodically

 COMMENTS

- The organism—difficult to eradicate with drug therapy
- Prognosis in dogs—guarded to grave
- Prognosis in cats—good if cutaneous lesions can be completely excised
- No zoonotic potential has been recorded.

Abbreviations

CBC, complete blood count; CNS, central nervous system; CSF, cerebrospinal fluid; GI, gastrointestinal; GMS, Gomori methenamine silver.

Suggested Reading

Hosaka S, Hosaka M. A case report of canine protothecosis. *J Vet Med Sci* 2004:66;593–597.

Pressler BM, Gookin JL, Sykes JE, et al. Urinary tract manifestations of protothecosis in dogs. *J Vet Intern Med* 2005;19:115–119.

Stenner VJ, Mackay B, King T, et al. Protothecosis in 17 Australian dogs and a review of the canine literature. *Med Mycol* 2007;45:249–266.

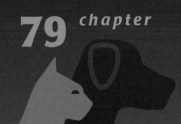

79 *chapter*

Pseudorabies Virus Infection

DEFINITION/OVERVIEW

- Rare but highly fatal viral disease of dogs and cats—usually have a history of contact with pigs
- Characterized by sudden death, often without signs—If signs occur, they include hypersalivation, intense pruritus, and CNS signs.

ETIOLOGY/PATHOPHYSIOLOGY

- Pseudorabies virus (suid herpesvirus, Aujeszky's disease, mad itch of pigs)—an α-herpesvirus
- Dogs and cats—become infected when they contact infected pigs, eat contaminated uncooked meat or offal from pigs, or eat infected rats

SIGNALMENT/HISTORY

- Domestic and exotic dogs and cats of any age or breed—contact with a farm
- May also be seen in other domestic species—cattle, sheep, goats, and pigs

CLINICAL FEATURES

- Usually sudden death
- Acute onset of:
  - Hypersalivation
  - Dyspnea
  - Fever
  - Vomiting
  - CNS signs, including depression, lethargy, ataxia, seizures, recumbency, coma, and death
- Intense pruritus and self-mutilation are features of the disease.

DIFFERENTIAL DIAGNOSIS

- Rabies—in various forms; affected dogs and cats will attack anything that moves; there is usually no intense pruritus with rabies; sudden death is usually not a feature of rabies
- Canine distemper—no hypersalivation, sudden death, or personality change; other multisystemic signs present
- Toxicity exposure (organophosphate, lead, strychnine, inorganic arsenic)—no pruritus or personality changes; history of exposure; other signs consistent with exposure

 ## DIAGNOSTICS

- CBC, serum biochemical profile, urinalysis—no characteristic changes
- CSF—increased protein and mononuclear pleocytosis
- Serologic assay—available, but antibodies develop after acute disease is over so may not be present at the time of death
- Definitive diagnostic test—direct FA on brain tissue
- Histologic examination—intranuclear inclusion bodies in glial and ganglion cells of brain
- PCR—used in Japan to identify one case in a cat
- Viral isolation at necropsy—from brain tissue

 ## THERAPEUTICS

- No known effective treatment, except supportive care and prevention of self-mutilation

Drugs of Choice

- No specific drugs available

Precautions/Interactions

- Transmission from infected cats and dogs to other cats and dogs does not seem to occur, so there should be no risk to other in-contact pets.

 ## COMMENTS

- Clinical course in cats typically lasts 24–36 hours, followed by death (60% of cases). Others (40%) last longer than 36 hours but also are invariably fatal.

- Mild potential for human infection; take precautions when treating infected animals and handling infected tissues and fluids

Abbreviations

CBC, complete blood count; CNS, central nervous system; CSF, cerebrospinal fluid; FA, fluorescent antibody; PCR, polymerase chain reaction.

Suggested Reading

Vandevelde M. Pseudorabies. In: Greene CE, ed. *Infectious Diseases of the Dog and Cat*. Philadelphia: WB Saunders, 2006:183–186.

Pythiosis

chapter 80

DEFINITION/OVERVIEW

- An infectious disease causing primarily either a chronic pyogranulomatous lesion of the stomach or intestines, or nonhealing wounds and invasive masses that contain ulcerated nodules and draining tracts in the skin of dogs and cats

ETIOLOGY/PATHOPHYSIOLOGY

- *Pythium insidiosum*—an aquatic pathogen
- Infective form—thought to be a motile biflagellate zoospore
- Zoospore is released into warm water and attracted chemotactically to damaged tissue and animal hair—animals likely infected when they enter or ingest contaminated water
- Distribution—occurs mainly in tropical or semitropical regions of the world
- Distribution—in the United States, occurs mainly in states bordering the Gulf of Mexico, but also reported in Oklahoma, Arkansas, Missouri, Kentucky, Tennessee, North and South Carolina, Virginia, Indiana, New Jersey, Arizona, Illinois, and even northern California
- Usually—only one body system (skin or GI tract) in any one patient affected at a time
- Cats—skin usually affected; retrobulbar, periorbital, or nasopharyngeal regions and tail head or footpads
- Dogs—skin and GI tract equally affected
- GI tract—usually gastric outflow tract affected, including the proximal small intestine, but also the ileocolic junction and colon
- Local thromboembolic events or vascular invasion—may lead to bowel wall ischemia and GI tract perforation or hemoabdomen (especially in dogs)
- Skin lesions—single or multiple cutaneous or subcutaneous lesions involving the extremities, tail head, ventral neck, perineum, or medial thigh (dogs)

SIGNALMENT/HISTORY

- Dogs more than cats; large-breed dogs (hunting, field trial breeds) working near water
- Labrador retrievers—over-represented

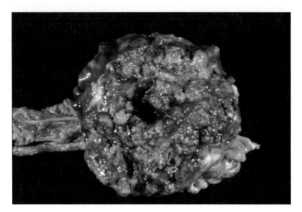

■ **Figure 80-1** Gross specimen of the gastric outflow tract of the stomach of a dog with pythiosis. Note the profound stomach wall thickening from the pylogranulomatous process.

- German shepherd dogs—may be predisposed to cutaneous form
- Mainly—dogs <3 years of age
- Sex distribution—more males affected than females

 ## CLINICAL FEATURES

Gastrointestinal Tract Pythiosis

- Emaciation—common
- Abdominal mass—often palpable
- Affected dogs—often bright and alert, in spite of severe weight loss
- Fever—occasionally
- Systemic signs—may develop if intestinal obstruction, infarction, or perforation occurs (Fig. 80-1)

Cutaneous Pythiosis

- Nonhealing wounds—characterized by poorly defined nodules that ulcerate and drain a serosanguinous or purulent exudate from multiple tracts

 ## DIFFERENTIAL DIAGNOSIS

Gastrointestinal Tract Pythiosis

- Intestinal mass and/or obstruction caused by foreign body, chronic intussusception, neoplasia (lymphosarcoma, carcinoma, other GI tract neoplasias), histoplasmosis; IBD; and other infections (prototheCosis, basidiobolomycosis)

Cutaneous Pythiosis

- Other fungal infectious diseases (oomycotic pathogens such as *Lagenidium*, zygomycosis caused by *Basidiobolus* or *Conidiobolus* spp., cryptococcosis, coccidioidomycosis, sporotrichosis, eumycotic mycetoma, and phaeohyphomycosis)
- Bacterial diseases (actinomycosis, nocardiosis, leprosy, mycobacteriosis, botryomycosis, and brucellosis) and other infectious causes (prototecosis, nodular leishmaniasis)
- Noninfectious pyogranulomatous diseases (foreign body reactions, idiopathic nodular panniculitis, sebaceous nodular adenitis, and canine cutaneous sterile pyogranuloma/granuloma syndrome, cutaneous neoplasia)
- Systemic vasculitis and cutaneous embolic disease

 DIAGNOSTICS

- CBC—eosinophilia, leukocytosis, and anemia of chronic disease may occur
- Serum biochemical profile—hypoalbuminemia and hyperglobulinemia may occur in chronically affected animals
- Electrolyte abnormalities (hypokalemia, hyponatremia, hypochloridemia, metabolic alkalosis)—in dogs with gastric outflow obstruction
- Imaging—abdominal radiographs and ultrasound examination may reveal GI tract obstruction, bowel wall thickening, and mesenteric lymph node enlargement
- Serology—ELISA and particularly immunoblot analysis (offered by Pythium Laboratory, LSU, Baton Rouge, Louisiana) is sensitive and specific. ELISA also can be used to monitor therapy efficacy.
- Histopathologic examination of biopsy specimen of GI tract and skin lesion—suggestive only but not definitive for pythiosis; need immunohistochemistry to confirm identity of hyphae in lesion
- Culture—tissue samples; ship overnight at room temperature to experienced laboratory (LSU)
- PCR—is available to identify cultured organisms or organisms in tissue biopsy samples (LSU)

 THERAPEUTICS

- Treatment of choice—aggressive surgical excision of all infected tissues
- Often not possible to remove all infected tissue—disease too advanced by the time a diagnosis is made
- Dogs often improve after obstructive GI tract lesion is resected, even if significant disease is still grossly evident.
- After surgery—Medical therapy with antifungal agents for 2–3 months will decrease likelihood of recurrence.

TABLE 80-1 Drug Therapy for Pythiosis					
Drug	Species	Dose (mg/kg)	Route	Interval (h)	Duration (months)
Itraconazole[a]	D	10	PO	24	4–6
Terbinafine (Lamisil)	D	5–10	PO	24	4–6
Amphotericin B lipid complex	D	2–3	IV	3 times weekly	1–4[b]
	C	0.5–1	IV	3 times weekly	1–4[b]

[a]Used in combination with terbinafine.
[b]To a total dose of 25–30 mg.
D, dogs; C, cats.

Drugs of Choice

- Itraconazole combined with terbinafine (Lamisil; Novartis Pharmaceuticals)—drug protocol of choice; efficacy is 20–25% in nonresectable or partially resectable lesions; continue for 4–6 months.
- Amphotericin B lipid complex—shown to be effective in a limited number of dogs; recommended if patient cannot tolerate oral drugs (Table 80-1)

Precautions/Interactions

- Azole drugs—should not be given to animals with hepatic disease; monitor for hepatic toxicity by monitoring ALT monthly throughout treatment course
- Amphotericin B lipid complex—can cause nephrotoxicity (monitor urine repeatedly for the appearance of hyaline casts); other side effects include fever, anorexia, vomiting during infusion

 COMMENTS

- Re-evaluation of ELISA serology 2–3 months after surgery or 3 months after medical management; excellent prognostic indicator
- Examination for reoccurrence of GI tract lesion with abdominal ultrasound is useful.
- Prognosis—guarded to poor unless a complete resection is possible
- Fewer than 25% of affected animals are cured with medical therapy alone.
- No zoonotic potential, although humans can become infected (very rare) from a common environmental source; no evidence of direct transmission from animals to humans

Abbreviations

ALT, alanine aminotransferase; CBC, complete blood count; ELISA, enzyme-linked immunosorbent assay; GI, gastrointestinal; IBD, inflammatory bowel disease; LSU, Louisiana State University; PCR, polymerase chain reaction.

Suggested Reading

Berryessa NA, Marks SL, Pesavento PA, et al. Gastrointestinal pythiosis in 10 dogs from California. *J Vet Intern Med* 2008;22:1065–1069.

Grooters AM. Pythiosis, lagenidiosis, and zygomycosis in small animals. *Vet Clin North Am Small Anim Pract* 2003:33;695–720.

Grooters AM, Foil CS. Miscellaneous fungal infections. In: Greene CE, ed. Infectious Diseases of the Dog and Cat. Philadelphia: WB Saunders, 2006:637–643.

81 *chapter*

Q Fever

DEFINITION/OVERVIEW

- A systemic infection causing abortion in cats and CNS disease in dogs

ETIOLOGY/PATHOPHYSIOLGY

- *Coxiella burnetii*—zoonotic rickettsia
- Infection—most commonly by inhalation or ingestion of organisms while feeding on infected body fluids (urine, feces, milk, or parturient discharges), tissues (especially placenta), or carcasses of infected animal reservoir hosts (cattle, sheep, goats)
- Can occur after tick exposure (many species of ticks implicated)
- Lungs—main portal of entry to systemic circulation
- Organism replicates in vascular endothelium, causing widespread vasculitis.
- Vasculitis results in necrosis and hemorrhage in lungs, liver, and CNS.
- Severity—depends on the pathogenicity of the strain of organism
- An extended latent period exists after recovery until chronic immune complex phenomena develop.
- Organism reactivated out of the latent state during parturition, resulting in large numbers entering the placenta, parturient fluids, urine, feces, and milk
- Endemic worldwide; most cases in the United States occur in western states

SIGNALMENT/HISTORY

- Cats and dogs
- History of contact with farm animals or ticks

CLINICAL FEATURES

- Fever
- Lethargy
- Depression

- Anorexia followed by ataxia, seizures, and other neurologic signs (dogs)
- Splenomegaly is often the only clinical finding.
- Abortion, especially in cats

 ## DIFFERENTIAL DIAGNOSIS

Dogs

- Differentiate from granulomatous meningoencephalomyelitis, protozoal encephalitis (toxoplasmosis, neosporosis), distemper, cryptococcosis or other infectious agents (meningitis, ehrlichiosis, RMSF), pug dog encephalitis, toxicities (lead poisoning, organophosphate, carbamate, strychnine), and neoplasia

Cats

- Other causes of abortion—infections (viral rhinotracheitis; panleukopenia; FeLV; toxoplasmosis; bacteria, including coliforms; streptococci; staphylococci; salmonellae), fetal defects, maternal problems (nutrition, genital tract abnormalities), environmental stress, and endocrine disorders (hypoluteidism)

 ## DIAGNOSTICS

- CBC, biochemical profile, urinalysis—nonspecific findings

Diagnostic Feature

- **Definitive diagnosis—made by isolation of organism or serology**
- Organism identification—Collect 2–3 ml of serum, refrigerate, and send on ice to test laboratory (New Mexico Department of Agriculture, Veterinary Diagnostic Services, Albuquerque, NM).
- Tissue samples (placenta)—Send to same test laboratory for animal inoculation.
- Serology—IFA and ELISA methods are available; a fourfold increase in IgG titer over a 4-week period is diagnostic; the use of newer serologic techniques that measure IgM on one sample has not been well documented in small animals.
- PCR—also performed by New Mexico Department of Agriculture laboratory; used to detect organisms in tissue culture or tissue specimens derived from the patient

 ## THERAPEUTICS

- Alert client of possible zoonotic risk.
- If treating in hospital, wear gloves and mask and maintain in an isolation facility.

TABLE 81-1 Drug Therapy for Q Fever in Dogs and Cats

Drug	Species	Dose (mg/kg)	Route	Interval (h)	Duration (weeks)
Doxycycline	D	10–20	PO, IV	12–24	2–6
	C	5–10	PO	12–24	2–4
Enrofloxacin	B	3–5	PO	12	2–6
Tetracycline	D	22	PO	8	2–6
	C	10–20	PO	8–12	2–3

D, dogs; C, cats; B, both dogs and cats.

Drugs of Choice

- Tetracycline
- Doxycycline—use in combination with enrofloxacin for extended periods in chronic infections
- Enrofloxacin—effective in vitro, but no clinical reports (Table 81-1)

Precautions/Interactions

- Tetracycline drugs are associated with yellowing of teeth in young animals; do not use in animals with renal failure.
- Doxycycline—may cause esophagitis and stricture
- Enrofloxacin—may cause cartilage defects in young animals
- Enrofloxacin—may cause retinal degeneration when used in cats with concurrent hepatic or renal disease or at high doses

 COMMENTS

- Difficult to determine success of therapy because many animals spontaneously improve
- Even asymptomatic cases should be aggressively treated because of the zoonotic potential.
- Utility of predicting success of therapy based on serologic improvement unknown
- The zoonotic potential cannot be overemphasized.
- By the time the diagnosis is made in a cat or dog, human exposure has occurred.
- Instruct owner and in-contact humans to seek medical advice immediately.
- Humans contract the disease by inhalation of infected aerosols.
- Children commonly infected from ingestion of raw milk, but they are usually asymptomatic
- Previous urban outbreaks in humans have been related to exposure to infected cats.
- Incubation period from time of contact to illness in humans is 5–32 days.
- Person-to-person transmission possible

Abbreviations

CBC, complete blood count; CNS, central nervous system; ELISA, enzyme-linked immunosorbent assay; FeLV, feline leukemia virus; IFA, immunofluorescence assay; Ig, immunoglobulin; PCR, polymerase chain reaction; RMSF, Rocky Mountain spotted fever.

Suggested Reading

Brouqui P, Badiaga S, Raoult D. Q fever outbreak in homeless shelter. *Emerg Infect Dis* 2004; 10:1297–1299.

Greene CE, Breitschwerdt EB. Q-fever. In: Greene CE, ed. *Infectious Diseases of the Dog and Cat.* Philadelphia: WB Saunders, 2006:242–245.

Komiya T, Sadamasu K, Kang MI, et al. Seroprevalence of *Coxiella burnetii* infections among cats in different living environments. *J Vet Med Sci* 2003;65:1047–1048.

Rabies

DEFINITION/OVERVIEW

- A severe, invariably fatal viral polioencephalitis of warm-blooded animals, including humans

ETIOLOGY/PATHOPHYSIOLOGY

- Rabies virus is a single-stranded RNA virus (genus, *Lyssavirus*; family, Rhabdoviridae).
- Virus enters the body through a wound (usually from a bite of rabid animal) or via mucous membranes and replicates in myocytes, then spreads to the neuromuscular junction and neurotendinal spindles; travels to the CNS via intra-axonal fluid within peripheral nerves; spreads throughout the CNS; then finally spreads centrifugally within the peripheral, sensory, and motor neurons.
- Affects nervous system (causing clinical encephalitis—either paralytic or ferocious rabies) and salivary glands (excessive salivation; saliva containing large quantities of virus)
- Once infected, clinical disease is virtually inevitable.
- Prevalence is low, except in enzootic areas, especially in underdeveloped countries, where vaccination rates of cats and dogs are low.
- Distribution is worldwide except in Australia, New Zealand, Hawaii, Japan, Iceland, and parts of Scandinavia.

SIGNALMENT/HISTORY

- All warm-blooded mammals can be infected.
- In the United States, four endemic strains within fox, raccoon, skunk, and bat populations exist.
- All endemic strains in the United States can be transmitted to dogs and cats.

CLINICAL FEATURES

- Quite variable—with atypical presentation being the rule rather than exception
- Classically, three progressive stages of disease—prodromal, ferocious, and paralytic; 90% of rabid cats have the ferocious form
- Often first signs are changes in behavior:
  - Seeking solitude
  - Apprehension
  - Nervousness
  - Anxiety
  - Unusual shyness or aggressiveness
- Then behavior becomes more erratic:
  - Biting
  - Snapping
  - Licking
  - Chewing at a wound site
  - Biting at cage
  - Wandering and roaming
  - Excitability
  - Irritability
  - Viciousness
  - Changes in tone of bark
  - Dilated pupils unresponsive to light; anisocoria
- Progression to more clinical signs of:
  - Disorientation
  - Incoordination
  - Seizures
  - Finally, paralysis
- Excess salivation or frothing at the mouth—may be exacerbated by mandibular and laryngeal paralysis, with a dropped jaw, and inability to swallow (Fig. 82-1)
- Fever—may or may not be present
- Death—occurs in all infected dogs and cats within 7–10 days of onset of clinical signs

 DIFFERENTIAL DIAGNOSIS

- Seriously consider rabies—in any unvaccinated (against rabies) dog or cat showing unusual mood or behavioral changes or unaccountable neurologic signs, especially in endemic areas
- Suspected cases—should be handled with considerable care to limit the number of individuals exposed

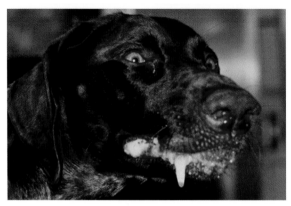

■ **Figure 82-1** A dog with rabies. Note the slightly dropped jaw, excessive salivation, and manic look (courtesy of Dr. A. Delahunta, Cornell University).

- Any neurologic disease causing diffuse signs—other infectious causes such as canine distemper (no hypersalivation or sudden death; other multisystemic signs present), toxoplasmosis, neosporosis, pseudorabies (no intense pruritus with rabies usually; sudden death is usually not a feature of rabies), toxicity (organophosphate, lead, strychnine, inorganic arsenic), neoplasia, GME, polyradiculoneuropathy, hepatic encephalopathy, and head injury
- Other causes of laryngeal paralysis, choking, or hypersalivation

 # DIAGNOSTICS

- CBC, serum biochemical profile and urinalysis—no characteristic changes
- CSF—minimally increased protein and leukocyte counts may be seen

Diagnostic Feature

- **DFA test of nervous tissue—method of choice for definitive diagnosis; rapid and very sensitive test**
- DFA—brain, head, or entire body can be shipped to rabies-certified laboratory for processing; chill samples immediately, but do not freeze; use extreme care and caution when collecting, handling, and shipping these samples.
- DFA test on dermal tissue—skin biopsy of the sensory vibrissae of the maxillary area, including deeper subcutaneous hair follicles; approved for human diagnostics, but not for animal diagnostics; accurate if positive, but negative test does not rule out rabies
- Although skin testing may augment a clinical diagnosis, verification can only be achieved by a DFA test of nervous tissue.
- Rabies antibody titer—A serological antibody titer of 0.5 IU/ml is considered adequate for protection in vaccinated people and animals.

THERAPEUTICS

- Inform client—as to the seriousness of contact with a rabid animal
- As a veterinarian, you must insist—that clients see a physician immediately to initiate postexposure therapy; local public health officials must be notified as soon as possible; local and state regulations must be adhered to carefully and completely
- Advise clients—to carefully consider any other human exposure
- If there is doubt regarding the diagnosis—The animal should be quarantined in an approved site with appropriate signage and cage security and only designated people should have access.
- An apparently healthy dog or cat that bites or scratches a person—should be monitored for a period of 10 days; if no signs of illness occur in the animal within 10 days, the person has had no exposure to the virus; animals do not shed the virus for more than 3 days before development of clinical disease
- An unvaccinated dog or cat that is bitten or exposed to a known rabid animal—may need to be quarantined for up to 6 months or according to local or state regulations
- Once a diagnosis is as close to certain as possible, euthanasia with submission of appropriate tissues for a definitive diagnosis is indicated.
- Vaccination—Vaccinate according to standard recommendations and state and local requirements; all dogs and cats with any potential exposure to wildlife or other dogs; vaccinate after 12 weeks of age; then 12 months later; then every 3 years (killed vaccines in cats and dogs) or yearly for cats if a nonadjuvanted recombinant vaccine (Purevax Feline Rabies; Merial) is used.
- Rabies-free countries—entering dogs and cats may be quarantined; contact specific countries for requirements
- Disinfection—Any contaminated area, cage, food dish, or instrument must be thoroughly disinfected; use a 1:32 dilution (4 ounces per gallon of water) of household bleach to quickly inactivate virus; usually virus deposited on a dog or cat hair after a bite from a rabid animal will die after exposure to the air for 1 hour.

Drugs of Choice

- No drug treatment is indicated—Once a diagnosis is made, euthanasia is indicated.
- Vaccines (dogs and cats)—Vaccinate according to standard recommendations and state and local requirements; all dogs and cats with any potential exposure to wildlife or other dogs; vaccinate after 12 weeks of age; then 12 months later; then every 3 years using a vaccine approved for 3 years; use only inactivated or recombinant vector vaccines for cats.
- Rabies-free countries—Entering dogs and cats are quarantined for long periods, usually 6 months.
- Disinfection—Any contaminated area, cage, food dish, or instrument must be thoroughly disinfected; use a 1:32 dilution (4 ounces per gallon) of household bleach to quickly inactivate the virus.

Precautions/Interactions

- The seriousness of the zoonotic potential cannot be overemphasized.
- Local and state regulations must be adhered to carefully and completely.

 COMMENTS

- Prognosis—grave; almost invariably fatal
- Dogs and cats with clinical infection usually succumb within 1–10 days of onset of clinical signs, often within 3–4 days.

Abbreviations

CBC, complete blood count; CNS, central nervous system; CSF, cerebrospinal fluid; DFA, direct fluorescent antibody; GME, granulomatous meningoencephalitis; RNA, ribonucleic acid.

Suggested Reading

Barr MC, Olsen CW, Scott FW. Feline viral diseases. In: Ettinger SJ, Feldman EC, eds. *Veterinary Internal Medicine*. Philadelphia: WB Saunders, 1995:409–439.

Frymus T, Addie D, Belák S, et al. Feline rabies: ABCD guidelines on prevention and management. *J Feline Med Surg* 2009;11:585–593.

Greene CE, Rupprecht CE. Rabies and other *Lyssavirus* infections. In: Greene CE, ed. *Infectious Diseases of the Dog and Cat*. Philadelphia: WB Saunders, 2006:167–183.

Jenkins SR, Auslander M, Conti L, et al. Compedium of animal rabies prevention and control. *J Am Vet Med Assoc* 2004;224:216–222.

Leslie M, Auslander M, Conti L, et al. Compendium of animal rabies prevention and control, 2006. *J Am Vet Med Assoc* 2006;228:858–864.

Richards JR, Elston TH, Ford RB, et al. The 2006 American Association of Feline Practitioners Feline Vaccine Advisory Panel Report. *J Am Vet Med Assoc* 2006;229:1405–1441.

chapter 83

Reovirus Infection

DEFINITION/OVERVIEW

- A respiratory and intestinal viral infection of cats and dogs resulting in mild upper respiratory signs or diarrhea

ETIOLOGY/PATHOPHYSIOLOGY

- *Reovirus* (respiratory enteric orphan virus)—nonenveloped, double-stranded RNA virus
- Easily isolated—from the respiratory and enteric tracts
- Like rotavirus and coronavirus—affects mature epithelial cells on luminal tips of intestinal villi
- Damage to villi—villous atrophy and osmotic diarrhea
- Transmission—fecal/oral (GI) route; also inhalation (respiratory)

SIGNALMENT/HISTORY

- Young animals usually more severely affected

CLINICAL FEATURES

Dogs

- Conjunctivitis
- Rhinitis
- Tracheobronchitis
- Pneumonia, if secondary bacterial infection involved
- Diarrhea

Cats

- Mainly mild respiratory signs (conjunctivitis)
- Diarrhea

DIFFERENTIAL DIAGNOSIS

Dogs

- Other causes of acute small bowel diarrhea in an otherwise healthy young animal:
  - Infectious; parvovirus, coronavirus, rotavirus, calicivirus, distemper, giardiasis, cryptosporidiosis, hookworms, whipworms, roundworms, GI tract bacterial overgrowth, and clostridia
  - Toxicity—lead
  - Dietary indiscretion, allergy
  - IBD
  - Foreign body
  - Intussusception
- Other causes of canine infectious tracheobronchitis—*Bordetella bronchiseptica*, mycoplasma, CAV, CHV, distemper, CIV, CRC, and parainfluenza

Cats

- Other causes of mild upper respiratory disease—rhinotracheitis virus, calicivirus, *Chlamydia* spp., and mycoplasma

DIAGNOSTICS

- CBC and biochemistry panel—normal
- Viral isolation—very time consuming, but can be identified on electron microscopy (Fig. 83-1)

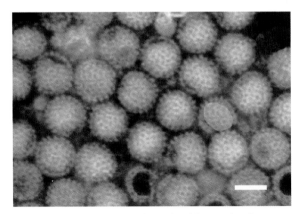

■ **Figure 83-1** Electron micrograph of reovirus particles isolated from a dog (bar = 50 nm).

- Even if virus is isolated from cat or dog with symptoms, this likely is not the primary pathogen.
- RT-PCR—available in some diagnostic facilities
- Histopathology—large intracyctoplasmic inclusion bodies

 ## THERAPEUTICS

- Antibiotics may be indicated if fever is present or diarrhea persists.
- Supportive care for osmotic diarrhea as needed
- Antiviral drugs are not indicated

Drugs of Choice

- N/A

Precautions/Interactions

- No vaccines are available.

 ## COMMENTS

- If reovirus is demonstrated to be present, search for the presence of other pathogens.

Abbreviations

CAV, canine adenovirus; CBC, complete blood count; CHV, canine herpes virus; CIV, canine influenza virus; CRV, canine respiratory coronavirus; GI, gastrointestinal; IBD, inflammatory bowel disease; RNA, ribonucleic acid; RT-PCR, real-time polymerase chain reaction.

Suggested Reading

Comins C, Heinemann L, Harrington K, et al. Viral therapy for cancer "as nature intended." *Clin Oncol* 2008;20:548–554.

Decaro N, Campolo M, Desario C, et al. Virological and molecular characterization of a mammalian orthoreovirus type 3 strain isolated from a dog in Italy. *Vet Microbiol* 2005;109:19–27.

Schiff LA, Nibert ML, Tyler KL. Orthoreoviruses. In: Knipe DM, Howley PM, eds. *Fields Virology*, 5th ed. Philadelphia: Lippincott Williams & Wilkins, 2007.

Respiratory Capillariasis (*Eucoleus*)

DEFINITION/OVERVIEW

- A nematode parasitic infection of both dogs and cats—mainly asymptomatic but can cause a chronic cough and wheezing respiratory sounds

ETIOLOGY/PATHOPHYSIOLOGY

- *Eucoleus aerophilus* (previously named *Capillaria aerophila*)—Trichuroidea parasite with bioperculate eggs
- Eggs—easily confused with those from other capillarids (*Eucoleus boehmi* of the nose and *Pearsonema plica* in the urinary bladder) and whipworms of dogs (*Trichuris vulpis*)
- Adult worms (long, up to 4cm)—embed in the mucosal lining of large airways, expelling eggs into the respiratory passages
- Eggs—coughed up the trachea and swallowed, to be passed in the feces
- Infection—occurs by ingesting L1 larvae
- Infections—can last as long as a year
- Direct life cycle—likely, although it is possible that earthworms are paratenic hosts
- PPP = about 40 days

CLINICAL FEATURES

- Fairly common infection in both cats and dogs
- Most infections are asymptomatic, rarely causing clinical signs
- Wheezing
- Chronic cough
- Weight loss is rare
- When complicated with bacterial pneumonia, can cause death

DIFFERENTIAL DIAGNOSIS

- A general differential diagnosis for cough includes such categories as:
  - Cardiovascular and congestive heart failure (pulmonary edema; enlarged heart, especially the left atrium; left-sided heart failure; pulmonary emboli; mitral valve insufficiency)
  - Allergic (bronchial asthma, eosinophilic pneumonia or granulomatosis, pulmonary infiltrate with eosinophilia)
  - Trauma (foreign body, irritating gases, collapsing trachea, hypoplastic trachea)
  - Neoplasia (not only of the respiratory tree but also associated structures such as ribs, lymph nodes, muscles)
  - Inflammatory (pharyngitis; tonsillitis; kennel cough from such agents as *Bordetella bronchoseptica*, parainfluenza virus, infectious laryngotracheitis virus, and mycoplasma; systemic fungal pneumonia; bacterial bronchopneumonia; aspiration; chronic pulmonary fibrosis; pulmonary abscess or granuloma; chronic obstructive pulmonary disease)
  - Parasites (*Oslerus* [*Filaroides*] *osleri*, *Filaroides hirthi*, *Filaroides milksi*, *Paragonimus kellicotti*, *Dirofilaria immitis*—heartworm disease in the dog, and *Aelurostrongylus abstrusus* in the cat)

 DIAGNOSTICS

Diagnositic Feature

- **Bioperculate eggs found in feces or tracheal wash fluids of both cats and dogs (Fig. 84-1)**

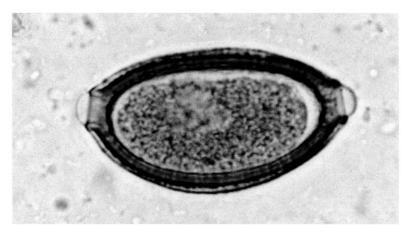

■ **Figure 84-1** Bioperculate egg found in the feces of an infected cat. In dog feces, the egg may be distinguished from those of *E. boehmi* by the fine lattice-work lines over the surface as opposed to the fine pitted surface of those of *E. boehmi*.

TABLE 84-1	Drug Therapy for Respiratory Capillariasis in Small Animals			
Drug	Dose (mg/kg)	Route	Interval (h)	Duration (days)
Ivermectin	0.2	PO, SC	Once	—
Fenbendazole	50	PO	24	10–14
Abamectin[a]	0.3	SC	Once	Repeat in 14

[a]Reported in cats only.

- Eggs—very similar to those of *Trichuris vulpis* (whipworms), found in infected dog's feces, and those of *E. boehmi* (nasal capillaria), which also may be found in feces
- Eggs are 58–79 × 29–40 μm in size; anastomosing ridges form a net-like pattern over the shell wall surface.
- Thoracic radiographs may show diffuse mild bronchoalveolar pattern but are not pathognomonic.

 THERAPEUTICS

- Asymptomatic cases do not require treatment.

Drugs of Choice

- Fenbendazole—treatment of choice in dogs; difficult to administer in cats over this time period
- Ivermectin—efficacy is unknown but is effective against nasal capillariasis and indications are that it is effective against other capillarids as well (Table 84-1)
- Abamectin—reported effective in treating a cat (Table 84-1)

Precautions/Interactions

- If using ivermectin, ensure dogs do not have microfilaremia before administering ivermectin.
- Ivermectin-sensitive collie breeds or collie-cross dogs may show neurologic signs with this dose of ivermectin.

 COMMENTS

- Pulmonary capillariasis is often found incidentally on routine fecal examinations.
- There is probably not a requirement to treat animals found to be infected with *E. aerophilus* on a routine fecal examination.

- It is the author's impression that the infection has become more uncommon with the advent of the wide use of monthly heartworm preventives.
- Infection is probably acquired from infected earthworms or the environment (eggs can persist for long periods)—One means of preventing reinfection would be to keep pets indoors.

Abbreviation

PPP, prepatent period.

Suggested Reading

Conboy G. Helminth parasites of the canine and feline respiratory tract. *Vet Clin Small Anim* 2009;39:1109–1126.

Rhinosporidium Infection

DEFINITION/OVERVIEW

- A rare chronic fungal infection of the mucous membranes of dogs (reported in two cats; rarely in horses, cows, and humans)
- Usually forms a cauliflower-like mass that protrudes from the nostril

ETIOLOGY/PATHOPHYSIOLOGY

- *Rhinosporidium seeberi*—thought to be associated with stagnant water and arid environments
- Distribution—worldwide
- Endemic areas—Argentina, Sri Lanka, and India
- In the United States—most infections reported from the southern states

SIGNALMENT/HISTORY

- Dogs mainly—no breed or sex predilection
- Cats—only one case report

CLINICAL FEATURES

- Cauliflower-like mass in the nasal cavity often seen protruding from the nostril
- Usually single and polypoid, but may be lobulated or sessile
- Surface often white or yellowish with superficial flecks, which are fungal sporangia
- Dog often present with:
  - Sneezing
  - Epistaxis
  - Stertorous breathing

DIFFERENTIAL DIAGNOSIS

- Nasal neoplasia
- Allergic inflammatory rhinitis
- Polyps
- Nasal foreign body
- Other fungal causes of rhinitis (aspergillosis)
- If epistaxis alone, rule out systemic causes of bleeding (coagulopathy, thrombocytopenia)

 DIAGNOSTICS

- CBC, serum biochemical panel, and urinalysis—usually normal
- Nasal radiographs—often normal because the mass is usually located in the anterior nasal cavity and does not invade turbinates
- CT or MRI scans—show a mass effect

Diagnostic Feature

- **Diagnostic method of choice—cytology of mass aspirate, impression smear, or biopsy of the nasal mass will reveals organisms (periodic acid–Schiff, GMS, and new methylene blue are the best stains) (Fig. 85-1)**

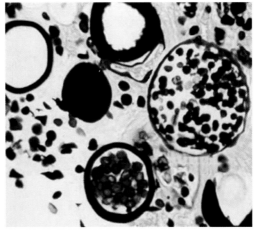

■ **Figure 85-1** *Rhinosporidium* spores present within a biopsy section of a nasal mass from a dog (GMS stain, 1000×).

THERAPEUTICS

- Surgical excision of mass—treatment of choice
- Approach—through the external nares or by rhinotomy
- Failure to remove all the mass—usually results in regrowth

Drugs of Choice

- Dapsone—has been used in one dog with favorable results, but not a complete cure and considerable side effects (dosage: 1.1 mg/kg, PO, q8–12h)
- Antifungal agents (ketoconazole, itraconazole)—consistently ineffective

Precautions/Interactions

- Dapsone—can cause hepatotoxicity, anemia, neutropenia, thrombocytopenia, GI signs, and skin reactions

COMMENTS

- Careful follow-up is necessary to identify regrowth after surgical removal.
- There is no known risk of direct transmission to humans in contact with infected dogs, but the organism is infectious to humans.

Abbreviations

CBC, complete blood count; CT, computed tomography; GI, gastrointestinal; GMS, Gomori's methamine silver; MRI, magnetic resonance imaging.

Suggested Reading

Abbitt B. Rhinosporidiosis. *Texas Vet* 2008;70:44.

Caniatti M, Roccabianca R. Scanziani E, et al. Nasal rhinosporidiosis in dogs: four cases from Europe and a review of the literature. *Vet Rec* 1998;142:334–338.

Wallin LL, Coleman GD, Froeling J, et al. Rhinosporidiosis in a domestic cat. *Med Mycol* 2001;39:139–141.

chapter 86

Rocky Mountain Spotted Fever

DEFINITION/OVERVIEW

- A tick-borne rickettsial disease affecting dogs; considered the most important rickettsial disease in humans
- Other as yet undefined rickettsial organisms may also cause clinical signs in dogs.

ETIOLOGY/PATHOPHYSIOLOGY

- *Rickettsia rickettsii*
- Antibodies to *Rickettsia akari* (causative agent of rickettsialpox in humans)—have been found in dogs in New York City, but it is not known if it causes disease in dogs
- Vector—American dog tick (*Dermacentor variabilis*), found east of the Great Plains; wood tick (*Dermacentor andersoni*), found from the Cascade Mountains to the Rocky Mountains
- Incidence of disease greatest during tick season—late March to end of September
- Prevalence—overall infection in ticks <2%; varies by geographic location
- Distribution—mainly in the eastern seaboard states (especially the Carolinas), Mississippi River Valley, and south-central states in the United States; also found in South America
- Transmission—via the saliva of the vector or blood transfusion
- Ticks—must attach for 5–20 hours to infect a host (humans, dogs, and cats) or reservoir hosts (rodents and dogs)
- Incubation period—2 days to 2 weeks
- Infection—organism invades and multiplies in vascular endothelium; causes widespread vasculitis in organs with endarterial circulation, leading to microvascular hemorrhage, platelet aggregation (thrombocytopenia), vasoconstriction, increased vascular permeability, increased plasma loss into the interstitial space (organ swelling), hypotension, and eventually DIC and shock

SIGNALMENT/HISTORY

- Purebred dogs—more prone to developing clinical illness than are mixed-breed dogs
- German shepherd dogs—more common

Historical Findings

- Fever—within 2–3 days of tick attachment
- Lethargy
- Depression
- Anorexia
- Swelling (edema)—lips, scrotum, prepuce, ears, and extremities
- Stiff gait—especially with scrotal or prepucial swelling
- Spontaneous bleeding—sneezing, epistaxis
- Respiratory distress
- Neurologic signs—ataxia, head tilt
- Ocular pain

 CLINICAL FEATURES

- Both clinical and subclinical illnesses occur.
- Clinical—variable in severity; lasting 2–4 weeks if untreated
- Ticks may still be present in acute cases.
- Pyrexia
- Cutaneous lesions—edema of face, limbs, prepuce, and scrotum (Fig. 86-1)
- Conjunctivitis
- Scleral injection (Fig. 86-2)
- Respiratory—dyspnea, exercise intolerance, and increased bronchovesicular sounds

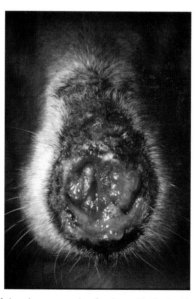

■ **Figure 86-1** Severe necrosis of the planum nasale of a dog with Rocky Mountain spotted fever.

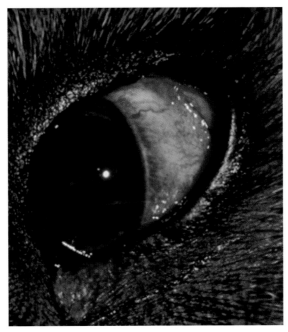

■ **Figure 86-2** Scleral injection in a dog with Rocky Mountain spotted fever (courtesy of Dr. R. Riis, Cornell University).

- Generalized lymphadenopathy
- Neurologic—vestibular dysfunction, altered mental status, and seizures
- Myalgia/arthralgia
- Petechiae
- Ecchymoses—ocular (Fig. 86-3), oral, and genital regions; in 20% of patients
- Hemorrhagic diathesis—epistaxis, melena, hematuria in severe cases
- Cardiac arrhythmias—sudden death
- DIC and death from shock—in severe acute cases

 DIFFERENTIAL DIAGNOSIS

- Canine ehrlichiosis—*Ehrlichia canis* and other *Anaplasmataceae*; not seasonal; clinically indistinguishable from RMSF (especially acute cases); differentiate with serologic testing; both respond to same treatment
- Immune-mediated thrombocytopenia—not usually associated with fever or lymphadenopathy; differentiate with serologic testing; may treat for both until results are known
- SLE—ANA test usually negative in RMSF; serologic testing is diagnostic
- Brucellosis—scrotal edema; serologic testing is diagnostic

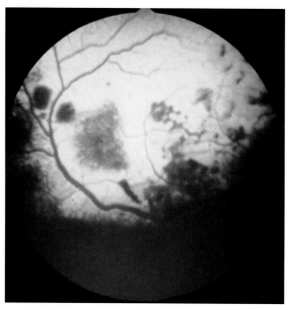

■ **Figure 86-3** Retinal hemorrhage and papilledema in a dog with Rocky Mountain spotted fever (courtesy of Dr. R. Riis, Cornell University).

DIAGNOSTICS

- CBC—thrombocytopenia (~40% of cases) partly due to antiplatelet antibody, megathrombocytosis, mild anemia (normochromic, normocytic), mild leukopenia (early in infection), and leukocytosis (and monocytosis) as disease becomes more chronic
- Serum biochemical profile—usually nonspecific changes; mild increases in ALT, ALP, BUN, creatinine, total bilirubin (rare); hypercholesterolemia consistently found (cause unknown); hypoalbuminemia (resulting from vascular endothelial damage); azotemia; hyponatremia, hypochloremia, and metabolic acidosis have all been reported
- Urinalysis—proteinuria, with or without azotemia, from glomerular/tubular damage; hematuria from coagulation defects
- Serologic tests—several exist, including microscopic immunofluorescence (Micro-IF) test, ELISA, and latex agglutination test:
  - Micro-IF test—most commonly used by diagnostic laboratories; measures IgG; levels may not be elevated when clinical signs first appear; take 2–3 weeks to rise; may be negative in very acute cases; perform paired titers 3 weeks apart; fourfold increase between acute and convalescent titers; avoid misdiagnosis because of considerable cross-reactivity with other rickettsial organisms; titers reach peak 3–5 months after infection, then decline (some can remain positive for 12 months even after treatment)

- ELISA—high sensitivity; can measure both IgG and IgM; therefore detects infection earlier than just measuring IgG alone
  - Latex agglutination test—higher specificity, lower sensitivity than Micro-IF test (false-negative results occur); single increased titer is diagnostic
- Direct immunofluorescence test—skin biopsies obtained by local anesthesia and punch biopsies from affected lesions; detect rickettsial antigens as early as 3–4 days postinfection
- CSF—often normal; may show an increase in protein and nucleated cells
- PCR on whole blood and tissue specimens—more sensitive than culture although might detect nonviable DNA; may detect DNA before seroconversion in some dogs; available at some academic institutions (North Carolina State University)

 THERAPEUTICS

- Most cases—treated as inpatient until stable
- Symptomatic—fluids and electrolyte solutions (dehydration and shock); blood transfusion (anemia); platelet-rich plasma or blood transfusion (hemorrhage from thrombocytopenia)
- Early antibiotic treatment—reduces fever and albumin extravasation and improves patient's attitude within 24–48 hours
- Platelet counts—repeat every 3 days after initiating treatment until within normal range; should return to normal within 2–4 days after initiating treatment
- Serologic titers—lower in treated than in untreated dogs; titers remain positive during convalescence

Drugs of Choice

- Doxycycline—drug of choice
- Prednisone—concurrent use; anti-inflammatory or immunosuppressive doses; given early in disease does not seem to be detrimental to the clinical recovery
- Alternative drugs:
  - Tetracyclines, chloramphenicol, and enrofloxacin—equally efficacious if used early
  - Oxytetracycline and tetracycline—effective and less expensive
  - Chloramphenicol—puppies <6 months of age; recommended to avoid yellow discoloration of erupting teeth caused by tetracyclines (Table 86-1)

Precautions/Interactions

- Tetracycline (or derivatives)—Do not use in patients <6 months of age because of permanent yellowing of teeth.
- Renal insufficiency—do not use tetracycline; doxycycline may be given (also excreted via the GI tract)
- Enrofloxacin—avoid in young dogs because articular damage can occur; GI upsets (vomiting, anorexia)

TABLE 86-1 Drug Therapy for Rock Mountain Spotted Fever in Dogs

Drug	Dose (mg/kg)	Route[a]	Interval (h)	Duration (days)
Doxycycline	10	PO, IV	12	10
Tetracycline	22	PO, IV	8	10
Enrofloxacin	3	PO, SC	12	10
Chloramphenicol	20	PO, IV	12	10

[a]Begin injectable therapy if patient is vomiting; change over to oral therapy once vomiting stops.

- Chloramphenicol—reduces titers to a greater extent than tetracyclines, so avoid use if serologic confirmation will be conducted after treatment; warn client of public health risk; directly interferes with heme and bone marrow synthesis; avoid use in dogs with thrombocytopenia, pancytopenia, or anemia

COMMENTS

- Prognosis—good in acute cases with appropriate and prompt therapy
- Response—occurs within hours of treatment
- Recovered dogs—are believed to be permanently immune to reinfection
- If treatment is not instituted until CNS signs occur or later in the disease process—mortality is high; patients with CNS signs may die within hours
- Prevention depends on controlling tick infestation on dogs—Use dips or sprays containing dichlorvos, chlorfenvinphos, dioxathion, propoxur, or carbaryl.
- Flea and tick collars (e.g., Preventic; Virbac Corp.), weekly insecticide baths (e.g., Ecto-Soothe [Virbac Corp.], Mycodex [Veterinary Products Lab.]), and/or monthly administrations of Revolution (selamectin; Pfizer), Sentinal (milbemycin/lufenuron; Novartis), Interceptor (milbemycin; Novartis), Frontline (fiprinol; Merial), or K9Advantix (imidacloprid/permithrin; Bayer) also protect against a number of species of ticks
- Environment—tick eradication impossible; organism maintained in rodents and other reservoir hosts
- Avoid—tick-infested areas
- Removal of ticks by hand—use gloves; ensure tick mouth parts are removed, because a foreign body reaction is likely to result if they are left in place
- Incidence of RMSF in humans—dropping in the United States; mid-1992 to mid-1993: 300 cases; earlier incidence: up to 1000 cases/year
- Source of infection for humans—from ticks that are transferred from dogs; not from dogs directly; when removing ticks from dogs
- Mainly—causes disease in young adults and children

Abbreviations

ALP, alkaline phosphate; ALT, alanine aminotransferase; ANA, antinuclear antibody; BUN, blood urea nitrogen; CBC, complete blood count; CNS, central nervous system; CSF, cerebrospinal fluid; DIC, disseminated intravascular coagulation; ELISA, enzyme-linked immunosorbent assay; GI, gastrointestinal; Ig, immunoglobulin; Micro-IF, microscopic immunofluorescence; PCR, polymerase chain reaction; RMSF, Rocky Mountain spotted fever; SLE, systemic lupus erythematosus.

Suggested Reading

Greene CE, Breitschwerdt EB. Rocky Mountain spotted fever, Murine Tryphuslike Disease, Rickettsialpox, Typhus, and Q fever. In: Greene CE, ed. *Infectious Diseases of the Dog and Cat*. Philadelphia: WB Saunders, 2006:232–245.

Kidd L, Maggi R, Diniz PP, *et al*. Evaluation of conventional and real-time PCR assays for detection and differentiation of Spotted Fever Group Rickettsia in dog blood. *Vet Microbiol* 2008;129:294–303.

Mikszewski JS, Vite CH. Central nervous system dysfunction associated with Rocky Mountain spotted fever infection in five dogs. *J Am Anim Hosp Assoc* 2005;41:259–266.

Rotavirus Infection

DEFINITION/OVERVIEW

- A rare intestinal viral infection of mammals, including cats and dogs, causing enteritis and diarrhea

ETIOLOGY/PATHOPHYSIOLOGY

- Rotavirus (from *rota* meaning wheel)—a nonenveloped, double-stranded RNA virus
- Relatively resistant—to environmental destruction
- Resistant to acid—allowing it to pass through the stomach to the intestinal tract
- Transmission—fecal/oral route
- Affects mature epithelial cells—on luminal tips of intestinal villi
- Villus damage—may lead to atrophy and osmotic diarrhea

SIGNALMENT/HISTORY

- Wide host range (main cause of diarrhea in children <2 years)
- Puppies (often <2 weeks old but usually <12 weeks)
- Kittens (<6 months) more susceptible to infection
- Animals deprived of colostrum may show more severe disease.

CLINICAL FEATURES

Dogs

- Usually subclinical
- Mild watery to mucoid diarrhea—occasionally
- Anorexia and lethargy—rare
- Fatalities in the very young—very rare

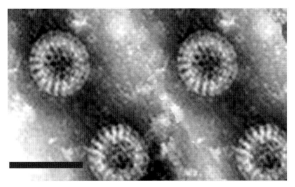

■ **Figure 87-1** Electron micrograph of rotavirus particles isolated from a dog. Note the wagon-wheel conformation that gives the virus its name (bar = 100 nm).

Cats

- Primarily subclinical or mild diarrhea
- Diarrhea more severe if concurrent infections or stress environment are present

 # DIFFERENTIAL DIAGNOSIS

- Other causes of acute small bowel diarrhea in an otherwise healthy young animal:
  - Infectious; parvovirus, coronavirus, rotavirus, calicivirus, distemper, giardiasis, FeLV, cryptosporidiosis, tritrichomoniasis, hookworms, whipworms, roundworms, GI bacterial overgrowth, and clostridia
  - Toxicity—lead
  - Dietary indiscretion, allergy
  - IBD
  - Foreign body
  - Intussusception

 # DIAGNOSTICS

- CBC and biochemical panel—usually normal or reflect dehydration and electrolyte abnormalities from diarrhea
- Viral detection—electron microscopy of negatively stained preparations of diarrheic feces will identify characteristic viral particles (wheel shape, 70-nm diameter) (Fig. 87-1)
- Detection of antigen in feces by ELISA and latex agglutination—commercially available in man (Rotazyme; Abbott Laboratories) but may be of low sensitivity for dog and cat rotaviruses

- Serologic examination (ELISA)—not recommended as most animals (85%) show exposure
- PCR—very sensitive but not currently commercially available
- Isolation on cell culture—time consuming, requires considerable expertise, and not all isolates grow

 ## THERAPEUTICS

- Symptomatic for diarrhea (fluids, electrolytes, NPO)
- Antibiotics are not indicated unless fever develops (use broad-spectrum agents).
- Antiviral drugs are not indicated.

Drugs of Choice

- N/A

Precautions/Interactions

- No vaccines are available.

 ## COMMENTS

- If outbreaks occur in very young animals in breeding situations, management practices should be scrutinized.
- Pay particular attention to environmental stress (temperature) and ability of animals to receive colostrum.
- Zoonotic potential—Rotaviruses are not host-specific, so infected animals pose a real risk to humans, particularly infants; in developing countries, causes life-threatening diarrhea in infants and young children.

Abbreviations

CBC, complete blood count; ELISA, enzyme-linked immunosorbent assay; FeLV, feline leukemia virus; GI, gastrointestinal; IBD, inflammatory bowel disease; NPO, nothing per os; PCR, polymerase chain reaction; RNA, ribonucleic acid.

Suggested Reading

Estes MK, Kapikian AZ. Rotavirus. In: Knipe DM, Howley PM, eds. *Fields Virology*, 5th ed. Philadelphia: Lippincott Williams & Wilkins, 2007:1917–1974.

McCaw DL, Hoskins JD. Canine viral enteritis. In: Greene CE, ed. *Infectious Diseases of the Dog and Cat*. Philadelphia: WB Saunders, 2006:63–73.

Roundworms (Ascariasis)

chapter 88

DEFINITION/OVERVIEW

- Large nematode parasites (10–12 cm long)—Adults live in the small intestine of dogs and cats.
- Infection—can lead to small intestine distention and interference with gut motility and digestion, especially in very young animals

ETIOLOGY/PATHOPHYSIOLOGY

- *Toxocara canis*—dogs
- *Toxocara cati*—cats
- *Toxascaris leonina*—dogs and cats
- For *T. canis*—Dogs may ingest eggs containing larvae, which hatch in the duodenum.
- Larvae—may migrate to the liver and lungs, resulting in pathology in young animals
- In adult hosts—Larvae are widely distributed and become encapsulated in tissues (especially skeletal muscle and kidneys).
- In bitches—Encapsulated, sequestered larvae form a source of infection for pups (transplacental and transmammary).
- Larvae—appear in milk as early as day 5 of lactation
- Transplacental transmission occurs to the fetus—Infected animals may be born with a developing worm burden, leading to abdominal distention and pain (can occur before eggs appear in the feces).
- Eggs—can appear in feces as early as 3 weeks of age
- Older pups and kittens—may become infected by ingesting infective eggs disseminated on the premises by dams with postgestational infections
- In dogs under 3 months of age (and occasionally adults)—Larvae that have migrated to the lungs break out into the airways, migrate up the trachea, and are swallowed, to develop to adults in the GI tract.
- *T. cati* life cycle—similar to that of T. canis, except transplacental infection does not occur
- Transtracheal migration following egg ingestion—probably occurs more commonly in adult cats

- Paratenic hosts—may be an important reservoir of infection for cats
- *T. leonina*—Infection can occur by ingestion of eggs or by ingesting a paratenic host (rodents) infected with dormant infective larvae.

 ## SIGNALMENT/HISTORY

- Dogs and cats—all ages, although clinical disease most severe in young pups and kittens

 ## CLINICAL FEATURES

Dogs

- *T. canis*—Parasitic pneumonia from tracheal migration of a large burden of prenatally acquired larvae can result in high mortality in pups (first 48–72 hours of life).
- Emaciation
- Digestive disturbances
- Abdominal distention
- Mucoid diarrhea and vomiting—sometimes containing adult worms
- Death—can occur in 2- to 3-week-old pups if burdens are high
- Less severe burdens
  - Unthriftiness
  - Rough hair coat
  - Pot-bellied appearance (Fig. 88-1)
  - Intermittent diarrhea
  - Anemia
  - Intestinal loops containing adults easily palpable
- Aberrant migrations by adults from the GI tract—may cause obstruction or rupture of the common bile duct, gallbladder, and pancreatic duct or migration to distant sites (spinal column)
- Neurologic signs—restlessness, twitching to convulsions (mechanism unknown)
- GI tract—Local hypersensitivity response has been reported, causing acute vomiting, hemorrhagic enteritis, or chronic eosinophilic enteritis (German shepherd dogs).
- Somatic larval migration—rarely causes clinical signs, but results in nodular lesions in kidneys, liver, lung, and myocardium
- *T. leonina*—least pathogenic; usually causes no clinical signs other than mild diarrhea and periodic vomiting

Cats

- *T. cati*—similar to those in dogs, but less severe; potbelly, intermittent diarrhea, unthriftiness
- Vomiting and coughing (but not neurologic signs)

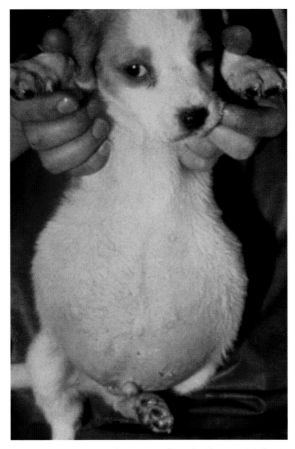

■ **Figure 88-1** Typical potbellied appearance of a puppy infected with *T. canis* infection.

- Intestinal loops containing adults easily palpable
- *T. leonina* is the least pathogenic roundworm, usually causing no clinical signs other than mild diarrhea and periodic vomiting.

 DIFFERENTIAL DIAGNOSIS

Dogs

- Causes of potbellied appearance in puppies:
  - Ascites
  - Hepatomegaly
  - Splenomegaly
  - Renomegally

- Causes of diarrhea in the puppy:
  - Dietary indiscretion
  - Allergy
  - Drugs (antibiotics)
  - Toxins—lead
  - Parasites (*Giardia* spp., cryptosporidiosis, GI parasitism with hookworms or *Strongyloides* spp.)
  - Infectious agents (salmonellosis, enteric calicivirus, reovirus, CPV, coronavirus, canine distemper, CHV, campylobacter, clostridiosis)
  - GI tract bacterial overgrowth (coliforms)
  - Systemic organ dysfunction (renal, hepatic, pancreas, cardiac)

Cats

- Causes of diarrhea in the kitten:
- Dietary indiscretion
- Allergy
- Drugs (antibiotics)
- Toxins—lead
- Parasites (*Giardia* spp., cryptosporidiosis, tritrichomoniasis, GI tract parasitism with hookworms or *Strongyloides* spp.)
- Infectious agents (panleukopenia, salmonellosis, enteric calici virus, reovirus, FeLV, feline calicivirus)
- GI tract bacterial overgrowth (coliforms)
- Systemic organ dysfunction (renal, hepatic, pancreas, cardiac)

DIAGNOSTICS

- *T. canis*—shows marked eosinophilia, mild leukocytosis with eosinophilia, anemia; hepatic enzyme elevations occur in larval migration
- *T. cati*—eosinophilia with mild leukocytosis; no anemia
- Fecal flotation (or less sensitive fecal smear)—characteristic eggs of each parasite (Fig. 88-2)

THERAPEUTICS

- To limit environmental contamination—Pups should be routinely treated with an anthelmintic (such as pyrantel pamoate) at 2, 4, 6, and 8 weeks, and then placed on a monthly heartworm treatment with efficacy against ascarids.
- Kittens—Because the PPP is 8 weeks, kittens can be first at 6 weeks of age, although if hookworm infection is a concern, then treat with pyrantel pamoate beginning at

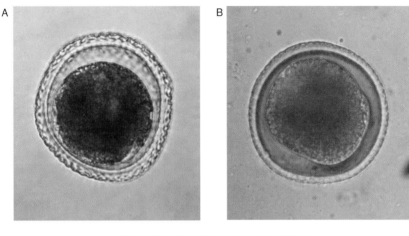

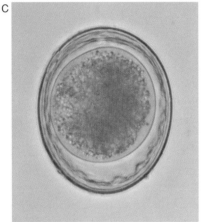

■ **Figure 88-2** The roundworm eggs of the (A) dog (*T. canis*), (B) cat
(*T. cati*), and (C) both dogs and cats (*T. leonina*). Note that the egg of *T. leonina* is ellipsoid and has a smooth shell that distinguishes it from those of other *Toxocara* spp.

2 weeks of age, and like dogs, put onto monthly heartworm preventative with efficacy against ascarids.

- Control and prevention—CAPCVET (http://www.capcvet.org) recommendations advise treating dogs and cats monthly to prevent acquiring new infections; fecal exams 2–4 times in the first year and 1–2 times per year thereafter to ensure client compliance; prevent predation; prompt removal of feces from litter boxes or yards; enforce leash laws.
- Treat bitch or queen with adulticide/larvacide anthelmintic (fenbendazole)—decreases subsequent litter and mature maternal infections
- Severely debilitated pups—IV fluids and nutritional support while parasiticidal drugs are used
- Pups with parasite-induced pneumonia—Treat severe inflammatory response (due to worm death from parasiticide drug treatment) in the lungs: prednisone (0.25 mg/kg, PO, q12h, for 5 days).

Drugs of Choice

Adulticide/Larvacide Anthelmintics

- Fenbendazole (Panacur granules 22.2%; Intervet)—from day 40 of pregnancy to 2 weeks after birth results in ascarid-free pups
- Unsequestered larvae—treat with fenbendazole for 5 consecutive days (does not kill sequestered larvae)
- Sequestered larvae—treat from day 40 gestation to 2 weeks postgestation to protect pups born in subsequent litters
- Once larvae are in the fetus (after day 40 of gestation)—probably not killed when fenbendazole is administered to the bitch
- Ivermectin (Ivomec; Merial)—Experimentally, large doses can markedly reduce pup infections (1 mg/kg, PO, q24h on days 20 and 42, or 0.5 mg/kg, PO, on days 38, 41, 44, and 47 of gestation to bitch).

Adulticide Anthelmintics

Pups <4 Weeks of Age
- Piperazine (Pipfuge and others)—starting in the second week of life, repeat every 3 weeks until pup is 3 months of age
- Praziquantel/pyrantel/febantel (Drontal Plus; Bayer)—monthly after pups reach 3 weeks of age and weigh over 2 pounds

Pups and Dogs >4 Weeks of Age
- Piperazine (Pipfuge and others)
- Milbemycin oxime (Interceptor or Sentinel; Novartis)
- Moxidectin (Advantage Multi; Bayer)—in dogs over 7 weeks, cats over 9 weeks of age
- Praziquantel/pyrantel/febantel (Drontal Plus; Bayer)
- Pyrantel (Nemex tablets and suspension; Pfizer)
- Ivermectin and pyrantel (Heartguard Plus; Merial)
- Fenbendazole (Panacur Granules 22.2%; Intervet)
- Dichlorvos (Task Tabs; Boehringer Ingelheim)
- Toluene and dichlorophene (Happy Jack Trivermicide Worm Capsules; Happy Jack Inc)
- Diethylcarbamazine (Filaribits; Pfizer) (Table 88-1)

Cats
- Because *T. cati* larvae do not cross the placenta—only necessary to treat cats every 3 weeks for the first 3–4 months of life
- Piperazine (Pipfuge and others)
- Pyrantel (Nemex tablets and suspension [Pfizer] or Drontal [Bayer])
- Dichlorvos, toluene/dichlorophene, milbemycin, moxidectin, emodepside (Profender; Bayer) and selamectin also work in cats.

TABLE 88-1 Drug Therapy of Roundworm Infections in Cats and Dogs					
Drug	Species	Dose (mg/kg)	Route	Interval (h)	Duration (days)
Fenbendazole (Panacur)	D	50	PO	24	3[a]
Piperazine (Pipfuge)	B	110	PO	Once	[b]
Praziquantel/pyrantel/febantel (Drontal) Plus	D	[c]	PO	Once	[d]
Milbemycin oxime (Interceptor, Sentinel)	D	0.5	PO	Once	[d]
Selamectin (Revolution)	B	6	Topical	Once	[d]
Moxidectin (Advantage Multi)	B	2.5-6.5 (D) 2 (C)	Topical	Once	[d]
Emodepside (Profender)	C	3	Topical	Once	[d]
Pyrantel (Nemex or Drontal)	D	5	PO	Once	[d]
	C	5–10	PO	Once	[d]
Ivermectin/pyrantel (Heartgard Plus)	D	5	PO	Once	[d]
Dichlorvos (Task Tabs)	B	11	PO	Once	[d]
Toluene/dichlorophene (Happy Jack)	B	[e]	PO	Once	[d]
Diethylcarbamazine (Filaribits)	D	6.6	PO	24	Life span[f]

[a] Repeat in 3 weeks in pups >4 weeks of age. Give from day 40 of pregnancy to 2 weeks after birth in pregnant bitches for ascarid-free pups.
[b] Pups—start in 2nd week of life, repeat every 3 weeks until pup is 3 months of age. Cats—every 3 weeks.
[c] Dose—praziquantel (5–12 mg/kg), pyrantel (5–12 mg/kg), and febantel (25–62 mg/kg).
[d] Repeat monthly
[e] Dose—toluene (264 mg/kg), and dichlorophene (220 mg/kg).
[f] Filaribits is primarily given for heartworm prevention so is given daily for the dog's life.
B, cats and dogs; C, cats; D, dogs.

Precautions/Interactions

- Piperazine—At low doses (55 mg/kg), worms are not paralyzed long enough to be expelled; use higher doses (110 mg/kg).
- Pay particular attention—to manufacturer's recommendations regarding use of the drugs in pregnant and young animals; for example:
  - Drontal Plus—not for puppies <3 weeks of age or <2 pounds
  - Heartgard Plus—not for puppies <6 weeks of age
  - Interceptor—not for puppies <6 weeks of age or <2 pounds
  - Sentinel—not for puppies <4 weeks of age or <2 pounds
  - Sentinel Flavor Tabs—not for puppies <4 weeks of age or 11 pounds
  - Revolution—use in animals >6 weeks of age
  - Task Tabs—not for puppies <10 days of age or <1 pound

- Check dogs for microfilaremia before using avermectin products.
- Pups may vomit 30–90 minutes after being given Task Tabs—should not affect efficacy
- Dichlorvos should not be given to animals with GI tract obstruction or liver problems.

 COMMENTS

- *Toxocara* eggs are extremely resistant remaining infective for years—virtually impossible to rid from soils in heavily contaminated situations
- Entomb eggs—cover runs with a concrete slab or bituminous asphalt
- Once installed—egg levels can be controlled by at least weekly cleaning of cement or asphalt
- Contaminated kennel areas—Physically clean surfaces using high-pressure washers, followed by 1% sodium hypochlorite (3 cups of bleach/gallon of water), followed by water rinsing. (NOTE: This does not kill the eggs, but merely removes their ability to stick to surfaces.)
- Prevent animals (particularly cats) eating potential paratenic hosts (rodents—*Toxocara* infection rates are high)
- Zoonotic potential—Visceral and ocular larva migrans may follow ingestion of infective eggs (especially in children).

Abbreviations

CHV, canine herpes virus; CPV, canine parvovirus; FeLV, feline leukemia virus; GI, gastrointestinal.

Suggested Reading

Bowman DD, ed. *Georgis' Parasitology for Veterinarians*, 9th ed. Philadelphia: WB Saunders, 2008.
Epe C. Intestinal nematodes: biology and control. *Vet Clin North Am Small Anim Pract* 2009;39: 1091–1107.

Salmonellosis

chapter 89

DEFINITION/OVERVIEW

- A bacterial disease that causes enteritis, septicemia, and abortions in both cats and dogs

ETIOLOGY/PATHOPHYSIOLOGY

- *Salmonella* spp.—gram-negative bacteria of many different serotypes
- The bacterium colonizes the small intestine (ileum), then invades enterocytes before entering and multiplying in the lamina propria and local mesenteric lymph nodes.
- Cytotoxin and enterotoxin are produced, causing inflammation and prostaglandin synthesis and leads to the development of a secretory diarrhea and mucosal sloughing.
- In uncomplicated enteritis, organisms are prevented from spreading from the mesenteric lymph nodes—Patients develop diarrhea, vomiting, and dehydration as a result of secretory diarrhea.
- If organisms spread from the lymph nodes to the circulation to produce bacteremia and septicemia, severe disease occurs.
- Focal extraintestinal infections—can result in abortion, joint disease, or endotoxemia with organ infarction, generalized thrombosis, DIC, and death
- Some patients recover from the septicemic form—suffer prolonged recovery as a result of their debilitated state
- The true incidence is unknown—Most infections are subclinical.

Dogs

- Most clinical disease seen in young or pregnant animals
- Fecal swab cultures from clinically normal domestic pets, pets in boarding kennels, and pets in veterinary hospitals showed incidences of 30%, 16.7%, and 21.5%, respectively.
- Common in racing greyhounds and sled dogs due to raw meat diets; presence of *Salmonella* does not necessarily imply infection but could reflect transient pass-through.

Cats

- Have a high natural resistance—especially older cats
- Stressed hospitalized animals—higher risk especially when treated with an oral antimicrobial drug prior to spay-neuter or declawing
- Fecal swab culture surveys of normal cats and cats from a research colony—incidences of 18% and 10.6%, respectively.
- Shelter cats—more likely to have *Salmonella* spp. in feces
- Pandemics of salmonellosis in migrating songbirds (usually *S. typhimurium*) in spring—create epidemics in bird-hunting cats

 SIGNALMENT/HISTORY

- Host factors that increase the likelihood of dogs or cats developing clinical illness:
  - Age (neonatal/young)
  - Overall health status (debilitated older animals; treatment with immunosuppressive drugs or antibiotics for other diseases are used when patient is exposed to virulent drug-resistant *Salmonella* spp. during hospital stay, concurrent GI parasitism)
- Environmental factors:
  - Coprophagia spreads infection
  - Dehydrated (dry) pet food can harbor organism (semimoist not as likely)
  - Contaminated foods (pig ear dog treats)
  - Dense populations (research colonies, boarding facilities)
- Hunting/stray animals—scavenge for food (exposure to organism in food, dead animals, infected raw meat, song birds)
- Hospitalized animals—increased nosocomial exposure coupled with increased stress of hospitalization and concurrent treatments with antimicrobials and immunosuppressive drugs
- Historically—Patients may have diarrhea, vomiting, fever, and anorexia.
- Vaginal discharge/abortion—may occur in dogs
- Chronic persistent febrile illness with persistent fever, anorexia, malaise without diarrhea—possible

Dogs

- Most infections—subclinical (carrier state: *Salmonella* spp. shed in feces)
- Clinical forms—varying from mild, to moderate, to severe are seen in neonatal/immature puppies and pregnant bitches
- Most adult carrier dogs—clinically normal

Cats

- Adult cats—highly resistant to clinical disease
- Neonatal/immature and immunocompromised animals—susceptible to disease

CLINICAL FEATURES

Dogs

- Gastroenteritis:
  - Anorexia
  - Malaise/lethargy
  - Depression
  - Fever
  - Diarrhea containing mucus and blood
- As disease progresses—the patient becomes more dehydrated, with:
  - Abdominal pain
  - Tenesmus
  - Pale mucous membranes
  - Mesenteric lymphadenopathy
  - Weight loss
- Gastroenteritis with bacteremia and septicemia, septic shock, or endotoxemia:
  - Pale mucous membranes
  - Weakness
  - Cardiovascular collapse
  - Tachycardia
  - Tachypnea.
  - Death preceded by multiple organ failure
- Focal extraintestinal infections—Conjunctivitis, metritis/abortion, cellulitis, and pyothorax have been reported.

Cats

- May exhibit a syndrome of a chronic febrile illness (without gastrointestinal signs):
  - Persistent fever
  - Prolonged illness with vague, nonspecific clinical signs and leukogram with a left shift
- Recovering patients—may exhibit chronic intermittent diarrhea for 3–4 weeks; may shed *Salmonella* spp. in stool for 6 weeks or longer

DIFFERENTIAL DIAGNOSIS

- All causes of diarrhea, including systemic or metabolic disease, as well as specific intestinal disorders, should be considered.
- Other causes of acute enterocolitis—dietary indiscretion, chronic IBD, HGE, neoplasia (especially GI tract lymphoma), drugs (antibiotics), toxins (lead), parasites (cryptosporidiosis, tritrichomoniasis, whipworms), infectious agents (parvovirus;

FIP; rickettsia, including salmon poisoning; GI tract bacterial overgrowth; *Campylobacter* spp.; clostridial enterotoxicosis; histoplasmosis; leishmaniasis; other rare infections—pythiosis), systemic organ dysfunction (renal, hepatic, pancreatic), and metabolic (hypoadrenocorticism, hyperthyroidism—cats)

DIAGNOSTICS

- CBC—variable; depends on stage of illness
  - Initially neutropenia—often with left shift and toxic neutrophils
  - Nonregenerative anemia
  - Lymphopenia
  - Thrombocytopenia
- Serum biochemical profile—hypoalbuminemia and electrolyte abnormalities with secretory diarrhea (metabolic acidosis, hypokalemia)
- Fecal/rectal culture—positive (requires special media); best performed on fresh feces to maximize culture results
- PCR—available but not widely used on a commercial basis
- Fecal leukocytes—usually present
- Blood cultures (perform if fever is present)—can be positive but not very sensitive
- Joint fluid—culture may be positive
- Subclinical carrier state—fecal culture intermittently positive often >6 weeks
- Use of antimicrobials in patient before sampling—may produce false-negative culture results

THERAPEUTICS

- Degree of care—depends largely on severity of diarrhea and whether systemically ill or not
- Uncomplicated gastroenteritis cases without bacteremia—treat as outpatients
- Bacteremia/septicemia/severe diarrhea—parenteral crystalloid fluid and electrolyte therapy based on degree of dehydration, shock, acid–base status, and ongoing fluid losses
- Consider colloid therapy (plasma, hetastarch)—when serum albumin <2 g/dl
- Once vomiting and diarrhea abate—Consider oral fluids containing hypertonic sugar solutions for secretory diarrhea.
- Limit movement of patient (isolate)—because patient can excrete large numbers of organisms in stool during acute diarrhea stage
- Maintain good hygiene—of associated animal health care workers (including clients)
- Restrict food until in recovery—then offer highly digestible, low-fat diet

Drugs of Choice

Asymptomatic Carrier State

- Antimicrobials—contraindicated because:
  - Increases the risk of resistance developing to the drugs
  - Prolongs the convalescent excretion period
- Quinolone drugs—clear carrier state in humans but unknown in animals

Uncomplicated Gastroenteritis

- Antimicrobials—not indicated
- Locally acting intestinal absorbents and protectants—mainstay of therapy

Neonates, Aged, and Debilitated Animals

- Antimicrobials—indicated, but important to base selection on culture and sensitivity results because *Salmonella* spp. are notoriously resistant to many agents
- TMS
- Amoxicillin
- Enrofloxacin
- Norfloxacin
- Chloramphenicol (Table 89-1)

Precautions/Interactions

- TMS—multiple adverse reactions, including:
  - KCS—monitor tear production weekly throughout treatment
  - Hepatotoxicity—anorexia, depression, icterus; monitor alanine ALT if prolonged therapy
  - Megaloblastic–folate acid deficiency anemia—especially in cats after several weeks; supplement with folinic acid (2.5 mg/kg/day)

TABLE 89-1 Drug Therapy for Salmonellosis in Dogs and Cats					
Drug	Species	Dose (mg/kg)	Route	Interval (h)	Duration (days)
Trimethoprim-sulfadiazine	B	15	PO, IV	12	10
Amoxicillin	B	10–20	PO	8	10
Enrofloxacin	B	5	PO, SC	12	7
Norfloxacin	B	22	PO	12	7
Chloramphenicol	D	15–25	PO, SC	8	7
	C	10–15	PO, SC	12	7

D, dogs; C, cats; B, both dogs and cats.

- Immune-mediated polyarthritis, retinitis, glomerulonephritis, vasculitis, anemia, thrombocytopenia, urticaria, toxic epidermal necrolysis, erythema multiforme, and conjunctivitis—remove from drug
- Renal failure and interference with renal excretion of potassium (leading to hyperkalemia)
- Salivation, diarrhea, and vomiting (cats)
- May interfere with thyroid hormone synthesis (dogs)—check T_3 and T_4 after 6 weeks
- Use chloramphenicol and TMS with caution in neonates and pregnant patients.
- Chloramphenicol—may cause a reversible nonregenerative anemia and myelosuppression
- Fluoroquinolones—avoid use in pregnant, neonatal, or growing animals (medium-sized dogs <8 months of age; large or giant breeds <12 to 18 months of age) because of cartilage lesions

COMMENTS

- Repeat a fecal culture monthly for 3 months to detect development of carrier state.
- Monitor for secondary spread to other animals.
- Avoid predisposing factors (host, environmental, etc.) described previously.
- Spread of infection to other animals and humans in the household not uncommon, resulting in chronic bouts of diarrhea, especially during times of stress.
- Prognosis for uncomplicated gastroenteritis is excellent; usually self-limiting, but patients can become chronic shedders of bacteria.
- Prognosis for severe disease is poor if left untreated; aggressive therapy usually produces a cure.
- Raw meat diets (especially chicken) offer dangers of infection with *Campylobacter*, *Salmonella*, and *Clostridium perfringens*.

Abbreviations

ALT, alanine aminotransferase; CBC, complete blood count; DIC, disseminated intravascular coagulation; FIP, feline infectious peritonitis; GI, gastrointestinal; HGE, hemorrhagic gastroenteritis; IBD, inflammatory bowel disease; KCS, keratoconjunctivitis sicca; PCR, polymerase chain reaction; TMS, trimethoprim-sulfadiazine.

Suggested Reading

Brain PH, Barrs VR, Martin P, et al. Feline cholecystitis and acute neutrophilic cholangitis: clinical findings, bacterial isolates and response to treatment in six cases. *J Feline Med Surg* 2006;8:91–103.
Cherry B, Burns A, Johnson GS, et al. *Salmonella typhimurium* outbreak associated with veterinary clinic. *Emerg Infect Dis* 2004;10:2249–2251.

Greene CE. Salmonellosis. In: Greene CE, ed. *Infectious Diseases of the Dog and Cat*. Philadelphia: WB Saunders, 2006:355–361.

Strohmeyer RA, Morley PS, Hyatt DR, et al. Evaluation of bacterial and protozoal contamination of commercially available raw meat diets for dogs. *J Am Vet Med Assoc* 2006;228:537–542.

Wright JG, Tengelsen L, Smith KE, et al. Multidrug-resistant *Salmonella typhimurium* in four animal facilities. *Emerg Infect Dis* 2005;11:1235–1241.

90 *chapter*

Salmon Poisoning

DEFINITION/OVERVIEW

- A rickettsial infection of dogs living in costal regions of northern California, Oregon, Washington, and southern British Columbia of Canada as a result of the distribution of *Oxytrema silicula,* the aquatic snail intermediate host
- Causes a systemic illness characterized by vomiting, diarrhea, and fever

ETIOLOGY/PATHOPHYSIOLOGY

- *Neorickettsia helminthoeca*—a rickettsial organism with a trematode vector, *Nanophyetus salmonincola*
- Dogs become infected by ingesting raw fish (usually of the salmonid family) that have eaten the trematode vector or by ingesting the vector or organism directly from water.
- The organism invades the small intestinal epithelium and associated lymphoid tissue and spleen.

SIGNALMENT/HISTORY

- Only dogs infected
- No age, sex, or breed predilection
- History of ingestion of raw fish caught in an endemic region
- Incubation period = 2–14 days

CLINICAL FEATURES

- Fever—initially
- Anorexia, lethargy
- Weight loss

- Diarrhea and vomiting—may occur in about 75% of cases
- Diarrhea—becomes progressively more severe and may consist mainly of blood at the time of death
- Lymphadenopathy—especially cervical and prescapular; abdominal lymphadenopathy may be present on ultrasonography in dogs without peripheral lymphadenopathy
- Nasal and ocular discharge—less common

DIFFERENTIAL DIAGNOSIS

- Gastroenteritis from ingestion of garbage, foreign bodies, toxins; infectious (distemper, parvovirus); IBD; systemic organ dysfunction (nephropathy, hepatopathy, pancreatitis); and HGE
- Diarrhea—can be so severe that sometimes it is misdiagnosed as parvovirus

DIAGNOSTICS

- CBC—Lymphopenia, thrombocytopenia, and neutrophilia with a left shift are the most common findings.
- Serum biochemical profile—Hyponatremia, hypocalcemia, hypoalbuminemia, and elevated alkaline phosphatase activity are the most common findings.
- Clotting function—elevated in a small proportion of dogs
- Aspirate cytologic specimen of enlarged lymph nodes—may reveal intracytoplasmic rickettsial bodies (Giemsa stain) associated with histiocytic hyperplasia and lymphoid reactivity
- Fecal examination—reveals operculated eggs of the trematode *Nanophyetus salmonincola* usually present (Fig. 90-1)
- Abdominal ultrasonography—may reveal mesenteric lymphadenopathy even when peripheral lymphadenopathy is absent
- PCR—available, but may not add much more diagnostic sensitivity

THERAPEUTICS

- Most require hospitalization for supportive fluid therapy and close monitoring of electrolytes, acid–base status, and body temperature.
- Basic measures to control diarrhea

Drugs of Choice

- Doxycycline
- Other tetracyclines are also effective—tetracycline, oxytetracycline, or minocycline

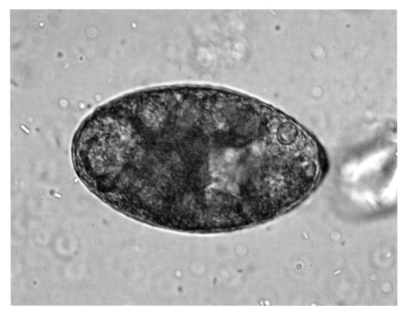

■ **Figure 90-1** Operculated egg of *N. salmonincola* from a fecal sample taken from a dog with salmon poisoning.

- If tetracyclines cannot be used—Penicillins, chloramphenicol, and sulphonamides are usually also effective (although, in one study, penicillins and chloramphenicol showed less efficacy).
- Praziquantel—to kill the fluke *Nanophyetus salmonincola* (Table 90-1)
- *N. salmonincola* does not cause severe clinical disease—treating for it will limit spread of eggs

Precautions/Interactions

- In a vomiting dog—best to start therapy with injectable oxytetracycline or doxycycline until the vomiting is controlled; then switch to an orally administered drug

TABLE 90-1 **Drug Therapy for Salmon Poisoning in Dogs**				
Drug	Dose (mg/kg)	Route	Interval (h)	Duration (days)
Doxycycline	10	PO, IV	12	7
Tetracycline	22[a]	PO	8	5
Oxytetracycline	10[a]	PO, IV	8	5
Minocycline	10	PO, IV[b]	12	7
Praziquantel	20–30	PO	Once	—

[a]Reduce dose in renal failure.
[b]Give by slow IV injection; rapid injection can cause hypotension, shock, and urticaria if given too rapidly.

- Doxycycline—contraindicated in pregnant or lactating bitches
- Minocycline—give by slow IV injection because too rapid injection can cause hypotension, shock, and urticaria
- Tetracyclines—can cause discoloration of teeth in young animals; reduce dose in renal failure

COMMENTS

- The sooner therapy is instituted after ingestion of raw fish, the better the prognosis.
- Warn clients—If other dogs may have eaten raw fish from the same area, they should receive a course of doxycycline and praziquantel.
- Prognosis—Without treatment, infected dogs usually die within 5–10 days.
- Prognosis—with early appropriate treatment, should see marked improvement of clinical signs within 24 hours; prognosis is good

Abbreviations

CBC, complete blood count; HGE, hemorrhagic gastroenteritis; IBD, inflammatory bowel disease; PCR, polymerase chain reaction.

Suggested Reading

Gorham JR, Foreyt WJ. Salmon poisoning disease. In: Greene CE, ed. *Infectious Diseases of the Dog and Cat*. Philadelphia: WB Saunders, 2006:198–203.

Sykes JE, Marks S, Mapes RM, et al. Salmon poisoning disease in dogs: 29 cases. *J Vet Intern Med* 2010;24:504–513.

DEFINITION/OVERVIEW

- Enteric protozoa of carnivores causing no disease in the definitive host (carnivores), but the cysts sequestered in the muscle of domestic herbivores (cattle) are of some economic importance
- The importance of the organism to small animal clinicians (finding *Sarcocystis* oocysts in the feces of dogs and cats)—understanding their significance

ETIOLOGY/PATHOPHYSIOLOGY

- *Sarcocystis* spp.—like other coccidia, are obligate intracellular protozoa that infect and reproduce in enterocytes of many carnivores (including cats and dogs)
- Unlike other coccidia—*Sarcocytis* requires a second host (intermediate host) to complete the life cycle.
- Intermediate hosts—domestic (cattle and sheep) and various wild herbivores
- Intermediate hosts acquire infection—oocysts from contaminated pasture
- Cysts—develop within muscle (and nervous tissue) of the herbivorous intermediate hosts causing economic downgrade of the carcass at slaughter
- Dogs and cats—become infected by eating cysts sequestered in the meat of a herbivorous intermediate host
- *Sarcocystis*—of no pathogenic consequence to definitive hosts (dogs and cats); muscle cyst stages can have a pathogenic effect on some intermediate hosts (cattle)

SIGNALMENT/HISTORY

- Dogs and cats—eating raw or undercooked meat
- Prevalence—can be >50% in stray dogs in some countries

CLINICAL FEATURES

- None
- Owners and veterinarians—may be concerned with finding *Sarcocystis* oocysts in feces of a pet

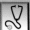 **DIFFERENTIAL DIAGNOSIS**

- None
- Need to differentiate the *Sarcocystis* oocysts from those of other coccidia

 DIAGNOSTICS

- Fecal flotation—small (9–16 mm) sporulated oocysts or sporocysts of *Sarcocystis* (Fig. 91-1)
- Individual species—possible to tell apart based on morphology of oocysts

 THERAPEUTICS

- No effective drug treatment known
- Because the organism is nonpathogenic to dogs and cats, and infection terminates spontaneously, drug therapy is not warranted.

Drugs of Choice

- None

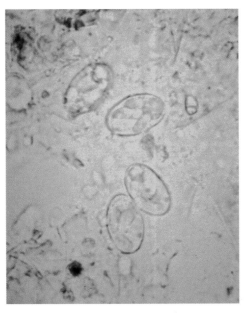

■ **Figure 91-1** Oocysts of *Sarcocystis* in the feces of a dog (1000×).

Precautions/Interactions

■ None

 COMMENTS

■ Owners should avoid feeding pets raw, uncooked meat.
■ Fresh meat in retail food stores—can be infected with *Sarcocystis* cysts, which can remain viable for several days under refrigeration
■ Frozen (for >3 days) or well-cooked meat—loses its infectivity to cats and dogs
■ Prevent contact of infected dogs and cats with the feed supply (grain or pasture lands) of herbivores—to reduce the contamination of feed with sporocysts

Suggested Reading

Dubey JP, Linday DS, Lappin MR. Toxoplasmosis and other intestinal coccidial infections in cats and dogs. *Vet Clin North Am Small Anim Pract* 2009;39:1009–1034.

Sarcoptic Mange

chapter 92

DEFINITION/OVERVIEW

- Nonseasonal, intensely pruritic, highly contagious parasitic skin disease of dogs and cats cause by infestation with the mite *Sarcoptes scabiei*

ETIOLOGY/PATHOPHYSIOLOGY

- Mites burrow through the stratum corneum and cause intense pruritus by mechanical irritation, production of irritating by-products, and secretion of allergenic substances that produce a hypersensitivity reaction.
- Mites can transiently affect a species other than the host species via direct contact.
- Highly contagious within the host species

SIGNALMENT/HISTORY

- Animals of all ages and breeds
- Exposure to a carrier often 2–6 weeks before development of symptoms
- Risk factors can include—living in a cattery and multiple cat households; living outside, boarded at kennel; visits to veterinarian's office or groomers, animal shelter
- Usually a history of nonseasonal extremely intense pruritus

CLINICAL FEATURES

- Alopecia and erythematous rash—pinnae, elbows, hocks, ventral abdomen, and chest
- Lesions on ear margins—vary from barely perceptible scaling to alopecia or crusts; ear canals not affected
- Chronic—periocular and truncal alopecia; secondary crusts, excoriations, and pyoderma; diffuse papular eruption
- Possible peripheral lymphadenopathy

- Frequently bathed dogs will often have chronic pruritus with minimal skin lesions ("scabies incognito").
- Dogs—often minimal or no response to anti-inflammatory doses of steroids
- Multiple dog households—More than one dog usually shows signs.

 DIFFERENTIAL DIAGNOSIS

- Food allergy
- Atopy
- Malassezia dermatitis
- Flea-allergic dermatitis
- Dermatophytosis
- Pyoderma
- Demodicosis
- Contact allergy
- Pelodera dermatitis
- Pruritic impetigo

 DIAGNOSTICS

- ELISA technique—identify *Sarcoptes*-infested dogs; detection of circulating IgG antibodies against *Sarcoptes* antigens available, yet high false-positive results in dogs successfully treated for scabies mites and false-negative results in young dogs and in dogs receiving corticosteroids; not widely used
- Positive pinnal-pedal reflex—rubbing the ear margin between the thumb and forefinger should induce the animal to scratch with the ipsilateral hind leg; occurs in 75–90% of cases
- Superficial skin scrapings—not always effective; if negative but a high clinical suspicion exists, treat with a scabicide to definitively rule out sarcoptic mange
- Fecal flotation—occasionally reveals mites or ova
- Favorable response to scabicidal treatment—often an effective method for tentative diagnosis
- Any dog with nonseasonal pruritus that responds poorly to steroids should be treated with a scabicide (even if skin scrape results are negative) to definitively rule out sarcoptic mange.

 THERAPEUTICS

- Scabicidal dips—the entire dog must be treated; treatment failures often linked to owner's reluctance to apply dip to the patient's face and ears; do not let the patient get wet between treatments

- All in-contact dogs, cats, rabbits—should be treated, even those with no clinical signs; may be asymptomatic carriers
- Thoroughly clean and treat environment; mites can survive for up to 3 weeks off a host animal
- Corticosteroids may be used concurrently with miticidal therapy.

DRUGS

- Ivermectin—highly effective; 0.2–0.4 mg/kg SC every 1–2 weeks for 4 treatments; do not use in ivermectin sensitive breeds (Collies, Shetland Sheepdogs, white German Shepherds, Australian Shepherds, Old English Sheepdogs); effective for *Sarcoptes scabiei* infestation (dogs)
- Selamectin (Revolution; Pfizer) is the only systemic treatment licensed for canine scabies; best results obtained when apply product 6–12 mg/kg topically every 2 weeks for 3–4 treatments (dogs and cats)
- Moxidectin (Cydectin; Wyeth) at 200 μg/kg, PO or SC, q2wks for 2 treatments is a less used option for sarcoptid mite infestation.
- Milbemycin (Interceptor)—effective when used at 0.75 mg/kg, PO, q24h; may be effective at 2 mg/kg, PO, every week for 3 weeks (dogs)
- Amitraz (Mitaban) dip—250 ppm; may be effective at every 1–2 weeks for 3 treatments; make sure entire body is covered, including the face and ears (dogs)
- Whole-body rinse solution—2–3% solution of lime sulfur (LymDip) apply for 5–6 weeks; make sure entire body is covered, including the face and ears (best treatment option for cats; approved for dogs and cats)
- Fipronil spray—at 3 ml/kg, applied as a pump spray to the entire body 3 times at 2-week intervals, or 6 ml/kg applied as a sponge-on once weekly for 4–6 weeks
- Topical antiseborrheic therapy in conjunction with scabicidal therapy helps speed clinical resolution of the lesions.
- Systemic antibiotics—may be needed for 21 days or longer to resolve any secondary pyoderma
- Antihistamines or low-dose glucocorticoids (0.5 mg/kg, q12h, for 1st week of treatment)—if mites were identified; may make pruritus diminish more quickly

 COMMENTS

- Bedding should be disposed of and the environment thoroughly cleaned and treated with parasiticidal sprays/foggers/bombs (flea insecticides for the environment are effective).
- Ivermectin—Use with extreme caution in collies, Shetland sheepdogs, old English sheepdogs, Australian shepherds, white German Shepherds, and their crossbreeds; toxicity is more likely to occur in herding-type breeds.
- May take as long as 4–6 weeks for the intense pruritus and clinical signs to resolve, owing to the hypersensitivity reaction

- Topical treatments are prone to failure, owing to incomplete application of the treatment solution.
- Reinfection can occur if the contact with infected animals continues.
- Always consider mites as a possible cause of pruritus in allergic dogs that cease to respond to steroid therapy.
- Approximately 30% of dogs with *Sarcoptes* infections will also react to house dust mite antigens.
- Zoonosis—People who come in close contact with an affected animal may develop a pruritic, papular rash on their arms, chest, or abdomen; human lesions are usually transient and should resolve spontaneously after the affected animal has been treated; if the lesions persist, clients should seek advice from their dermatologist.

Abbreviations

ELISA, enzyme-linked immunosorbent assay; SC, subcutaneously

Suggested Reading

Feather L, Cough K, Flynn RJ, et al. A retrospective investigation into risk factors of sarcoptic mange in dogs. *Parasitol Res* 2010;107:279–283.

Pin D, Densignor E, Carlotti DN, et al. Localized sarcoptic mange in dogs: a retrospective study of 10 cases. *J Small Anim Pract* 2006;47:611–614.

chapter 93

Spirocerca lupi

DEFINITION/OVERVIEW

- Nematode parasite—adult worms are found in fibrous nodules within the walls of the esophagus and stomach of dogs
- Cause vomiting or regurgitation, aortic aneurysm (rarely aortic rupture), cervical spondylitis, esophageal osteosarcoma, pulmonary hypertrophic osteoarthropathy, and aberrant migration of adults to unusual sites within the thorax (subcutis, heart)
- Common in Israel (where it seems to be re-emerging), South Africa, Greece—rare in North America (mideastern states; Alabama)

ETIOLOGY/PATHOPHYSIOLOGY

- *Spirocerca lupi*—Adults (within the esophageal or gastric wall nodules) deposit very small (15 × 30 mm) eggs containing an embryo into the esophageal luminal tract, to be passed in feces.
- Eggs—eaten by intermediate hosts (coprophilic beetles); develop to L3 infective larvae
- Transmission—dogs infected by ingesting L3 larvae in paratenic hosts (lizards, chickens, mice)
- Dogs—larvae migrate via the adventitia of visceral arteries and mature in the thoracic aorta, to the walls of the stomach and caudal esophagus
- Spondylitis of the thoracic vertebrae—pathognomonic lesion
- Aortic aneurysm—develops in about 50% of infected dogs (very rarely, aortic rupture)
- Chronic infections—result in large, calcified fibrous nodules within the esophagus walls
- Neoplasia of the nodules—occurs occasionally
- PPP = 5–6 months

SIGNALMENT/HISTORY

- Median age of infection—5 years
- Infection in dogs <1 year of age—rare

- Large hunting-breed dogs—with access to intermediate hosts (mice, uncooked chicken, lizards) are overrepresented
- Most cases—diagnosed during the colder months (December through April in Israel)

 ## CLINICAL FEATURES

- Vomiting
- Regurgitation
- Salivary gland necrosis—resulting in enlarged, hard, painful salivary glands
- Associated signs—retching; vomiting; regurgitation of saliva
- Pyrexia
- Weakness
- Respiratory abnormalities
- Anorexia
- Melena
- Paraparesis—less common

 ## DIFFERENTIAL DIAGNOSIS

- Other causes of regurgitation—megaesophagus (idiopathic, myasthenia gravis, polymyositis, hypoadrenocorticism, hypothyroidism, lead toxicity), esophagitis, esophageal diverticulum, vascular ring anomaly, esophageal neoplasia, hiatal hernia, esophageal foreign body, and sialadenitis
- Other causes of vomiting—dietary; toxins (lead, ethylene glycol), IBD, metabolic (diabetes mellitus, renal disease, hepatic disease, acidosis, heat stroke, hypoadrenocorticism), gastric abnormalities (neoplasia, obstruction, atrophic gastritis, ulcers, dilatation/volvulus), gastroesophageal junction disorders (hiatal hernia), small intestine disorders (IBD, neoplasia, fungal, parasitic, viral, obstruction, paralytic ileus), large intestine disorders (colitis, obstipation, irritable bowel syndrome), abdominal disorders (pancreatitis, gastrinoma, peritonitis, steatitis, prostatitis, pyometra, diaphragmatic hernia, neoplasia), and neurologic disorders (psychogenic, motion sickness, vestibular lesions, head trauma, brain neoplasia)

 ## DIAGNOSTICS

- CBC—anemia (blood loss), 50% of cases
- Creatine kinase elevations—50% of cases
- Fecal flotation (sugar best)—identifies eggs in about 80% of infected dogs

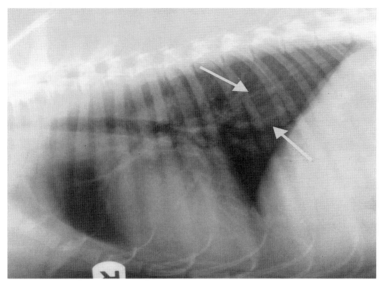

■ **Figure 93-1** Lateral radiograph of a dog with an esophageal granuloma (*between arrows*) caused by *S. lupi* (courtesy of Dr. Eran Lavy, Israel).

- Thoracic radiology—identifies caudal esophageal masses in about 50% of infected dogs (Fig. 93-1)
- Midthoracic vertebral spondylitis—on radiographic examination (33% of cases)

Diagnostic Feature

- **Esophageal endoscopy—most sensitive diagnostic procedure (100%)**
- Endoscopy—may show granulomas in various degrees of severity (Fig. 93-2) or tumors (Fig. 93-3) but endoscopic biopsies are not sensitive in showing neoplastic transformation

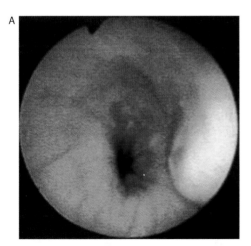
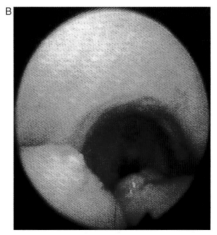

■ **Figure 93-2** Endoscopic views of esophageal granulomas caused by *S. lupi* in various forms of development (courtesy of Dr. Eran Lavy, Israel).

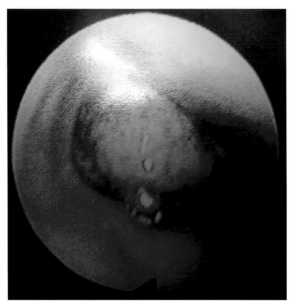

■ **Figure 93-3** Endoscopic view of esophageal neoplasm caused by *S. lupi* (courtesy of Dr. Eran Lavy, Israel).

 THERAPEUTICS

- Drug therapy—institute quickly
- If not treated—about 60% of dogs will die or be euthanized within a month of diagnosis if not treated
- Surgery to remove nodules has been successful.

Drugs of Choice

- Doramectin (Dectomax Injectable Solution, 10 mg/ml; Pfizer)
  - Regimen 1: 0.2 mg/kg, SQ every 14 days for 3 treatments—resolves clinical signs and nodules in most dogs, but further treatment with doramectin (0.5 mg/kg, PO, q24h for 6 weeks) may be required if nodules not fully resolved
  - Regimen 2: 0.4 mg/kg, SQ every 14 days for 6 treatments and then monthly until all esophageal granulomas are gone—2 years in some cases

Precautions/Interactions

- Doramectin is not labeled for use in the dog (cattle and pig wormer).

COMMENTS

- Sialidinitis will resolve with long-term treatment with doramectin.
- Prophylactic use of doramectin (0.4 mg/kg, SQ, q30d for 3 treatments)—markedly reduces egg production and clinical signs but does not completely prevent infection in all dogs

Abbreviations

CBC, complete blood count; IBD, inflammatory bowel disease; PPP, prepatent period.

Suggested Reading

Berry WL. *Spirocerca lupi* esophageal granulomas in 7 dogs: resolution after treatment with doramectin. *J Vet Intern Med* 2000; 14: 609–612.

Mazaki-Tovi M, Baneth G, Aroch I, et al. Canine spirocercosis: clinical, diagnostic, pathologic, and epidemiologic characteristics. *Vet Parasitol* 2002;107:235–250.

Van der Merwe LL, Kirberger RM, Clift S, et al. *Spirocerca lupi* infection in the dog: a review. *Vet J* 2008;176:294–309.

94 *chapter*

Sporotrichosis

DEFINITION/OVERVIEW

- A zoonotic fungal disease that may affect the integument or lymphatics; may cause systemic disease

ETIOLOGY/PATHOPHYSIOLOGY

- *Sporothrix schenckii*—ubiquitous dimorphic fungus living mainly in soil rich in decaying organic material
- Infection—occurs typically by direct inoculation such as puncture wounds associated with foreign bodies (dogs mainly) or introduced by scratches (cats)

SIGNALMENT/HISTORY

Dogs

- More commonly seen in hunting breeds because of increased likelihood of puncture wounds associated with thorns or splinters
- Historically, dogs initially presenting with clinical disease have had a poor response to antibiotic therapy.

Cats

- Intact males that roam outdoors and fight, because of the increased likelihood of puncture wounds and acquiring the disease from their opponents

CLINICAL FEATURES

Cutaneous Form

Dogs

- Associated with numerous nodules, which may drain or crust, typically affecting the head or trunk but can also be found on the limb (Fig. 94-1)

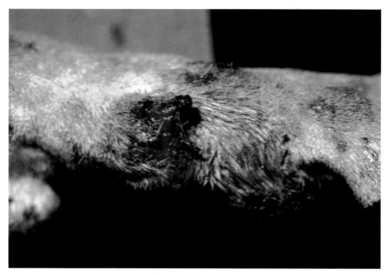

■ **Figure 94-1** Sporotrichosis in a dog. Note the crusted excoriated draining tract around the dew claw on the limb.

Cats

■ Lesions often initially appear as wounds or abscesses, mimicking wounds associated with fighting, found on the head, lumbar region, or distal limbs.

Cutaneolymphatic Form

■ Usually an extension of the cutaneous form; spreads via the lymphatics, resulting in new nodules and draining tracts or crusts; lymphadenopathy common

Disseminated Form

■ Associated with the systemic signs of fever, malaise, and anorexia
■ Consider underlying immunosuppressive disorder, which is a predisposing factor for systemic form (neoplasia)

    # DIFFERENTIAL DIAGNOSIS

■ Various bacterial and fungal diseases—consider when symptoms include a nodular granulomatous disease and draining tracts (e.g., blastomycosis, feline leprosy, histoplasmosis, cryptococcosis)
■ Neoplasia
■ Parasitic infections (*Demodex* or *Pelodera* spp.)

DIAGNOSTICS

- CBC, serum biochemical profile, and urinalysis usually normal unless in the systemically ill, in which there can be a leukocytosis with a left shift and monocytosis
- REMEMBER: This is a zoonotic disease that can be acquired across intact skin—take particular care when collecting samples from infected patients.

Diagnostic Feature

- **Cytologic examination of the exudate and staining—often the only test necessary to confirm disease (cats)—cigar-shaped to round yeast intracellularly or free in the exudates**
- Dogs—special fungal stains (PAS or GMS) may aid in the diagnosis; a negative finding does not rule out the disease
- Culture of deeply affected tissues—often requires surgery to obtain an adequate sample
- Important—to alert laboratory that sporotrichosis is on the differential diagnosis list
- Bacterial contamination of biopsy samples for culture—is common

THERAPEUTICS

- Warn owner of zoonotic potential of patient under treatment.

Drugs of Choice

SSKI

- Treatment of choice.
  - Dogs—40 mg/kg, PO, q8h with food
  - Cats—20 mg/kg, PO, q12h with food
- Treat for at least 2 months and continue for 30 days after the resolution of the clinical lesions.
- Dogs—If signs of iodism are noted (see following discussion of signs of iodism), discontinue treatment for 1 week; if symptoms are mild, reinitiate at the same dose; if severe, consider other drugs.
- Cats—iodism is more commonly seen in cats; if develops, discontinue and use other drugs

Ketoconazole and Itraconazole

- Dogs—ketoconazole: 15 mg/kg, PO, q12h, preferably with an acidic meal (e.g., tomato juice), until 1 month after clinical resolution, which should occur within about 3 months
- Cats—ketoconazole: 5–10 mg/kg, PO, q12–24h, or itraconazole 10 mg/kg/day until 1 month after clinical resolution

Precautions/Interactions

Signs of Iodism

- Dogs—dry hair coat, excessive scales, nasal or ocular discharge, vomiting, depression, or collapse
- Cats—depression, vomiting, anorexia, twitching, hypothermia, and cardiovascular collapse

Side Effects of Azole Therapy

- Dogs—anorexia, acute hepatopathy (follow hepatic enzymes to monitor), pruritus, alopecia, and lightening of the hair color reported
- Cats—GI disturbances, depression, fever, jaundice, and neurologic signs; may be necessary to alternate drugs

 COMMENTS

- Re-evaluate—every 2–4 weeks for clinical signs and side effects associated with treatment
- Although difficult—Try to determine the source of the original infection to prevent repeat infections.
- Consider—having male cats neutered to stop fighting behavior
- Unresponsive to therapy—not unexpected; consider alternative treatment or combined regimens (SSKI and ketoconazole)
- Zoonotic—Proper precautions and client education cannot be overemphasized; an absence of a break in the skin does not protect against acquiring the disease.
- Clinically healthy cats sharing a household with an infected cat may be a source of infection for people.

Abbreviations

CBC, complete blood count; GI, gastrointestinal; GMS, Gomori's methamine silver (stain); PAS, periodic acid–Schiff; SSKI, supersaturated potassium iodide.

Suggested Reading

Scott DW, Miller WH, Griffin CE. Muller and Kirk's Small Animal Dermatology, 5th ed. Philadelphia: WB Saunders, 1995.

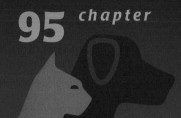

Staphylococcal/ Bacterial Pyoderma and Resistant

DEFINITION/OVERVIEW

- Common bacterial infections of the skin categorized based on depth of infection:
  - Surface (epithelium)—includes acute moist dermatitis ("hot spots" and skin fold pyoderma [intertrigo])
  - Superficial pyoderma (epidermis and follicles)—includes impetigo (puppy pyoderma), mucocutaneous pyoderma, superficial spreading pyoderma, and superficial folliculitis
  - Deep pyoderma (hair follicle rupture with extension into dermis and SC tissue)—includes muzzle folliculitis and furunculosis, nasal and pedal pyoderma, generalized deep pyoderma, bacterial granulomas ("acral lick dermatitis"), pressure point pyoderma, and pyotraumatic folliculitis and furunculosis
- Emerging bacterial infections also usually of the skin, but can cause deep infections include: methicillin-resistant staphylococcus, *Pseudomonas* spp., *Enterococcus* spp., and *Corynebacterium* spp., with staphylococcal infections being the most widespread and problematic at this time

ETIOLOGY/PATHOPHYSIOLOGY

- *Staphylococcus pseudintermedius*—most frequent cause
- Other species of staph include: *S. schleiferi* and *S. aureus*
- *Pasteurella multocida*—an important pathogen in cats
- Deep pyoderma (furunculosis)—may be complicated by gram-negative organisms (e.g., *E. coli*, *Proteus* spp., *Pseudomonas* spp.)
- Rarely caused by higher bacteria (e.g., Actinomyces, Nocardia, mycobacteria, Actinobacillus)
- Predisposing factors may include: systemic immunoincompetence (metabolic disease), trauma (pressure, licking, scratching, parasites), follicular damage (demodex mites, scratching), dermal damage (collagen disruption, extension of disease, etc.), physical factors (poor grooming, maceration of the skin, heat, humidity), inappropriate antibacterial therapy (too short a course, poor drug choice, inappropriate dose)

- Problematic resistant infections are mainly those that are methicillin (and other drugs in the class, including penicillin, amoxicillin, and oxacillin)-resistant Staphylococcal infections (MRSA) including the spp. *S. aureus*, *S. pseudintermedius*, and *S. schleiferi*.
- MRSA is thought to have developed because of overuse of antibiotics particularly broad spectrum antibiotics, such as cephalexin, cefazolin, cefadroxil, amoxicillin, penicillin, and even fluoroquinolones.
- Zoonotic potential—All three *Staphylococcus* spp. have the potential to cause disease in both humans and animals; one study found MRSP in 4.5% of healthy dogs and 1.2% of healthy cats.

 # SIGNALMENT/HISTORY

- Dogs—very common
- Cats—uncommon
- Breeds with short coats, skin folds, or pressure calluses
- German shepherds—develop a severe, deep pyoderma that may only partially respond to antibiotics and frequently relapses; similar problem noted in the Pit Bull breed in the interdigital regions
- Acute or gradual onset
- Variable pruritus—underlying cause may be pruritic (aeroallergens—atopic dermatitis) or the staphylococcal infection itself may be pruritic (bacterial hypersensitivity)

 # CLINICAL FEATURES

- Acute moist dermatitis ("hot spot")—self-induced traumatic skin disease with secondary bacterial infection, maceration of the skin may lead to folliculitis and furunculosis (facial region in large breed dogs)
- Intertrigo—skin fold dermatitis caused by maceration of tissue from chronic moisture/anatomical predisposition (facial folds, interdigital, perivulvar, axillae)
- Impetigo (nonfollicular subcorneal pustules)—puppy impetigo (poor nutrition, dirty environment, etc.) and Bullous impetigo in older dogs (large flaccid nonfollicular pustule often caused by *E. coli* or pseudomonas on the nose or glaborous skin; older patients may be immunocompromised)
- Mucocutaneous pyoderma—idiopathic ulcerative mucosal dermatitis with crusting and variable degrees of depigmentation; lesions often involve the lips, perioral, perivulvar, prepuce, anal regions
- Superficial pyoderma—usually involves the trunk; extent of lesions may be obscured by the hair coat; papules, pustules, epidermal collarettes, and hyperpigmented macules

- Superficial spreading pyoderma—arge coalescing epidermal collarettes on the lateral trunk; common in the Collie and Sheltie breeds; look for underlying metabolic disease
- Deep pyoderma—often affects the chin, bridge of the nose, pressure points, and feet; may be generalized; elicits a foreign body reaction due to ruptured hair follicle release of hair shaft antigen into the dermis
- Pseudomonas "post grooming furunculosis"—unique presentation of deep pyoderma initiated by bathing and/or grooming; acute, febrile, and extremely painful; combing, clipping, or overly aggressive bathing against the direct of growth of the hair may cause traumatic rupture of the hair follicle inciting a foreign body reaction; short-coated breeds predisposed; dorsal midline is often the most severely affected region; bacterial contamination of shampoos or equipment may be important in the etiology of this condition; lesions often occur within 24–48 hours after grooming
- Bacterial overgrowth syndrome—usually due to overgrowth of *Staphylococcus* spp. on the surface of the skin; bacterial toxins can have an allergenic role acting as superantigens triggering nonspecific inflammatory reactions; primary clinical signs are pruritus, erythema, and lichenification; cases often associated with malassezia overgrowth, have underlying diseases such as allergic skin disease or chronic glucocorticoid therapy. Topical shampoo therapy is absolutely vital to therapeutic success.

 DIFFERENTIAL DIAGNOSIS

- Atopic dermatitis
- Parasitic dermatitis (fleas, scabies, demodicosis, cheyletiellosis)
- Food allergy
- Neoplasia (cutaneous lymphoma)
- Metabolic (diabetes, superficial necrolytic dermatitis, idiopathic and iatrogenic hyperadrenocorticism, hypothyroidism)
- Cornification/ keratinization defects (seborrhea, vitamin A responsive dermatosis, sebaceous adenitis)
- Color dilution alopecias/ follicular dysplasias
- Immune-mediated diseases (Pemphigus, lupus erythematosus, vasculitis, etc.)
- Immunosuppression (glucocorticoids, chemotherapy, metabolic)
- Panniculitis
- Nodular dermatosis (e.g., histiocytosis)

 DIAGNOSTICS

- Identify risk factors—allergy (flea, atopy, food, contact); fungal infection (dermatophyte); endocrine diseases (hypothyroidism, hyperadrenocorticism, sex hormone imbalance); immune incompetency (glucocorticoids, young animals); seborrhea acne; schnauzer comedo syndrome

- Conformation—short coat, skin folds; trauma (pressure points, grooming, scratching, rooting behavior, irritants); foreign body (foxtail, grass awn)
- Superficial—normal or may reflect the underlying cause (e.g., anemia owing to hypothyroidism; stress leukogram and high serum alkaline phosphatase owing to Cushing disease; eosinophilia owing to parasitism)
- Generalized, deep—may show leukocytosis with a left shift and hyperglobulinemia; also changes related to the underlying cause

Diagnostic Tests

- Skin scrapings, trichogram, dermatophyte culture, intradermal allergy testing, hypollergenic food trial, endocrine tests—identify the underlying cause
- Skin biopsy
- Cytology—direct smear from intact pustule-neutrophils engulfing bacteria; differentiate bacterial infection from pemphigus foliaceus (acantholytic keratinocytes) and deep fungal infections (blastomycosis, cryptococcosis); tissue grains may identify filamentous organisms characteristic of higher bacteria
- Therapeutic diagnostic trials
- Culture and sensitivity—obtained as an aspirate from intact pustule, swab from the ventral surface of an epidermal collarette, tissue biopsy, or freshly expressed exudate from a draining tract or beneath a crust; may yield the pathogen

 THERAPEUTICS

- Severe, generalized, deep—may require IV fluids, parenteral antibiotics, or daily whirlpool baths
- Benzoyl peroxide or chlorhexidine shampoos—remove surface debris
- Whirlpool baths—deep pyodermas; remove crusted exudate; encourage drainage.
- Hypoallergenic diets—if secondary to food allergy; otherwise a high-quality, well-balanced dog food
- Avoid high-protein, poor-quality "bargain" diets and excessive supplementation.
- Fold pyodermas may require surgical correction to prevent recurrence.
- Superficial pyodermas—initially may be treated empirically with one of the recognized common therapeutic antibiotics
- Recurrent, resistant, or deep pyodermas—base antibiotic therapy on culture and sensitivity testing
- Multiple organisms with different antibiotic sensitivities—often best to choose antibiotic on basis of staphylococcal susceptibility, yet may need to find a medication to cover multiple pathogens in severe cases

- Steroids—will encourage resistance and recurrence when used concurrently with antibiotics

Drugs of Choice

- Systemic treatment options for MRSA species (based on culture and sensitivity testing)
    1. Chloramphenicol—often best choice
    2. Potentiated sulfonamides—often second best choice
    3. Amikacin—injectable, painful, potential for nephrotoxicity
    4. Doxycycline
    5. Clindamcyin—limited use
    6. Fluoroquinolones—limited use
    7. Vancomycin—sensitive to the vast majority of MRS spp. yet it is nephrotoxic in dogs
    8. Linezolid—excellent activity, oral or parenteral, low toxicity yet very expensive; controversy regarding veterinary use since it is often the only effective drug in "life-threatening" human cases
- Administer antibiotics for a minimum of 2 weeks beyond clinical cure; this is usually about 1 month for superficial pyodermas, and 2–3+ months for deep pyodermas.
- Routine bathing with benzoyl peroxide or chlorhexidine shampoos—may help prevent recurrences

Topical Treatment Options:

1. Mupirocin 2%—excellent penetration, mostly gram-positive sensitivity, bacteriostatic
2. Fusidic acid
3. Chlorhexidine gluconate—less irritating than benzoyl peroxide, good residual effect, good for gram positive, poor against pseudomonas
4. Benzoyl peroxide—oxidizing agent, caution: may bleach fabrics, lowers skin pH, can be drying, disrupts bacterial cell membranes
5. Ethyl lactate 10%—lowers skin pH
6. Retapamulin (Altabax)—excellent penetration, gram-positive bacteria, expensive

Precautions/Interactions

- Erythromycin, lincomycin, and oxacillin often induce vomiting; administer with small amount of food.
- Gentamicin and kanamycin—renal toxicity usually precludes their prolonged systemic use
- Trimethoprim-sulfa antibiotics—associated with keratoconjunctivitis sicca, fever, hepatotoxicity, polyarthritis, and hematologic abnormalities; may lead to low thyroid test results

- Chloramphenicol—use with caution in cats; may cause mild, reversible anemia in dogs (rare); hindlimb weakness noted in large-breed dogs (resolves when the medication is discontinued)
- Staphage lysate, staphoid AB, or autogenous bacterins—may improve antibiotic efficacy and decrease recurrence in a small percentage of cases

 COMMENTS

- Some cases that continue to relapse may be managed with subminimal inhibitory concentrations of antibiotics (long-term/low-dose).
- Padded bedding—may ease pressure-point pyodermas
- Topical benzoyl peroxide gel or mupirocin ointment may be helpful adjunct therapies.
- Likely to be recurrent or nonresponsive if underlying cause is not identified and effectively managed
- Impetigo—affects young dogs before puberty; associated with poor husbandry; often requires only topical therapy
- Superficial pustular dermatitis—occurs in kittens; associated with overzealous "mouthing" by the queen
- Pyoderma secondary to atopy—usually begins at 1–3 years of age
- Pyoderma secondary to endocrine disorders—usually begins in middle adulthood
- Dogs infected with MRS species—avoid contact with hospital patients (during hospital visitation programs); transmission is usually by direct contact with the nasal passages, throat, and skin or by indirect contact from walls, floors, counters, bedding, dishes.
- Therapy to decolonize bacteria from nasal passages, skin, or mucosa is not recommended, and usually ineffective when tried; most dogs will clear MRSA colonization spontaneously.
- To reduce the possibility of zoonotic spread:
  - Wash hands thoroughly with soap and water for at least 15 seconds (avoid bar soap).
  - Use an alcohol-based hand sanitizer (62% alcohol).
  - Use gloves when handling suspect patients.
  - Avoid reusing contaminated clothing (lab coats, neck ties, scrubs).
  - Do not share food with pets or use the same dishes.
  - Do not allow a pet to lick your face or open wounds.
  - Take extra caution with individuals who are immunocompromised.
  - Sterilize surgical equipment.
  - Sanitize all cages and equipment routinely (e.g., stethoscope).
  - Launder bedding at 140°F.
  - Clean the clinic surfaces on a routine basis (table surfaces, anesthetic machines, floors, walls, cages, keyboards, telephones, clippers, leashes, muzzles).

- Client education—several excellent sources on the internet (i.e., http://www .wormsandgermsblog.com has a handout called MRSP for Pet Owners and additional useful clinical information including client education handouts can be found at http://www.CCAR-ccra.org)

Abbreviations

MRSA, methicillin-resistant *Staphylococcus*; MRSP, methicillin-resistant *S. pseudintermedius*; SC, subcutaneous.

Suggested Reading

Fitzgerald JR. The *Staphylococcus intermedius* group of bacterial pathogens: species re-classification, pathogenesis, and the emergence of methicillin-resistance. *Vet Dermatol* 2009;20:490–495.

Streptococcal Infections

DEFINITION/OVERVIEW

- A bacterial infection causing a wide range of clinical entities depending on which organ is infected

ETIOLOGY/PATHOPHYSIOLOGY

- *Streptococcus* spp. is a gram-positive, nonmoltile coccal or spherical bacteria.
- Normal flora of the upper respiratory tract, oropharynx, lower genital tract, and skin
- Under appropriate conditions, capable of infecting all areas of the body, but primary infections involve the respiratory, circulatory, integumentary, urogenital, or central nervous systems
- Frequently a secondary invader of body tissues
- Classified by ability to RBCs and produce a zone around the bacterial colony on blood agar plates
- Hemolytic strains subdivide further by antigenic differences in cell wall carbohydrates into Lancefield serogroups A to H and K to T.
- Some groups more likely to be associated with disease, depending on species (e.g., group G associated with cats and dogs; group A with humans)
- *S. equi* subsp. *zooepidemicus*—identified recently to be associated with outbreaks of fatal hemorrhagic pneumonia in shelter dogs in the United States, especially those kenneled for long periods
- Produce exotoxins, streptolysins (hemolysins), streptokinase, deoxyribonucleases, and hyaluronidases

SIGNALMENT/HISTORY

- Very young—more prone to infection because of immature immune system, especially kittens born to primiparous queens

- Severity of disease—dependent on age, exposure, and immune response; virulence
- Opportunistic circumstances—wounds, trauma, surgical procedures, and concurrent viral infections
- Shelter dogs—higher incidence of exposure to *S. equi* subsp. *zooepidemicus*
- Maternal antibodies—generally protect puppies and kittens against clinical disease
- Carrier states—do occur

 CLINICAL FEATURES

- Vary—with site of infection and host immunocompetence
- Respiratory tract—weakness, cough, dyspnea, fever, and hemoptysis
- Urinary tract—hematuria, stranguria, and pollakiuria
- Local wound—purulent exudates with lymphadenopathy

Dogs

- Septicemia, endometritis, vaginitis, mastitis (Fig. 96-1), fading puppies, abortion, urinary tract infection, pneumonia, necrotizing fasciitis, streptococcal shock syndrome, acute hemorrhagic pneumonia leading to death

Cats

- Septicemia, peritonitis, cervical lymphadenitis, pharyngitis, tonsillitis, necrotizing fasciitis, and fading kitten

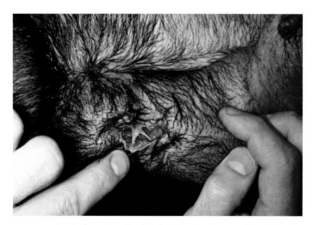

■ **Figure 96-1** The mammary gland of a rottweiler bitch with streptococcal mastitis, showing swelling, discoloration, and sinus development within the mammary gland.

DIFFERENTIAL DIAGNOSIS

- Other systemic infectious diseases causing fever, lymphadenopathy, and pneumonia, including viral (CIV and hemorrhagic pneumonia caused by *S. equi* subsp. *zooepidemicus* look very similar), bacterial, fungal, rickettsial, and protozoal infections

 # DIAGNOSTICS

- CBC—usually leukocytosis with neutrophilia and left shift (degenerative or regenerative)
- Cocci—may be found in circulating neutrophils in overwhelming sepsis
- Serum biochemical profile—may suggest a predisposing condition
- Urinalysis—pyuria, bacteruria
- Diagnosis—best made with culture of affected tissue, exudate, urine, blood, or needle aspirate to confirm causative organism
- Direct microscopy with Gram stain of exudates—reveals single gram-positive cocci or chains of organisms
- Thoracic radiographs—interstitial or alveolar pulmonary pattern with pneumonia
- UTI—radiodense uroliths (struvite) often present with streptococcal cystitis
- PCR—available in several commercial laboratories in the United States

 # THERAPEUTICS

- Drain and flush abscesses, debride necrotic tissue.
- Septic shock or deep infections (pneumonia, mastitis) causing systemic illness—fluid therapy support with intravenous antibiotic therapy

Drugs of Choice

- Base on culture and sensitivity results
- First choice—penicillin G or penicillin V
- Ampicillin
- Erythromycin
- Cephalexin
- *S. equi* subsp. *zooepidemicus*—Penicillins, cephalexin, or macrolide (erythromycin or azithromycin) are the drugs of choice (Table 96-1).
- Prophylactic treatment—all kittens born to a primiparous queen indicated by neonatal infections

TABLE 96-1 **Drug Therapy for Streptococcal Infections in Dogs and Cats**

Drug	Species	Dose (mg/kg)	Route	Interval (h)	Duration (days)
Penicillin G	B	10,000–20,000 U/kg	IM, SC	12–24	7
Penicillin V	B	10–30	PO	8	7
Ampicillin	B	10–40	PO, IV, SC	8	7–14
Erythromycin	D	5–20	PO	12–24	7
Azithromycin	B	10	PO	12	7–10
Cephalexin	B	10–40	PO	12	7

D, dogs; B, both dogs and cats.

Precautions/Interactions

- Erythromycin—may cause vomiting, abdominal discomfort, anorexia, and diarrhea; if occurs, stop medicating until symptoms abate, then restart at half the initial dose, giving medication with food, then raise to required dose if tolerates drug
- Cephalexin—may cause anorexia, vomiting, diarrhea, and hypersalivation

 # COMMENTS

- Avoid—overcrowding and poor environmental sanitation
- Prevention in newborns—dip navel and umbilical cord in 2% tincture of iodine
- Prevention in colonies—avoid overcrowding, maintain clean feeders, and segregate infected animals
- *Streptococci* isolated from humans—usually of human (group A) and not animal origin
- *S. canis* infections in people reported from dog bites and ulcers or wounds in contact with dogs
- Dogs and cats—can develop pharyngeal colonization with group A *Streptococcus* (with no clinical signs) acquired from an infected human; the pet may serve as a source of reinfection of humans; important to treat all family members, including the pets, in a household to break the reinfection cycle

Abbreviations

CBC, complete blood count; PCR, polymerase chain reaction; RBCs, red blood cells; UTI, urinary tract infection.

Suggested Reading

Byun J-W, Yoon S-S, Woo G-H, et al. An outbreak of fatal hemorrhagic pneumonia caused by *Streptococcus equi* subsp. *zooepidemicus* in shelter dogs. *J Vet Sci* 2009;10:269–271.

Messer JS, Wagner SO, Baumwart RD, Colitz CM. A case of canine streptococcal meningoencephalitis diagnosed using universal bacterial polymerase chain reaction assay. *J Am Anim Hosp Assoc* 2008;44:205–209.

Sura R, Hinckley LS, Risatti GR, and Smyth JA. Fatal necrotising fasciitis and myositis in a cat associated with *Streptococcus canis*. *Vet Rec* 2008;162:450–453.

Strongyloides

DEFINITION/OVERVIEW

- Nematode parasite—Adult worms infect the paramucosa of the small intestine of dogs and cats, causing diarrhea.
- Larval migration—may cause respiratory signs

ETIOLOGY/PATHOPHYSIOLOGY

- *Strongyloides stercoralis*—parasitizes humans, dogs, and cats
- Neonates—infected from larvae in colostrums
- Larvae migrate via lungs (possibly causing bronchopneumonia)—to small intestinal tract
- Female worms only—inhabit dogs and cats and lay eggs that hatch into L1 larvae
- Some L1 larvae molt to infective L3 larvae—can infect the host (autoinfection) before leaving in feces
- Transmission—infective L1 larvae via skin penetration and ingestion (usually in colostrum)
- Relatively host specific—with possible transmission to humans
- *Strongyloides tumefaciens*—adenomatous mass in colon of cats
- PPP = 2 weeks

SIGNALMENT/HISTORY

- Most disease—neonatal puppies and kittens after transcolostral transmission
- Most infections—occur in hot humid summer conditions
- Dogs and cats in kennel and cattery situations—higher prevalence

CLINICAL FEATURES

- Asymptomatic to watery diarrhea—main sign
- Severe debilitation—especially in neonates

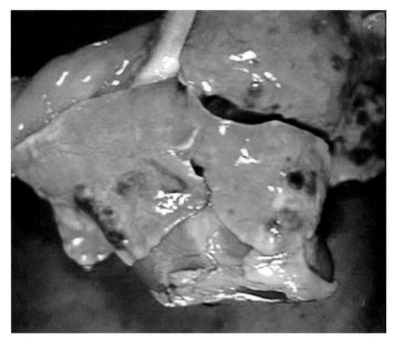

■ **Figure 97-1** Hemorrhagic lesions on the surface of a puppy's lungs infected with *Strongyloides* organisms.

- Dermatitis—intense pruritus and erythema at site of larvae skin penetration
- Cough—may develop a few days after skin penetration as larvae migrate through lungs (Fig. 97-1)
- Watery diarrhea (but may contain blood and mucus)—develops a few days after cough as parasites reach small intestine

 DIFFERENTIAL DIAGNOSIS

Dogs

- Causes of diarrhea in the puppy:
  - Dietary indiscretion
  - Allergy
  - Drugs (antibiotics)
  - Toxins—lead
  - Parasites (*Giardia* spp., cryptosporidiosis, GI parasitism with hookworms or *Strongyloides* spp.)
  - Infectious agents (salmonellosis, enteric calici virus, reovirus, CPV, coronavirus, canine distemper, CHV, *Campylobacter* spp., clostridiosis)
  - GI tract bacterial overgrowth (coliforms)
  - Systemic organ dysfunction (renal, hepatic, pancreas, cardiac)

Cats

- Causes of diarrhea in the kitten:
  - Dietary indiscretion
  - Allergic
  - Drugs (antibiotics)
  - Toxins—lead
  - Parasites (*Giardia* spp., cryptosporidiosis, tritrichomoniasis, GI tract parasitism with hookworms or *Strongyloides* spp.)
  - Infectious agents (panleukopenia, salmonellosis, enteric calici virus, reovirus, FeLV, and feline calicivirus)
  - GI tract bacterial overgrowth (coliforms)
  - Systemic organ dysfunction (renal, hepatic, pancreas, cardiac)

 # DIAGNOSTICS

- CBC—normal; may see mild nonregenerative anemia, and stress leukogram
- Biochemistry profile—normal
- Fecal flotation or direct smear—eggs (50–60 mm by 30–35 mm)—must use very fresh feces because eggs usually hatch before examination can occur
- Serology (in IFAT and ELISA format)—has been used to diagnose the parasite in some parts of the world

Diagnostic Feature

- **L1 larvae—most common diagnostic form in feces either by fecal flotation or Baermann's technique (Fig. 97-2)**
- L1 larvae—380 mm long, large genital rudiment, esophagus with three distinct sections, and a long, straight tail

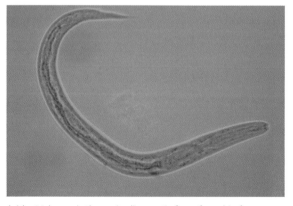

■ Figure 97-2 *Strongyloides* L1 larvae is the main diagnostic form found in feces.

TABLE 97-1 Drug Therapy for Strongyloidiasis in Dogs					
Drug	Dose (mg/kg)	Route	Interval (h)	Duration (days)	Repeat Interval (weeks)
Ivermectin (Ivomec)	0.2	SC, PO	Once	—	4
Fenbendazole (Panacur)	50	PO	24	5	4

- Differentiate *Strongyloides* spp. L1 larvae from *Ancylostoma* spp. L1 larvae—incubate fecal specimen in Baermann's apparatus for 48 hours—*Strongyloides* larvae will develop into unique filariform infective larvae (long, cylindrical esophagus, split tail).

THERAPEUTICS

- Isolate infected animals from noninfected animals and avoid human contact.
- After treatment, examine feces monthly for at least 6 months to ensure treatment success.
- One post-treatment fecal examination is not enough to ensure treatment success because of the intermittent nature of fecal larvae shedding.
- Treat not only affected pups, but dams also.

Drugs of Choice

- Ivermectin (Ivomec 1% Injectable or Ivomec 0.27% Sterile Solution; Merial)
- Fenbendazole (Panacur Granules 22.2%; Intervet—use in adults and bitches (Table 97-1)

Precautions/Interactions

- This dose of ivermectin is extralabel use—ensure heartworm-negative before treatment
- Do not use this dose of ivermectin in collie dogs or collie-like breeds.

COMMENTS

- Warn owners of zoonotic nature of *Strongyloides* spp.
- *Strongyloides stercoralis*—may produce dermatitis, severe abdominal discomfort, and diarrhea in humans
- May cause death in immunosuppressed individuals
- Frequent cleaning of cages (every 24 hours) and monthly administration of ivermectin—needed to clear kennels of infection

- Alternate anthelmintic—between ivermectin and fenbendazole to prevent resistance from developing
- Using wire-bottom cages in colony situations—no guarantee of preventing infection
- Cage cleaning—high-pressure washers followed by 1% sodium hypochlorite (3 cups of bleach/gallon of water) followed by water rinsing

Abbreviations

CBC, complete blood count; CHV, canine herpes virus; CPV, canine parvovirus; FeLV, feline leukemia virus; GI, gastrointestinal; IFAT, indirect fluorescent antibody test; ELISA, enzyme-linked immunosorbent assay; PPP, prepatent period.

Suggested Reading

Bowman DD, ed. *Georgi's Parasitology for Veterinarians*, 8th ed. Philadelphia: WB Saunders, 2003: 197–201.

Itoh N, Kanai K, Hori Y, et al. Fenbendazole treatment of dogs with naturally acquired *Strongyloides stercoralis* infection. *Vet Rec* 2009;164;559–560.

Junior AF, Goncalves-Pires MR, Silva DA, et al. Parasitological and serological diagnosis of *Strongyloides stercoralis* in domesticated dogs from southeastern Brazil. *Vet Parasitol* 2006;138:137–146.

Tapeworms
(Cestodiasis)

chapter 98

DEFINITION/OVERVIEW

- Helminth parasites in the class Cestodes—infect the small intestine of cats and dogs but cause few clinical signs

ETIOLOGY/PATHOPHYSIOLOGY

- *Taenia pisiformis*—dogs
- *Taenia taeniaeformis*—cats
- *Dipylidium caninum*—cats and dogs
- Transmission—predation of rabbits and rodents
- *D. caninum*—flea vectored, with flea maggots ingesting tapeworm eggs in dog or cat feces
- Transmission—occurs when dogs and cats ingest the adult flea
- Tapeworms—attach to the small intestinal mucosa, causing virtually no pathological condition or clinical signs, other than mild perianal pruritus
- The sight of tapeworm segments crawling from the anus or around the perianal fur of a pet, or in its feces, is often repugnant to owners (Fig. 98-1).

SIGNALMENT/HISTORY

- Cats and dogs of all ages—exposure to fleas or ingesting the viscera of rodents or rabbits

CLINICAL FEATURES

- Chains or segments in feces or attached to perianal fur
- Perianal pruritus (*D. caninum*) manifested by dragging anus on ground

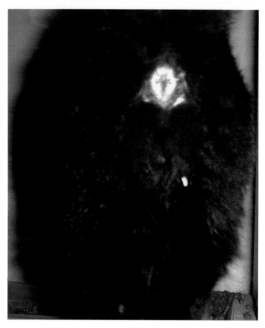

■ **Figure 98-1** Tapeworm segment on the perianal region of a cat.

DIFFERENTIAL DIAGNOSIS

- Anal sac impaction, sacculitis or abscess, perianal fistulas, and anal sac neoplasia
- Perianal pruritus—food hypersensitivity, flea allergy dermatitis, atopy, tail-fold pyoderma, and seborrheic skin disorders affecting the perineum

DIAGNOSTICS

- *D. caninum*—Scotch tape pressed to the perianal skin for egg capsules containing eggs (Fig. 98-2) ~50 mm in diameter, pale yellow, hexacanth embryo
- Even if owners report or you see tapeworm segments on the perianal fur—eggs may not be found using this method.
- *Taenia*—eggs spherical, brown, ~30 mm, hexacanth embryo (Fig. 98-3); segments are square with a single lateral pole (Fig. 98-4)

THERAPEUTICS

- Outpatient
- Discuss flea control (*D. caninum*)

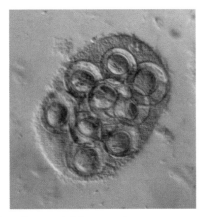

■ **Figure 98-2** Egg packet of *D. caninum* containing several eggs.

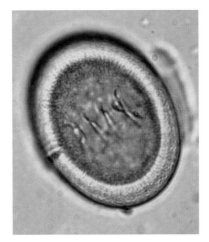

■ **Figure 98-3** Egg of *T. pisiformis*; brown spheroid egg containing hexocanth embryo with hooks.

Drugs of Choice

Dogs

- Fenbendazole (Panacur Granules 22.2%; Intervet)
- Praziquantel (Droncit; Bayer)
- Praziquantel/pyrantel/febantel (Drontal Plus; Bayer)
- Epsiprantel (Cestex; Pfizer)

Cats

- Praziquantel (Droncit; Bayer)
- Praziquantel/pyrantel (Drontal; Bayer)
- Epsiprantel (Cestex; Pfizer) (Table 98-1)

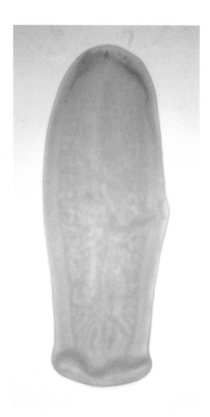

■ **Figure 98-4** The square segment of *T. pisiformis* with a single lateral pore.

TABLE 98-1 Drug Therapy for Tapeworm Infections in Dogs and Cats					
Drug	Species	Dose (mg/kg)	Route	Interval (h)	Duration (d)
Fenbendazole (Panacur)	D	50	PO	24	3
Praziquantel (Droncit)	B	5–7.5	PO, SC, IM	Once	—
Praziquantel/pyrantel/febantel (Drontal Plus)	D	a	PO	Once	—
Epsiprantel (Cestex)	B	5.5	PO	Once	—
Praziquantel/pyrantel (Drontal)	C	b	PO	Once	—

a Praziquantel (22.7), pyrantel (22.7), febantel (113.6).
b Praziquantel (18.2), pyrantel (72.6).
B, both dogs and cats; C, cats; D, dogs.

Precautions/Interactions

- Praziquantel or epsiprantel—Do not use in puppies or kittens <4 weeks old.

 ## COMMENTS

- Careful attention to flea control using preparations such as:
  - Dinotefuran, pyriproxyfen (Vectra for cats) and permethrin (Vectra 3D; Summit VetPharm)
  - Selamectin (Revolution; Pfizer)
  - Lufenuron (Program or Sentinal; Novartis)
  - Imidacloprid (Advantage; Bayer); also combined with permethrin or moxidectin (Advantage Multi.
  - Fipronil (Frontline; Merial)
  - Metaflumizone amitraz (Promeris for dogs and cats; Fort Dodge Animal Health)
  - Nitenpyram (Capstar; Novartis)
  - Permethrin (Proticall; Schering-Plough)
  - Permethrin pyriproxyfen (Virbac Long Acting Knockout Spray; Virbac)
  - Spinosad (Comfortis; Eli Lilly)
- *D. caninum* may be infective to children.

Suggested Reading

Bowman DD. In: *Georgis' Parasitology for Veterinarians*, 8th ed. Philadelphia: WB Saunders, 2003:138–148.

Georgi JR. Tapeworms. *Vet Clin North Am Small Anim Pract* 1987;17:1285–1306.

Tetanus

DEFINITION/OVERVIEW

- Disease caused by a bacterium found in soil and as part of the normal bacterial flora of mammalian intestinal tracts
- When it contaminates necrotic anaerobic wounds, germinating spores in the wound produce a potent exotoxin (tetanospasmin).

ETIOLOGY/PATHOPHYSIOLOGY

- *Clostridium tetani*—obligate anaerobic spore-forming, gram-positive rod
- Distribution—worldwide
- Very resistant—to disinfectants and environmental exposure
- Tetanospasmin—blocks release of neurotransmitters by entering the axon of the nearest motor nerves at the neuromuscular end plate, migrates up axon to neuronal cell body within spinal cord, and then ascends to the brain
- Hematogenous tetanospasmin—can enter the brain through an intact blood–brain barrier to cause intracranial signs before development of generalized limb rigidity
- Early involvement of facial musculature after hematogenous spread—due to shortness of cranial nerve motor axons (relative to those of limbs)
- Tetanospasmin—inhibits glycine and GABA release (neurotransmitters of inhibitory interneurons of the brain and spinal nerves)
- May also cause autonomic dysfunction—resulting in increased vagal tone.
- Tetanospasmin binding to inhibitory neuron presynaptic sites—irreversible
- Recovery—depends on growth of new axon terminals

SIGNALMENT/HISTORY

- Dogs—small wounds, often unseen
- Association—with foreign bodies
- Hunting breeds—higher prevalence near horse farms, where *C. tetani* reaches high levels
- Cats—very resistant; large obvious wounds with extensive contamination

CLINICAL FEATURES

- Dogs—the most common initial clinical sign: ocular and facial abnormalities

Localized

- Rigidity—of muscle(s) or entire limb closest to wound site
- Thoracic limb—often fixed extended elbow; carpus flexed or extended; spreads to include opposite extremity and eventually involves entire CNS
- Pelvic limb—held rigidly extended out behind; often associated with infection in female reproductive tract
- Localized—may spontaneously resolve if infection source removed and partial immunity to tetanospasmin present

Generalized

- Initially, stiff gait with outstretched or dorsally curved (cats) tail
- Difficulty walking progressing to stretched out "sawhorse" appearance (Fig. 99-1)
- Difficulty lying down
- Difficulty opening jaw and eating
- Eventually, difficulty breathing
- Eyelids retract, enophthalmos and prolapsed third eyelids (Fig. 99-2)
- Forehead skin wrinkles (Fig. 99-3)
- Ears erect or pulled back, grinning (commissure of lips retracted)

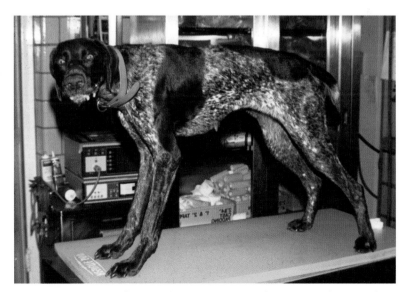

■ **Figure 99-1** Dog with generalized tetanus showing classical "sawhorse" stance (courtesy of Dr. A. Delahunta, Cornell University).

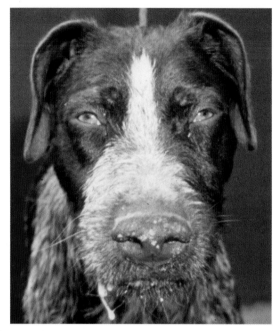

■ **Figure 99-2** Facial features of a dog with tetanus can show prolapse of the third eyelid and retraction of the ears (courtesy of Dr. A. Delahunta, Cornell University).

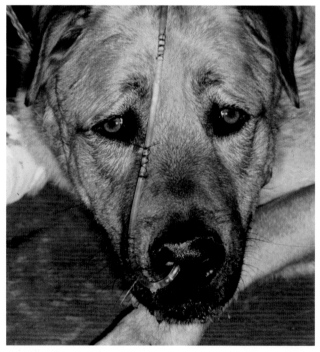

■ **Figure 99-3** This dog shows the wrinkling of the forehead to give the apprehensive appearance of dogs with tetanus. Note the nasal oxygen tube, which may be helpful in dogs with respiratory depression from tetanus.

- Hypersalivation
- Tachycardia, laryngeal spasm
- Fever (from muscle rigidity)
- Dysuria
- Constipation
- Tetanic muscle spasms, especially when stimulated by noise or touch
- Clonic seizures; opisthotonus initially (animals often vocalize as muscle contraction painful), progressing to seizure and loss of consciousness
- Death—usually due to respiratory system compromise from laryngeal and respiratory muscle spasm

 ## DIFFERENTIAL DIAGNOSIS

- Intoxications (lead, strychnine poisoning); the dystonic reaction to neuroleptic drugs (atropine, acepromazine); rabies; meningitis-encephalitis; immune-mediated polymyositis; spinal trauma; eclampsia
- Examine carefully—looking for foot injury/trauma (footpad, nails, interdigital), foreign bodies in conjunction with puncture wounds; contaminated fractures of long bones and distal extremities
- Intoxications—lead, strychnine, organophosphate, carbamate, and 1080 poison usually show GI signs and less severe muscle spasm

 ## DIAGNOSTICS

- Diagnosis—made mainly on history, presence of wound and clinical appearance
- CBC—mild leukopenia initially then leukocytosis
- Serum biochemistry panel—AST and CK elevations (muscle spasms)
- Anti-tetanus antibody—often provides false-negative results but a positive result helps confirm diagnosis
- Wound culture for *C. tetani*—unrewarding as high contamination risk; must use anaerobic transport medium (do not refrigerate)

 ## THERAPEUTICS

- Warn owners—of lengthy hospital stay (and subsequent costs), complications in generalized cases
- Localized or mild cases—good survival if treated aggressively

Drugs of Choice

- Therapy involves a combination of—anti-toxin, local wound treatment, antibiotics, sedation, nursing care, and autonomic agents

Anti-toxin

- ATS—binds circulating tetanospasmin (will not eliminate bound toxin to neurore-ceptors)
- Anaphylaxis reactions—possible (see Precautions/Interactions)
- No need to repeat injection—Therapeutic levels of anti-tetanus serum persist for 14 days.
- Risk for anaphylaxis—increases on subsequent injections

Local Wound Treatment

- Administer ATS before surgical manipulation of wound to counteract toxin release into circulation.
- Remove any foreign material and necrotic tissue.
- Irrigate wound with hydrogen peroxide (increases oxygen tension in tissue, inhibits growth of obligate anaerobes).

Antibiotics

- Penicillin G
- Tetracycline
- Metronidazole and clindamycin are also effective.

Sedation

- A combination of phenothiazine and barbiturates controls reflex spasm and convulsions but maintains consciousness.
- Chlorpromazine
- Pentobarbital

Nursing Care

- Dark, quiet environment—with minimal stimulation
- Soft bedding or air/water bed—protects against decubital ulcers
- Encourage to eat, drink unassisted—Homogenize food so it can be sucked in through clenched teeth.
- Maintain hydration—parenteral balanced isotonic fluids
- PEG tube—if megaesophagus or hiatal hernia develop, or severely debilitated
- Urinary catheterization (sterile system essential) and periodic enemas—may be required
- Tracheostomy—if laryngeal obstruction from laryngeal spasm develops
- Hyperthermia—control with parenteral fluids, fans, alcohol on footpads

TABLE 99-1	**Drug Therapy for Tetanus in Dogs**			
Drug	**Dose (mg/kg)**	**Route**	**Interval (h)**	**Duration (days)**
Anti-tetanus equine serum	100–1,000[a]	IV	Once	—
Penicillin G	20,000–100,000[b]	IV	8	10–14
Tetracycline	22	PO, IV	8	10–14
Metronidazole	10	PO, IV	8	14
Chlorpromazine	0.5–2	PO, IV, IM	8	As needed
Pentobarbital	3–15	IV	3–4	To effect
Glycopyrrolate	0.005	SC, IV	—	To effect
Atropine	0.05	SC	—	To effect
Epinephrine	0.1[c]	IV	Once	To effect

[a] Units per kilogram to a maximum dose of 20,000 U given slowly over 10 minutes.
[b] Units per kilogram.
[c] Milliliters per kilogram of 1:10,000 dilution.

Autonomic Agents

- Bradycardia—may occur when chlorpromazine and pentobarbital are used together
- If heart rate drops below 60 beats/minute—give glycopyrrolate or atropine

Precautions/Interactions

- To test for anaphylaxis from ATS administration—0.1 to 0.2 ml given SC or ID, 30 minutes before IV dose; wheal at injection site indicates anaphylactic reaction may occur
- Treat anaphylaxis—epinephrine (Table 99-1)

 COMMENTS

- Use glucocorticoids and antihistamine—only if necessary
- Careful nursing care and attention to details—Most generalized tetanus cases show improvement after 1 week and fully recover after 3–4 weeks.
- Tetanus toxoid—not recommended for dogs and cats

Abbreviations

AST, aspartate aminotransferease; ATS, anti-tetanus equine serum; CBC, complete blood count; CK, creatine kinase; CNS, central nervous system; GABA, gamma-aminobutyric acid; GI, gastrointestinal; PEG, percutaneous endoscopic gastrostomy.

Suggested Reading

Burkitt JM, Sturges BK, Jandrey KE, et al. Risk factors associated with outcome in dogs with tetanus: 38 cases (1987–2005). *J Am Vet Med Assoc* 2007; 230: 76–83.

Greene CE. Tetanus. In: Greene CE, ed. *Infectious Diseases of the Dog and Cat*. Philadelphia: WB Saunders, 2006:395–402.

Linnenbrink T, McMichael M. Tetanus: pathophysiology, clinical signs, diagnosis, and update on new treatment modalities. *J Vet Emerg Crit Care* 2006;16:199–207.

Sprott KR. Generalized tetanus in a Labrador retriever. *Can Vet J* 2008;49:1221–1223.

Tick Bite Paralysis

chapter **100**

DEFINITION/OVERVIEW

- Flaccid lower motor neuron paralysis caused by salivary neurotoxins from certain species of female ticks

SIGNALMENT/HISTORY

- In North America, ticks include:
  - *Dermacentor variabilis* (common wood tick—distributed over eastern two thirds of country and into California and Oregon)
  - *Dermacentor andersoni* (Rocky Mountain wood tick—distributed from the Cascade Mountains to the Rocky Mountains)
  - *Amblyomma americanum* (lone star tick—distributed from Texas and Missouri to the Atlantic Coast)
  - *A. maculatum* (Gulf Coast tick—found in the high temperatures and humidity of the Atlantic and Gulf of Mexico seaboards)
- In Australia—*Ixodes holocyclus* secretes a far more potent neurotoxin than the North American ticks; incidence of disease is much more common in Australia.
- *I. holocyclus*—injects salivary neurotoxins
- Neurotoxin—probably interferes with the depolarization/acetylcholine release mechanism in the presynaptic nerve terminal, leading to reduction in the release of acetylcholine
- One adult tick is sufficient to cause neurologic signs—a large larval or nymphal tick infestation can also induce signs
- Signs—occur 6–9 days after tick attachment
- Not all adult female ticks produce neurotoxin—not all tick-infected animals develop signs.
- Overall incidence is low in the United States—occurs mainly in the warmer months and regions of the southern states
- Incidence—higher in Queensland, Australia (only other country where the disease exits) than in United States
- Australia—dogs and cats
- United States—dogs; cats appear to be resistant

517

- History—exposure of animal while walking in woods a week or so before the onset of signs
- Onset of signs is gradual—initial unsteadiness and weakness in pelvic limbs

 CLINICAL FEATURES

Non-*Ixodes* Tick (American Ticks)

- Once neurologic signs appear—rapidly ascending lower motor neuron paresis progressing to paralysis occurs
- Recumbency occurs 1–3 days after onset—hyporeflexia to areflexia and hypotonia to atonia
- Pain sensation preserved
- Cranial nerve dysfunction—not a prominent feature
- May note facial weakness and reduced jaw tone—sometimes dysphonia and dysphagia early in course
- Respiratory paralysis—uncommon in the United States
- Urination and defecation—usually normal

Ixodes Tick (Australian)

- Neurologic signs—much more severe and rapidly progressive
- Ascending motor weakness—can progress to paralysis within a few hours
- Signs—ptyalism, megaesophagus, and vomiting or regurgitation characteristic
- Sympathetic nervous system affected—mydriatic and poorly responsive pupils; hypertension; tachyarrhythmias; high pulmonary capillary hydrostatic pressure; and pulmonary edema
- Caudal medullary respiratory center affected—additive to the peripheral pulmonary changes, causing progressive fall in respiratory rate without a change in the tidal volume, resulting in hypoxia, hypercapnia, and respiratory acidosis
- Asymetrical focal neurologic deficits—such as unilateral facial paralysis, anisocoria, unilateral loss of the cutaneous trunci reflex, and Horner's syndrome has been reported in both cats and dogs; associated with tick attachment on the head ipsilateral to the side of the facial paralysis
- Respiratory muscle paralysis—much more prevalent
- Progression to dyspnea, cyanosis, and respiratory paralysis within 1–2 days if not treated

 DIFFERENTIAL DIAGNOSIS

- Botulism—history of ingestion of toxin source (dead birds); more cranial nerve involvement and autonomic signs than tick bite paralysis in the United States

- Coonhound paralysis—may follow a raccoon bite, systemic illness, or vaccination; cranial nerve involvement usually limited to facial and pharyngeal/laryngeal paresis; no autonomic signs; often shows diffuse hyperesthesia
- Acute polyneuropathy—no ticks present or history of exposure
- Distal denervating disease—tick bite paralysis usually more diffuse
- Myelopathy—generalized or multifocal
- Rabies—no ticks present or history of exposure; no vaccination against rabies; other behavioral signs

DIAGNOSTICS

- CBC and other laboratory parameters—usually within normal range, except arterial blood gases in severely affected patients —low PaO_2, high $PaCO_2$, and low blood pH

Diagnostic Feature

- **Most important diagnostic procedure is to search for ticks—remove immediately**
- Electrodiagnostics—normal insertion activity and an absence of spontaneous myofiber activity (no fibrillation potentials or positive sharp waves); lack of motor unit action potentials; motor nerve stimulation is followed by either a dramatic decrease in amplitude or a complete absence of compound muscle action potentials

THERAPEUTICS

- Hospitalize—until tick is found and removed or administer treatment to kill hidden ticks
- Supportive care—until patient begins to show signs of recovery
- Oxygen therapy if hypoventilation and hypoxia present—may require artificial ventilation if respiratory failure ensues

Drugs of Choice

- United States—if ticks not found, dip patients in insecticidal bath; often only treatment needed
- Australia—able to obtain hyperimmune serum (0.5–1 mg/kg, IV); given depending on severity of signs; if severe, can also give phenoxybenzamine, an α-adrenergic antagonist (1 mg/kg, IV, diluted in saline, given slowly over 20 min), which appears to be beneficial in relieving the sympathetic effects of the tick toxin; acepromazine (0.1 to 0.2 mg/kg, IV, up to 2 mg total dose) can be used as an alternative because it also has α-adrenergic antagonist effects

Precautions/Interactions

- Drugs that interfere with neuromuscular transmission—contraindicated (e.g., tetra-cyclines, aminoglycosides, and procaine penicillin)
- Atropine—contraindicated in advanced stages of disease or with marked bradycardia from *Ixodes* tick bite

 COMMENTS

- Non-*Ixodes* tick—once tick is removed, recovery is rapid with minimal nursing care required; recovery usually complete within 1–3 days
- *Ixodes* ticks—signs will often progress despite tick removal; thus aggressive treatment to neutralize toxin is indicated; prognosis often guarded and recovery can be pro-longed; more cats than dogs have adverse systemic reactions to tick antitoxin serum which can be markedly reduced with the routine use of atropine prior to antiserum administration
- To reduce risk of disease—Owners should check for ticks within 2–3 days of possible exposure.
- Treatment—weekly insecticide baths (Ecto-Soothe Shampoo [Virbac]; Adams Flea and Tick Shampoo and Mycodex products [Veterinary Products Laboratories]) or the use of insecticide-impregnated collars (Preventic; Virbac) help
- Some monthly topical parasiticides (Frontline [Merial]; K9Advantix [Bayer]; Revo-lution [Pfizer]) also protect against a number of species of ticks.
- Zoonosis—Ticks are not transmitted from dogs to humans, although humans can suffer tick bite paralysis (especially in Australia).
- Be aware—Tick species that can cause tick bite paralysis are also capable of transmit-ting certain rickettsial diseases RMSF, *Erhlichia* spp.).

Abbreviations

CBC, complete blood count; RMSF, Rocky Mountain spotted fever.

Suggested Reading

Atwell RB, Campbell FE. Reactions to tick antitoxin serum and the role of atropine in treatment of dogs and cats with tick paralysis caused by *Ixodes holocyclus*: a pilot survey. *Aust Vet J* 2001;79:394–397.

Holland CT. Asymmetrical focal neurological deficits in dogs and cats with naturally occurring tick paralysis (*Ixodes holocyclus*): 27 cases (1999–2006). *Aust Vet J* 2008;86:377–384.

Ticks and Tick Control

chapter **101**

DEFINITION/OVERVIEW

- Dogs and cats may be parasitized by hard ticks of the family Ixodidae.
- Ectoparasites that feed only on the blood of their hosts; arthropods; closely related to scorpions, spiders, and mites
- Transmitted microbial pathogens: protozoa, helminths, fungi, bacteria, rickettsiae, and viruses
- May cause toxicosis, hypersensitivity, paralysis, and blood loss anemia

ETIOLOGY/PATHOPHYSIOLOGY

- Hard ticks—four life stages: egg, larva, nymph, and adult; larvae and nymphs must feed to repletion before detaching and molting; as adult female ixodid ticks engorge, they may increase their weight by more than 100-fold; after detachment females may lay thousands of eggs
- Blood loss anemia—from heavy infestations
- Damage to the integument—Tick mouth parts cut through the host's skin; bites are generally painless; local irritation and infection may occur.
- Salivary secretion of neurotoxins—may lead to systemic signs (tick paralysis); local action may cause impaired hemostasis and immune suppression
- Pathogens—acquired when ticks feed on infected reservoir hosts (often rodents and small feral mammals); sometimes transovarial transmission occurs and infected eggs hatch and produce infected larvae; greatest potential for systemic disease occurs when infections acquired in early life stages are transmitted to new hosts when the next stage feeds; may affect virtually any organ system
- Transmission of pathogens and toxins—often requires periods of attachment from hours to days; the essentially painless bite allows adequate feeding times

SIGNALMENT/HISTORY

Geographic Distribution

- Strong geographic specificities exist for some tick species; thus geographic prevalence of associated diseases.
- Tick ranges are expanding and therefore tick parasitism, infections vectored by ticks, and emergence of new tick-borne diseases and coinfections are expanding.
- *Ixodes scapularis*—Lyme disease; midwest, northeast, and parts of the southeast United States
- *Ixodes pacificus*—western coastal states of the United States
- *Rhipicephalus sanguineus*—found throughout the continental United States; but canine ehrlichiosis and babesiosis most common in the southeast
- *Dermacentor variabilis*—Eastern seaboard and west coast
- *Amblyomma americanum*—Midwest, south-central, and southeast mainly but also parts of the northeastern United States; strong range expanasion

Species

- Dogs and cats
- Cats are thought to be quite efficient at removing ticks, but tick attachment and subsequent tick-vectored diseases, such as Lyme disease, anaplasmosis, and cytauxzoonosis, have been diagnosed in cats.

Risk Factors

- Large hunting breeds (dogs)—considered to be at high risk because they are likely to come in contact with environments harboring questing ticks
- Domestic animals—can be in close contact with ticks owing to encroachment of ticks into suburban environments and expansion of suburban environment into surrounding forests, prairies, and coastline areas

CLINICAL FEATURES

- Attached ticks or tick feeding cavities may be seen on the skin.
- Irritation secondary to bite
- Petechiation secondary to transmitted infectious organisms (e.g. *Rickettsia richettsii* causes necrotizing vasculitis, others such as *Ehrlichia canis, Anaplasma platys,* thrombocytopenia)
- Blood loss anemia (direct effect)); thrombocytopenia, anemia, inclusion bodies in neutrophils, monocytes, RBCs secondary to infectious organisms transmitted

- Limb/joint abnormalities secondary to infectious organisms transmitted (*Borrelia burgdorferi* and other organisms implicated in oligo- and polyarthritis)
- Cardiac—varying degrees of heart block secondary to infectious organisms transmitted (*B. burgdorferi*)
- Neurotoxin-induced paralysis, CNS signs develop secondary to infectious organisms transmitted (*R. rickettsii*)

 # DIAGNOSTICS

- Attached ticks or tick-feeding cavities from which ticks have detached may be seen on the skin
- Associated tickborne diseases (borreliosis, ehrlichiosis, babesiosis, RMSF, and others)—vary with the organ system(s) affected; use rapid in-house diagnostic assays to detect most of these tick-borne diseases
- Irritation caused by ticks and subsequent self-trauma—may lead to pyotraumatic dermatitis ("hot spots") in dogs
- Tickborne diseases—evaluate epidemiologic considerations for each disease, history of tick parasitism, and complete clinical examination

 # THERAPEUTICS

- Outpatient—after removal of ticks
- Removal—do as soon as possible to limit time available for neurotoxin or pathogen transmission; grasp ticks close to the skin with fine-pointed tweezers and gently pull free; species with short, strong mouth parts (e.g., *Dermacentor* spp.) usually pull free with host skin attached; species with long, fragile mouth parts (e.g., *Ixodes* spp.) often leave fragments of mouth parts embedded in the feeding cavity
- Wash feeding cavity with soap and water—generally sufficient to prevent local inflammation or secondary infection
- Inform client—that application of hot matches, Vaseline, or other materials not only fails to cause tick detachment but allows for longer periods of attachment and feeding

Prevention/Avoidance

- Avoid environments that harbor ticks—may be difficult except for pets kept strictly indoors
- Tick control—essential to realize that this does not always equal control of tickborne diseases; often the goal is the perceived absence of ticks on the host animal
- Pets—Owners report complete tick control, even though there may be some period of attachment and tick feeding or live ticks may spend some time crawling on the animal after they have been exposed to lethal levels of an acaricide; immature ticks

of some species (*R. sanguineus* and *I. scapularis*) may be undetected because of their minute size.
- Tickborne pathogens—may be transmitted very rapidly (viruses) or may require several hours (*Rickettsia rickettsii*) or days (*Borrelia burgdorferi*)

Insecticides and Acaricides

- In the United States—The EPA licenses agents as effective against various species of pests.
- Control—inferred as providing control of diseases carried by that species; although this may be correct in some or all cases, veterinarians should be sophisticated enough to require demonstration of efficacy in prevention of disease transmission before accepting a disease-control claim at face value; challenging because ticks are widely dispersed in the environment, spend a relatively short time on their hosts, possess great reproductive capacities, and have long lifetimes
- Acaricidal collars (Preventic; Virbac) and spot treatment (Frontline; Merial)—have gained wide use; ease of application is as important as efficacy; direct marketing to pet owners of veterinarian-dispensed products has been a major factor in shifting tick control away from OTC formulations
- Disease transmission interruption studies have been published for the products containing fipronil, amitraz, and permethrin. Rapid killing and clinical repellence essential to prevent or interrupt tick feeding. At approximately 4 weeks after product application, efficacy in prevention of transmission of *B. burgdorferi* to dogs was 75–87.5% for fipronil (found in Frontline Topspot) and 100% for permethrin (found in K9 Advantix and Vectra 3D); Amitraz (found in Preventic Collar and Promeris) was 100% effective at 7 days postapplication.
- Bathing, spraying, or powdering with appropriate organophosphate or pyrethrin-containing products has become far less common with the advent of new convenient and effective products.

 COMMENTS

Conditions

- Canine babesiosis—vectored by *R. sanguineus*, caused by protozoan parasite *Babesia canis*, infects canine RBCs, leading to sludging in capillaries and destruction in the spleen
- RMSF—vectored by *Dermacentor variabilis*, caused by *R. rickettsii*, invades vascular endothelial tissues, leading to necrotizing vasculitis
- Canine monocytic ehrlichiosis—vectored by *R. sanguineus*, caused by *Ehrlichia canis*, infects mononuclear cells and platelets
  - Cyclic thrombocytopenia—caused by *A. platys*, the only intracellular pathogen of platelets

- Granulocytic anaplasmosis—caused by *A. phagocytophilum* vectored by *I. scapularis* and *I. pacificus*; infects granulocytes; *E. ewingii* vectored by *A. americanum* also infects granulocytes and causes granulocytic ehrlichiosis.
- Lyme disease—vectored by *I. scapularis* and *I. pacificus*, caused by *B. burgdorferi*; dogs may develop fevers associated with arthritis or syndromes possibly leading to complete heart block, protein-losing nephropathy, and possibly neurologic abnormalities
  - American canine hepatozoonosis—caused by protozoal organism *H. americanum* after the dog ingests an infected *A. maculatum*
- Canine hepatozoonosis—caused by protozoal organism *Hepatozoon canis* after the dog ingests an infected *R. sanguineus*; cysts and pyogranulomas in the muscles and other tissues associated with myositis and renal failure, often leading to death in chronic cases
- Tick paralysis—caused by a neurotoxin; affects acetylcholine synthesis and/or liberation at the neuromuscular junction of the host animal; signs (typified by ascending flaccid paralysis often initially affecting the pelvic limbs) develop 5–9 days after tick attachment

Vaccines

- Currently for "prevention" of only Lyme disease; two types for dogs: whole-cell, killed bacterin (since 1990) and Osp A (since 1996)

Zoonotic Potential

- Ticks may parasitize many different species of mammals, birds, and reptiles at different stages in their developmental cycles; infections acquired in early life stages may be transmitted when ticks feed again in the next stage.
- Humans, if parasitized, may be exposed to babesiosis, RMSF, ehrlichiosis, borreliosis, or tick paralysis.

Abbreviations

EPA, Environmental Protection Agency; OTC, over-the-counter; RBCs, red blood cells; RMSF, Rocky Mountain spotted fever.

Suggested Reading

Blagburn BL, Spencer JA, Butler JM, et al. Prevention of transmission of *Borrelia burgdorferi* and *Anaplasma phagocytophilum* from ticks to dogs using K9 Advantix and Frontline Plus applied 25 days before exposure to infected ticks. *Int J Appl Res Vet Med* 2005;3:69–75.

Elfassy OJ, Goodman FW, Levy SA, et al. Efficacy of an amitraz-impregnated collar in preventing transmission of *Borrelia burgdorferi* by adult *Ixodes scapularis* to dogs. *J Am Vet Med Assoc* 2001;219:185–189.

Jacobsen R, McCall J, Hunter J, et al. The ability of fipronil to prevent transmission of *Borrelia burgdorferi*, the causative agent of Lyme disease to dogs. *Int J Appl Res Vet Med* 2004;3:39–45.

Toxoplasmosis

DEFINITION/OVERVIEW

- A multisystemic protozoal disease affecting both cats and dogs; affects nearly all mammals, with Felidae being the definitive host

ETIOLOGY/PATHOPHYSIOLOGY

- *Toxoplasma gondii*—an obligate intracellular coccidian protozoan parasite
- Infection—acquired by ingestion of tissue cysts or oocysts
- After infection—organism spreads to extraintestinal organs via blood or lymph, resulting in focal necrosis of many organs (heart, eye, central nervous system)
- Acute disseminated infection—rarely fatal
- Chronically—tissue cysts form to produce low-grade disease that usually is not clinically apparent unless immunosuppression or concomitant illness allows *T. gondii* to proliferate and cause an acute inflammatory response
- Clinical toxoplasmosis—often associated with other infections causing severe immunosuppression (e.g., canine distemper, FIP, FIV, FeLV)
- Severity and manifestations of disease—depend on location and degree of tissue injury caused by tissue cysts
- Distribution—worldwide
- Approximately 30% of cats and up to 50% of humans in some countries are serologically positive for *T. gondii*.
- Clinical disease—uncommon; most animals with toxoplasmosis are asymptomatic

SIGNALMENT/HISTORY

- Cats (particularly males)—more commonly clinically affected than dogs
- Historically—initially get nonspecific signs of lethargy, depression, and anorexia
- Weight loss
- Fever

- Ocular discharge, photophobia, and miotic pupils (cats)
- Respiratory distress
- Neurologic signs—ataxia, seizures, tremors, paresis/paralysis, and cranial nerve deficits
- Digestive tract signs—vomiting, diarrhea, abdominal pain, and jaundice
- Stillborn kittens
- Abortion

 # CLINICAL FEATURES

Cats

- Disease is most severe in transplacentally infected kittens—may be stillborn or die before weaning
- Surviving kittens:
  - Anorexia
  - Lethargy
  - High fevers unresponsive to antibiotics
  - Signs reflecting necrosis/inflammation of lungs (dyspnea, increased respiratory noises), liver (icterus, abdominal enlargement from ascites), and CNS (encephalopathic) (Fig. 102-1)
- Respiratory and gastrointestinal signs (postnatal):
  - Anorexia
  - Lethargy
  - High fevers unresponsive to antibiotics
  - Dyspnea
  - Weight loss
  - Icterus

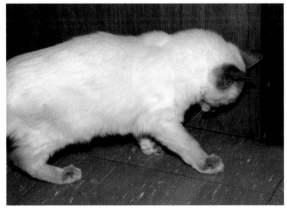

■ **Figure 102-1** A young kitten with toxoplasmosis showing ventral flexion of the neck due to muscle weakness from neurologic and muscular involvement.

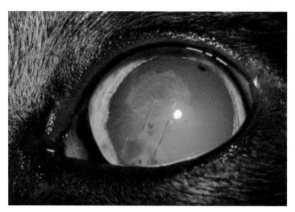

■ **Figure 102-2** Eye of a cat with ocular toxoplasmosis, showing nodular iritis and a fibrin clot within the anterior chamber, as a result of severe uveitis (courtesy of Dr. R. Riis, Cornell University).

- Vomiting
- Diarrhea
- Abdominal effusion
- Neurologic signs—seen in <10% of patients, blindness, stupor, incoordination, circling, torticollis, anisocoria, and seizures
- Ocular signs—common (approximately 80% of affected cats show intraocular inflammation); uveitis (aqueous flare, hyphema, mydriasis), iritis, detached retina, iridocyclitis, and keratic precipitates (Fig. 102-2)
- Rapid course—acutely affected patients with CNS and/or respiratory involvement
- Slow course—patients with reactivation of chronic infection
- Clinical syndromes are diverse but infection of pulmonary (97.7%), CNS (96.4), hepatic (93.3%), pancreatic (84.4%) and ocular (81.5%) tissues are most common.

Dogs

- Young—usually generalized infection:
  - Fever
  - Weight loss
  - Anorexia
  - Tonsillitis
  - Dyspnea
  - Diarrhea
  - Vomiting
- Older—usually localized infections; mainly associated with neural and muscular systems
- Neurologic—quite variable; usually reflecting diffuse neurologic inflammation; seizures, tremors, ataxia, paresis, paralysis, muscle weakness, and tetraparesis
- Ocular—rare; similar to those found in the cat
- Cardiac involvement—occurs; usually is not clinically apparent

DIFFERENTIAL DIAGNOSIS

Cats

- Intraocular disease (anterior uveitis)—FIP, FeLV, FIV, immune-mediated, trauma, lens-induced, and corneal ulceration with reflex uveitis
- Dyspnea (respiratory signs)—asthma, cardiogenic, pneumonia (bacterial, fungal, parasitic), neoplasia, heartworm disease, pleural disease (effusions), diaphragmatic hernia, and chest wall injury
- Neurologic signs (causes of meningoencephalitis)—viral (FIP, rabies, pseudorabies), fungal (cryptococcosis, blastomycosis, histoplasmosis), parasitic (cuterebriasis, coenurosis, aberrant heartworm migration), bacterial, and idiopathic disease (feline polioencephalomyelitis)

Dogs

- Often associated with other immunosuppressive diseases—for example, signs of distemper may be seen
- Neurologic—usually in very young dogs; differentiate from *Neospora caninum* (both produce CNS and neuromuscular disease) using serology or PCR
- Consider other conditions causing multifocal neurologic signs—infectious/inflammatory toxicity, metabolic diseases, neoplasia, GME, and hereditary and congenital defects

DIAGNOSTICS

- CBC—mild normocytic normochromic anemia
- Approximately 50% of infected cats have leukopenia (severe disease)—mainly as a result of lymphopenia; some have neutropenia alone, lymphopenia, and/or a degenerative left shift; leukocytosis may occur during recovery
- Serum biochemical profile—ALT and AST increased in most patients; approximately 25% of cats have icterus; most have hypoalbuminemia
- Cats that develop pancreatitis as a result of toxoplasmosis—mildly low serum calcium concentrations
- Urinalysis—mild proteinuria in a small proportion of cats; bilirubinuria (in icteric cats)
- Serology (ELISA)—IgM, IgG, and antigen serum titers give the most definitive information from one sample but no one serological test definitively confirms infection; a follow-up sample 3 weeks after the first will provide more complete information as to the type of infection (active, recent, or chronic).
- IgM—single serologic titer of choice for diagnosis of active infection; elevated 2 weeks postinfection (usually coincides with onset of clinical signs), persists for

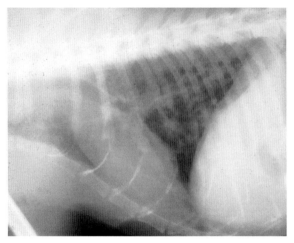

■ **Figure 102-3** Lateral thoracic radiograph of a cat with pulmonary toxoplasmosis. Note the patchy alveolar and interstitial pulmonary infiltrates.

a maximum of 3 months, then falls; a prolonged titer may indicate reactivation or delay in antibody class shift from IgM to IgG (a result of immunosuppression from FeLV or FIV infection or steroid therapy)
- IgG—rises 2–4 weeks postinfection and persist beyond a year
- A single high IgG titer is not diagnostic for active infection—a 4× increase in IgG titer over a 3-week period suggests active infection; most cats remain IgG positive for life
- Antigen—positive 1–4 weeks postinfection; however, as it remains positive during active or chronically persistent infection, measurement does not give much more information than antibody titers.
- PCR—on CSF, aqueous humor, or infected tissues can differentiate toxoplasmosis from neosporosis; not commercially available
- Radiographic examination—mixed pattern of diffuse patchy alveolar and interstitial pulmonary infiltrates especially in acute disease in cats (Fig. 102-3), with occasional pleural effusion; abdominal effusions and hepatomegaly
- CSF—elevated leukocyte count (both mononuclear cells and neutrophils) and protein in encephalopathic animals
- Cytologic examinaiton—tachyzoites, although rare, in body fluids (CSF, pleural or peritoneal effusions) during acute infection; BAL (pulmonary involvement) can reveal tachyzoites (Fig. 102-4)
- Fecal examination (Sheather's sugar solution)—Oocysts may be detected on routine fecal examinations in asymptomatic cats (<1% of cats shed cysts on any given day because cats only shed cysts for 1–2 weeks after first exposure) but are morphologically indistinguishable from *Hammondia* spp. and *Besnoitia* spp. (Fig. 102-5); PCR or mouse inoculation may distinguish species; oocysts are rarely shed during clinical disease.

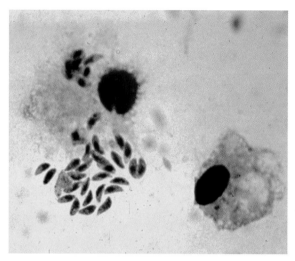

■ **Figure 102-4** Transtracheal wash from a cat with pulmonary toxoplasmosis. Note the banana-shaped tachyzoites in the process of rupturing out of the cell. (Wright–Giemsa stain, 1000×).

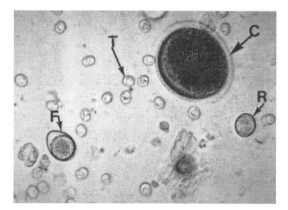

■ **Figure 102-5** A fecal preparation from a cat showing the relative sizes of *T. gondii* (*T*), *I. rivolta* (*R*), *I. felis* (*F*), and *T. cati* (*C*) (courtesy of Dr. J. P. Dubey, U.S. Department of Agriculture, Beltsville, MD).

 THERAPEUTICS

■ Patients with severe disease will require hospitalization and fluid and nutritional support while receiving antiprotozoal therapy.

Drugs of Choice

■ Clindamycin—for at least 2 weeks after clinical signs clear; will also inhibit oocyst shedding
■ Uveitis—1% prednisolone drops

TABLE 102-1 Drug Therapy for Toxoplasmosis

Drug	Species	Dose (mg/kg)	Route	Interval (h)	Duration (weeks)
Sytemic infections:					
Clindamycin	D	10–20	PO, IM	12	4
	C	10–12.5	PO, IM	12	4
Sulfadiazine[a]	B	30	PO	12	2
Pyrimethamine	B	0.5	PO	12	2
Trimethoprim-sulfadiazine	B	15	PO, IV	12	4
Azithromycin	B	7.5	PO	12	4
Prednisilone (1% ophthalmic drops)	B	[b]	Topically	8	2
Folinic acid[c]	B[d]	2.5	PO	24	2
Inhibit oocyst shedding:					
Clindamycin	C	50	PO, IM	24	2
	C	12.5–25	PO, IM	12	1–2[e]
Toltrazuril	C	5–10	PO	24	2[e]

[a] Use in combination with pyrimethamine.
[b] Give 2–3 drops in affected eye(s).
[c] If giving sulfonamide drugs.
[d] Especially cats
[e] Days, not weeks.
D, dogs; C, cats; B, both dogs and cats.

- Alternative to clindamycin—sulfadiazine in combination with pyrimethamine; TMS; azithromycin
- Folinic acid (2.5 mg/kg/day) or brewer's yeast (100 mg/kg/day)—correct bone marrow suppression caused by sulfadiazine/pyrimethamine therapy (Table 102-1)
- Toltrazuril—in cats, will inhibit oocyst shedding
- Ponazuril—been used in a dog to treat systemic infection with success
- Azithromycin—in cats, can be used to treat systemic infections

Precautions/Interactions

- Clindamycin and azithromycin—can cause GI signs (vomiting, anorexia, transient diarrhea); dose should be reduced or temporarily discontinued; reinitiate when signs stopped; give with food
- Sulfonamide and pyrimethamine—can cause vomiting, leukopenia, myelosuppression, fetal teratogenesis, myelodysplasia; reduce dose with hepatic insufficiency
- TMS—multiple adverse reactions including:
  - KCS—monitor tear production weekly throughout treatment

- Hepatotoxicity—anorexia, depression, icterus; monitor ALT if prolonged therapy
- Megaloblastic–folate acid deficiency anemia—especially in cats after several weeks; supplement with folinic acid (2.5 mg/kg/day)
- Immune-mediated polyarthritis, retinitis, glomerulonephritis, vasculitis, anemia, thrombocytopenia, urticaria, toxic epidermal necrolysis, erythema multiforme, conjunctivitis—remove from drug
- Renal failure and interference with renal excretion of potassium (leading to hyperkalemia)
- Salivation, diarrhea, and vomiting (cats)
- May interfere with thyroid hormone synthesis (dogs)—check T_3 and T_4 after 6 weeks

 ## COMMENTS

- Examine 2 days after initiating clindamycin treatment—Clinical signs (fever, hyperesthesia, anorexia, uveitis) should begin to resolve; uveitis should resolve completely within 1 week.
- Examine 2 weeks after initiating treatment—assess neuromuscular deficits; should partially resolve (some deficits permanent owing to CNS or peripheral neuromuscular damage) (Fig. 102-6)
- Examine 2 weeks after owner-reported resolution of signs—consider discontinuing treatment; some neuromuscular deficits permanent
- Prognosis—guarded in cats needing therapy because response is inconsistent.
- Worse prognosis in neonates and the severely immunocompromised

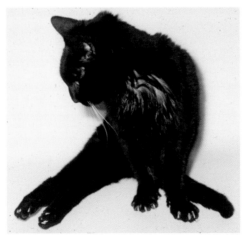

■ **Figure 102-6** A cat that has survived treatment for toxoplasmosis, displaying residual hind limb atrophy and rigid contracture.

- Prevent cats from eating raw meat, bones, viscera, or unpasteurized milk (especially goat milk) or from eating mechanical vectors (flies, cockroaches)—meat may be eaten if well cooked.
- Prevent—cats from free roaming to hunt prey (birds, rodents) or from entering buildings where food-producing animals are housed

Zoonotic Potential

- Healthy cat with a positive *T. gondii* antibody titer—poses little danger to its owner
- Cats with no antibody titer—are at more risk of becoming infected, shedding oocysts in the feces, and constitutes the highest public health risk to humans
- To avoid contact with oocysts or tissue cysts:
  - Do not feed raw meat.
  - Wash hands and surfaces (cutting boards) after preparing raw meat.
  - Boil drinking water if the source is unreliable.
  - Keep sandboxes covered to prevent cats defecating in them.
  - Wear gloves when gardening.
  - Wash hands and vegetables before eating to avoid contact with oocyst soil contamination.
  - Empty cat litterboxes daily (oocysts need at least 24 hours to become infective).
  - Disinfect litterboxes with boiling water.
  - Control stray cat population to avoid oocyst contamination of environment.
  - Pregnant women should avoid contact with cats excreting oocysts in feces, soil, cat litter, and raw meat (meat cooked to 150°F will kill *T. gondii*).
- Parasitemia during pregnancy—can cause spread of tachyzoites to the fetus; probably does not happen unless first-time infection of dam occurs during pregnancy (as with humans)
- Placental transmission—rare

Abbreviations

ALT, alanine aminotransferase; AST, aspartate aminotransferase; BAL, bronchoalveolar lavage; CBC, complete blood count; CNS, central nervous system; CSF, cerebrospinal fluid; ELISA, enzyme-linked immunosorbent assay; FeLV, feline leukemia virus; FIP, feline infectious peritonitis; FIV, feline immunodeficiency virus; GI, gastrointestinal; GME, granulomatous meningoencephalopathy; Ig, immunoglobulin; KCS, keratoconjunctivitis sicca; PCR, polymerase chain reaction; TMS, trimethoprim-sulfadiazine.

Suggested Reading

Dubey JP, Lappin MR. Toxoplasmosis and neosporosis. In: Greene CE, ed. *Infectious Diseases of the Dog and Cat*, 3rd ed. Philadelphia: WB Saunders, 2006:754–775.

Dubey JP, Lindsay DS, Lappin MR. Toxoplasmosis and other intestinal coccidial infections in cats and dogs. *Vet Clin Small Anim Pract* 2009;39:1009–1034.

chapter 103

Trichinosis

DEFINITION/OVERVIEW

- Nematode infection—Adults infect the small intestine of a wide range of carnivores (including dogs and humans) and omnivores (pigs), causing little GI disease.
- Larvae—sequest in skeletal muscle throughout the body
- Of major zoonotic importance—Humans obtain infection by eating poorly cooked meat containing sequestered larvae from a wide range of animals (pigs, bears, seals, horses).
- Zoonosis—causes severe myositis and sometimes death in humans
- In China—Eating dog meat is an important source of trichinosis in humans.
- Distribution—worldwide

ETIOLOGY/PATHOPHYSIOLOGY

- *Trichinella spiralis*—Dogs and cats become infected by eating L1 larvae sequestered in the muscle of other animals.
- *Trichinella native*—reported to cause a nonhealing ulcerative skin lesion in a cat
- Sources of infection—wild caught rodents or the carcasses of carnivores (mainly cats), or foxes, opossum, raccoons, and wild pigs (dogs)
- L1 larvae—molt to adults in the small intestine
- Adult worms—produce large numbers of "prelarvae," which are injected into the intestinal mucosa
- Prelarvae—migrate via lymphatics initially, then the blood stream to skeletal muscles, where they coil up and develop to L1 in cyst-like structures
- L1 larvae—remain infective in the muscle for months to years
- Dogs—Only a very few larvae are needed for infection.
- Ingestion of large numbers of larvae—results in same degree of muscle sequestration as very small infections because most infecting larvae in large infections pass right through the GI tract without developing to adults
- Infection rate in dogs—higher than in pigs in some studies

SIGNALMENT/HISTORY

- Hunting dogs (including those that foxhunt)—high rate of infection
- Puppies—more susceptible to infection than older dogs

 CLINICAL FEATURES

- Mild GI upset—vomiting, diarrhea
- Myalgia, muscle stiffness—mild and rarely observed
- Cardiac infection—syncopy due to conduction disturbances
- Cats—nonhealing ulcerative skin lesion

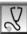 **DIFFERENTIAL DIAGNOSIS**

- Other causes of mild transient gastroenteritis—dietary indiscretion, early IBD, drugs (antibiotics), parasites (giardiasis, trichomoniasis, whipworms), infectious agents, partial foreign body (hairballs in cats)

 DIAGNOSTICS

- CBC—eosinophilia during acute stage of infection; may persist for several weeks in severe infections
- Identification of the small adults (female: 3 mm, male 1.5 mm) in the feces—may require examination of feces collected over time (Fig. 103-1)

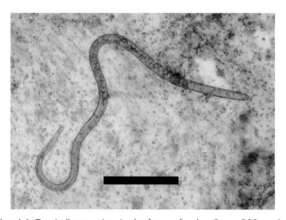

■ **Figure 103-1** A male adult *T. spiralis* organism in the feces of a dog (bar =300 mm).

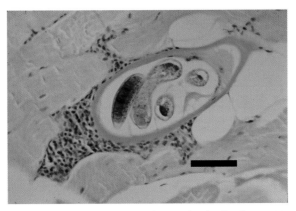

■ **Figure 103-2** A cyst containing a *T. spiralis* larvae in the muscle of a dog (bar =100 mm).

- Adults and larvae in feces—distinguished from the larvae of *Crenosoma, Angiostrongylus,* and *Filaroides* spp. by the stichosome esophagus (both adults and larvae), copulatory lobes (male), and presence of prelarvae within the uterus (female)
- May identify prelarvae in blood (100 mm as opposed to the ~300 mm of larvae of *Dirofilaria immitis* and *Dipetalonema reconditum*)—by modified Knott's technique
- Muscle biopsy—L1 larvae with characteristic stichosome esophagus in "cysts" (Fig. 103-2)

THERAPEUTICS

- No specific treatment required—for GI tract signs or myalgia
- Albendazole—shown to significantly reduce muscle larval forms
- Because of the efficacy of albendazole—Fenbendazole is likely to be efficacious with no side effects.

Drugs of Choice

- Fenbendazole (Panacur Granules 22.2%; Intervet).
- Albendazole (Valbazen suspension 11.36%; Pfizer) (Table 103-1)

TABLE 103-1 **Drug Therapy for Trichinosis in Dogs and Cats**				
Drug	Dose (mg/kg)	Route Route	Interval (h)	Duration (days)
Fenbendazole (Panacur)	50	PO	24	10
Albendazole (Valbazen)	50[a]	PO	12	7

[a]May cause myelosuppression at this dose in dogs and cats.

Precautions/Interactions

- Albendazole—has been shown to cause myelosuppression in cats and dogs at these doses
- If use albendazole—monitor CBC for signs of pancytopenia

 COMMENTS

- Although not a serious health problem in dogs or cats—may act as a source of infection to other species (pigs) that are eaten by humans
- Humans could become infected directly—from the feces of infected dogs and cats (in theory)

Abbreviations

CBC, complete blood count; GI, gastrointestinal tract; IBD, inflammatory bowel disease.

Suggested Reading

Saari S, Airas N, Nareaho A, et al. A nonhealing ulcerative skin lesion associated with Trichinella nativa infection in a cat. *J Vet Diagn Invest* 2008;20:839–843.
Sleeper MM, Bissett S, Craig L. Canine trichinosis presenting with syncope and AV conduction disturbance. *J Vet Intern Med* 2006;20:1228–1231.

Trichomoniasis

chapter

104

DEFINITION/OVERVIEW

- Enteric pear-shaped motile flagellated protozoa similar to *Giardia* organisms that inhabits the large intestine of cats, dogs, and humans
- One species causes diarrhea in cats.

ETIOLOGY/PATHOPHYSIOLOGY

- *Pentatrichomonas hominis* (family: trichomonads)—inhabits the large intestine of cats, dogs, and humans
- Nonpathogenic in dogs and cats—except very rarely, when it may become an opportunistic pathogen
- *Tritrichomonas foetus*—causes diarrhea in cats; experimental infections of cats with bovine *T. foetus* isolates (which cause infertility and abortion in cattle) suggest that the isolate that causes large-bowel diarrhea in cats is different from the *T. foetus* isolate that affects cattle
- *T. foetus* prevalence in cats—~30% in show cats but very low in feral or indoor cats
- Pathogenic factors leading to infected cats developing diarrhea—endogenous bacterial flora, adherence of parasite to host epithelium, and cytotoxin and enzyme elaboration
- Parasites colonize the terminal ileum, cecum, and colon—leads to large bowel-diarrhea

SIGNALMENT/HISTORY

- High population density (catteries, shelters)—may be a risk factor for infection
- Coinfection with *Giardia* spp.—common
- Young cats—usually <1 year (range: 3 months to 13 years)

CLINICAL FEATURES

- Intermittent large-bowel diarrhea
- Diarrhea occasionally contains blood and mucus.
- Anus may become edematous, erythematous, and painful in very young cats.
- Rectal prolapse if anal irritation becomes severe
- Diarrhea improves with antibiotic treatment but reoccurs when treatment stops.
- Median length of time of diarrhea—9 months with resolution in most cats by 2 years; persistence of infection after diarrhea has resolved is common

 ## DIFFERENTIAL DIAGNOSIS

- Dietary indiscretion, IBD, neoplasia (especially GI lymphoma), drugs (antibiotics), toxins (lead), parasites (cryptosporidiosis, *Giardia* spp., hookworms, roundworms), infectious agents (FIP, salmonellosis, GI bacterial overgrowth, clostridia), systemic organ dysfunction (renal, hepatic, pancreatic, cardiac), and metabolic (hyperthyroidism)

 ## DIAGNOSTICS

- Direct fecal smear—low sensitivity
- Method—Dilute fresh feces 50:50 in saline, coverslip, examine at 40× objective with condenser lowered to increase contrast.

Diagnostic Feature

- **Distinguish from *Giardia* spp. (concave ventral disc, spiral forward motion)— *T. foetus* has jerky forward motion, is spindle-shaped, and has undulating membranes (Fig. 104-1).**
- *T. foetus* trophozoites—are not seen on fecal flotation
- *T. foetus* trophozoites—will not survive refrigeration
- Fecal protozoal culture—use in-house culture system (In Pouch TF; Biomed Diagnostics)
- Method—Inoculate with 0.05 g of fresh feces, incubate at room temperature, examine for motile trophozoites daily for 12 days.
- *Giardia* spp. and *P. hominis*—Do not grow after 24 hours in In Pouch culture system.
- PCR—more sensitive than fecal culture above but not commercially available

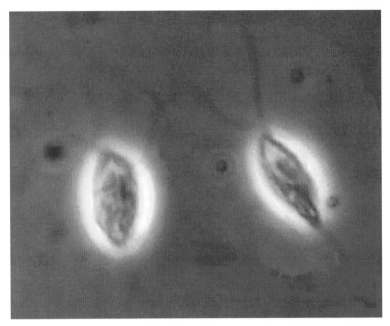

■ **Figure 104-1** *T. foetus* tachyzoites in the feces from a kitten. Note the undulating membrane protruding from the posterior of the tachyzoite which partly distinguishes it from *Giardia* spp.

 THERAPEUTICS

■ Essential to rule out coexisting disease (cryptosporidiosis, giardiasis), especially if diarrhea persists after specific treatment

Drugs of Choice

■ *P. hominis*—metronidazole (20 mg/kg, PO, q12h for 7 days)
■ *T. foetus*—failed all attempted drug treatment protocols to date
■ Most cats spontaneously resolve their diarrhea—but may take years

Precautions/Interactions

■ Glucocorticoids may exacerbate clinical disease.

 COMMENTS

■ Possible zoonotic transmission should be discussed with owner.
■ Treatment may decrease the severity of diarrhea but may also cause prolongation of time to resolution of diarrhea.

Abbreviations

CBC, complete blood count; FIP, feline infectious peritonitis; GI, gastrointestinal; IBD, inflammatory bowel disease; PCR, polymerase chain reaction.

Suggested Reading

Foster DM, Gookin JL, Poore MF, et al. Outcome of cats with diarrhea and *Tritrichomonas foetus* infection. *J Am Vet Med Assoc* 2004;15:888–892.

Gookin JL, Stebbins ME, Hunt E, et al. Prevalence of and risk factors from feline *Tritrichomonas foetus* and *Giardia* infection. *J Clin Microbiol* 2004;42:2707–2710.

Stockdale HD, Dillon AR, Newton JC, et al. Experimental infection of cats (*Felis catus*) with *Tritrichomonas foetus* isolated from cattle. *Vet Parasitol* 2008;154:156–161.

Trichosporonosis

DEFINITION/OVERVIEW

- A systemic or localized fungal infection causing granulomas usually on the nose; also can cause systemic infections in cats

ETIOLOGY/PATHOPHYSIOLOGY

- *Trichosporon* spp.—yeast-like saprophytic fungi of the family Cryptococcaceae
- Not considered to be primary pathogens—infect animals that are immunosuppressed, are receiving multiple broad-spectrum antibiotics, or have neoplasia
- In severely immunosuppressed host—Fungus invades mucosal surfaces of the GI, urinary, and respiratory tracts, with subsequent dissemination.
- Cats—Infections are characterized by pyogranulomatous inflammation of the mucosa, submucosa, and subcutaneous tissue.

SIGNALMENT/HISTORY

- Usually older cats
- Although immunosuppression has not been documented in most feline cases, it has been suspected.

CLINICAL FEATURES

- Nasal mass (Fig. 105-1).
- Mass sometimes protrudes from the nostril (similar to that with *Cryptococcus neoformans*)
- Fever
- Inspiratory stridor
- Regional lymphadenopathy—uncommon
- Subcutaneous lesions—secondary to a cat bite (one reported case)
- Chronic cystitis—hematuria and dysuria

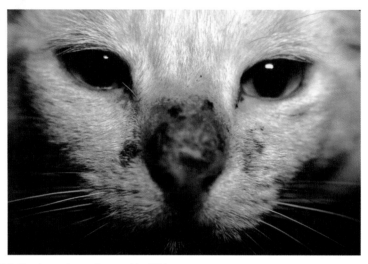

■ **Figure 105-1** Nasal mass in a cat caused by *Trichosporon* spp.

DIFFERENTIAL DIAGNOSIS

- Other causes of nasal masses:
  - Other fungal infections—*C. neoformans*, *Aspergillus*, and *Penicillium*
  - Neoplasia
  - Nasal polyps

DIAGNOSTICS

Diagnostic Feature

- **Requires—histologic confirmation on biopsied tissue**
- Culture of mucosal surfaces not adequate—Normal microflora of these areas may include *Trichosporon*.
- Culture biopsy material—Sabouraud's or Mycosel agar at 25°C for several days
- Culture—cream-colored, yeast-like colonies with blastoconidia that do not have a capsule when stained with mucin stains (unlike *C. neoformans*)
- PCR—developed to detect *Trichosporon* spp. although not commercially available

THERAPEUTICS

- Benzimidazoles—drugs of choice
- *Trichospora* spp.—demonstrate resistance to amphotericin B

TABLE 105-1 **Drug Therapy for Trichosporonosis in Cats**				
	Dose (mg/kg)	Route	Interval (h)	Duration (weeks)
Itraconazole (Soranox)	10	PO	12	4
Fluconazole (Diflucan)	10–25[a]	PO	12	4

[a]Up to a maximum dose of 200 mg/cat/day.

Drugs of Choice

- Itraconazole (Sporanox; Janssen)
- Fluconazole (Diflucan; Pfizer) (Table 105-1)

Precautions/Interactions

- Itraconazole—can cause vomiting, diarrhea, inappetence, elevations in hepatic enzymes, peripheral edema, fever, hypertension, and skin rash
- Monitor ALT—if rises, stop drug for 2 weeks and restart at 50% original dose
- Fluconazole—can cause similar side effects to itraconazole but less hepatotoxic in cats

 COMMENTS

- It is essential to examine the cat for underlying immunosuppressive conditions and direct therapy toward these if found.
- Zoonotic risk—none demonstrated to date

Abbreviations

ALT, alanine aminotransferase; GI, gastrointestinal; PCR, polymerase chain reaction.

Suggested Reading

Greene CE, Chandler FW. Trichosporosis. In: Greene CE, ed. *Infectious Diseases of the Dog and Cat.* Philadelphia: WB Saunders, 2006:634–636.
Sugita T, Mishikawa A, Shinoda T. Rapid detection of species of the opportunistic yeast *Trichosporon* by PCR. *J Clin Microbiol* 1998;36:1458–1460.

Tularemia

DEFINITION/OVERVIEW

- An acute systemic bacterial infection of cats (rarely dogs) that can result in septicemia, generalized lymphadenopathy, splenomegaly, hepatomegaly, lingual ulcers, and icterus

ETIOLOGY/PATHOPHYSIOLOGY

- *Francisella tularensis*—small gram-negative facultative intracellular coccobacilli found mainly in wild rabbits and rodents
- North America—most cases described from Missouri, Alaska, Oklahoma, Illinois, Utah, Maine, South Dakota, Tennessee, Kansas, and Colorado
- Europe—increased numbers of outbreaks
- Peak occurrence—June to August
- Infection—occurs by ingestion of tissue or body fluids of infected animal or contaminated water or by bite of a blood-sucking insect (ticks, flies, mites, midges, fleas, and mosquitoes)
- Dogs resistant
- Only a few bacteria needed to infect cats through skin, airways, or conjunctiva
- Large number of bacteria needed to infect—via GI tract
- Once inoculated—organisms spread via lymphatics to regional lymph nodes, then blood stream (septicemia), causing acute disease 2–7 days after infection
- *F. tularensis*—considered a potential biological warfare agent; occurrence of a cluster of pneumonia cases in companion animals may indicate animals as sentinels and the potential risk for human disease

SIGNALMENT/HISTORY

- Cats mainly; dogs relatively resistant
- Higher prevalence in outdoor/hunting cats
- Exposure to infected lagomorphs and rodents
- Contact with biting insects

CLINICAL FEATURES

- Serologic surveys—suggest many animals exposed but few develop clinical disease
- In acute disease:
  - Fever
  - Anorexia
  - Lethargy
  - Lymphadenopathy (especially cervical and submandibular)
- Later—hepatomegaly with icterus
- Splenomegaly
- Multifocal ulcers—sometimes with white pseudomembrane along glossopalantine arches and tongue

DIFFERENTIAL DIAGNOSIS

- Any acute systemic disease causing fever, lymphadenopathy, malaise, oral ulceration, and often a fatal outcome, including:
  - Lymphoma
  - Bubonic plague (*Yersinia pestis*)
  - FIP
  - FeLV
  - FPV
  - Bacterial sepsis
  - Endotoxemia

DIAGNOSTICS

- CBC—initially panleukopenia followed by leukocytosis, left shift, toxic neutrophils, and thrombocytopenia as DIC develops
- Biochemical panel—elevated bilirubin, ALT
- Decreased glucose—late in infection
- Coagulation parameters—reflect DIC
- Serologic examination—Animal may die before antibody titer rises.
- Gram stain of lesions—difficult to see organism as they are small gram-negative organisms (Fig. 106-1)

Diagnostic Features

- **Culture—Use blood, pleural fluid, lymph node aspirate into special medium (containing cysteine, usually on chocolate agar), because not recoverable on routine laboratory media.**
- DFA assay—of clinical material and tissues provides the most rapid and accurate assay for infection

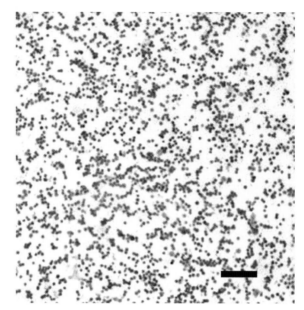

■ **Figure 106-1** *F. tularensis* are very small gram-negative coccobacilli that are difficult to find in lesions because they stain poorly (bar =10 mm).

 # THERAPEUTICS

- Aggressive treatment for septicemia and DIC—indicated with IV fluids, plasma, and heparin

Drugs of Choice

- Little information available on efficacy of antimicrobials, because usually fatal before treatment can begin
- Amoxicillin (20 mg/kg, IM or SC, q12h) combined with gentamicin (4.4 mg/kg, IM or SC, q24h) until a clinical response is achieved (Table 106-1)
- Fluoroquinolones may show some efficacy as might doxycycline.

TABLE 106-1	Drug Therapy for Tularemia in Dogs and Cats			
Drug	**Dose (mg/kg)**	**Route**	**Interval (h)**	**Duration**
Amoxicillin	20	IM, SC	12	[a]
Gentamicin[b]	4.4	IM, SC	24	[a]
Enrofloxacin	10–15	PO, IM, IV, SC	12	[a]

[a] Until a clinical response is achieved.
[b] Give in combination with amoxicillin.

Precautions/Interactions

- The organism is infectious to humans (only 100 organisms inhaled or splashed on a conjunctiva will cause infection).
- Extreme care must be taken on handling infected animals/tissues; send tissues out for culture, or body out for autopsy; do not perform these in the veterinary clinic.
- Monitor renal function, mainly by examining urine sediments, while administering gentamicin especially in dehydrated animals.

COMMENTS

- Prognosis poor—if not treated very early or if lymph nodes are palpable
- Most human cases of tularemia—result from tick-borne infections rather than contact with infected rodents or rabbits
- Some human cases—develop from cat scratches and bites, with initial lesion developing at the site of the injury
- Human cases acquired from dogs—rarely include injury but have been reported from dogs licking humans (an excellent reason not to let dogs lick the mouths of humans)
- In endemic areas—cats should be neutered to prevent roaming, limit hunting behavior, prevent exposure to contaminated water, and treated for ectoparasites

IMPORTANT: Zoonosis potential is high—gloves, gowns, face masks should be worn when handling a suspected case, which should be isolated from others in the hospital.

Abbreviations

ALT, alanine aminotransferase; CBC, complete blood count; DFA, direct fluorescent antibody; DIC, disseminated intravascular coagulation; FeLV, feline leukemia virus; FIP, feline infectious peritonitis; FPV, feline panleukopenia virus; GI, gastrointestinal.

Suggested Reading

Foley JE, Nieto NC. Tularemia. *Vet Microbiol* 2010;140:332–338.
Greene GE, DeBay BM. Tularemia. In: Greene CE, ed. *Infectious Disease of the Dog and Cat*. Philadelphia: WB Saunders, 2006:446–451.

Tyzzer's Disease

DEFINITION/OVERVIEW

- Bacterial infection of dogs and cats initially proliferating within the GI tract, then spreading via hepatic portal vein to the liver to cause hepatic colonization with multifocal periportal hepatic necrosis

ETIOLOGY/PATHOPHYSIOLOGY

- *Clostridium piliformis* (formally *Bacillus piliformis*)—gram-negative obligate intracellular bacterium
- Organisms—initially proliferate in intestinal epithelial cells before spreading to liver
- In liver—multifocal hepatic necrosis
- Sudden death—occurs after a short (24–48 hours) illness
- Occasional spread to other organs—focal myocarditis and enteric lymphadenitis

SIGNALMENT/HISTORY

- Dogs and cats—any age, although young at higher risk
- Other risk factors—contact with rodents, immunosuppression

CLINICAL FEATURES

- Rapid onset
- Lethargy
- Depression
- Anorexia
- Abdominal discomfort
- Hepatomegaly
- Terminally—hypothermia
- Death within 24–48 hours
- Small amounts of pasty feces—diarrhea infrequent

DIFFERENTIAL DIAGNOSIS

- Other causes of acute hepatitis:
  - Infectious canine hepatitis
  - FIP
  - Toxoplasmosis
  - Suppurative cholangitis
  - DIC
  - RMSF
  - Acute hemorrhagic necrotizing pancreatitis
  - Leptospirosis
  - Idiosyncratic hepatotoxin (drugs and chemicals)

 DIAGNOSTICS

- Diagnosis usually made at necropsy—hepatic necrosis with filamentous organisms within cytoplasm of hepatocytes (Fig. 107-1); widely disseminated lesions, including severe myocarditis, hepatitis, enterocolitis, intestinal leiomyositis, and adrenal cortical adenitis have been reported in a dog
- ALT—markedly elevated if taken shortly before death

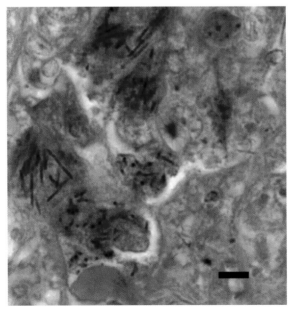

■ **Figure 107-1** Filamentous organisms of *C. piliformis* (the etiologic agent of Tyzzer's disease) in the cytoplasm of hepatocytes (Giemsa stain; bar =5 mm).

- Serologic examination—to identify latent infections in rodent colonies
- Serology—could be used to investigate illness in dogs and cats
- Organism isolation—requires mice, embryonating eggs, or cell culture inoculation

 # THERAPEUTICS

- None effective

Drugs of Choice

- None

Precautions/Interactions

- None

 # COMMENTS

- Avoid contact of cats and dogs with rodents.
- Examine causes of immunosuppression.

Abbreviations

ALT, alanine aminotransferase; DIC, disseminated intravascular coagulation; FIP, feline infectious peritonitis; GI, gastrointestinal tract; RMSF, Rocky Mountain spotted fever.

Suggested Reading

Jones BR, Greene CE. Tyzzer's disease. In: Greene CE, ed. *Infectious Diseases of the Dog and Cat*. Philadelphia: WB Saunders, 2006:362–363.
Young JK, Baker DC, Burney DP. Naturally occurring Tyzzer's disease in a puppy. *Vet Pathol* 1995;32:63–65.

Urinary Capillariasis (Pearsonema)

108

DEFINITION/OVERVIEW

- A parasitic infection of the bladder and occasionally the renal pelvis of dogs and cats

ETIOLOGY/PATHOPHYSIOLOGY

- *Pearsonema* (previously *Capillaria*) *plica* (dogs and cats) and *Pearsonema feliscati* (cats)—capillarid parasite that invades the mucosa and submucosa of the urinary bladder, renal pelvis, and ureters (rarely), causing a mild inflammatory response
- *P. plica*—produces ova with bipolar plugs in urine; after earthworms ingest embryonated ova, the parasite develops into the infective stage
- Ingestion of infective earthworms—results in a patent infection in dogs
- PPP = 58–88 days
- *P. feliscati*—life cycle poorly understood
- Infection of cats—thought to occur by ingestion of eggs or possibly some undetermined paratenic host

SIGNALMENT/HISTORY

- In the United States, infection is rare.
- In Australia, prevalence is up to 35%.

Dogs

- No predilection reported
- High prevalence (up to 50%) in natural hosts (foxes and raccoons) in southeastern United States may predispose to infection in dogs in this region.
- In kennels—Dirt surfaces may predispose to high infection rates.

553

Cats

■ Affected cats >8 months of age

CLINICAL FEATURES

■ Usually asymptomatic, except in heavy infections
■ Pollakiuria
■ Hematuria
■ Stranguria
■ Dysuria

DIFFERENTIAL DIAGNOSIS

■ Consider—other causes of lower urinary tract disease (calculi, bacterial infection, trauma, and neoplasia)
■ Differentiated from other conditions—finding parasite eggs in urine

DIAGNOSTICS

■ CBC, serum biochemical profile—normal
■ Urinalysis—Ova with bipolar plugs (60 mm to slightly smaller than those of *Trichuris vulpis*) in urine sediment are diagnostic (Fig. 108-1).
■ Consider the possibility of fecal contamination of urine with *T. vulpis* (dogs) or other *Capillaria* spp. ova if the urine was free-catch.
■ Note also that a false diagnosis of trichuriasis may be made if feces are contaminated with urine containing *P. plica* ova.

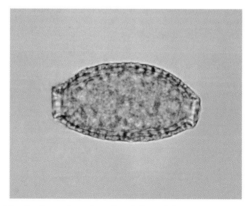

■ **Figure 108-1** The ova of *P. plica* from the urine of an infected dog.

TABLE 108-1 Drug Therapy for *P. plica* Infection in Dogs and Cats				
Drug	Dose (mg/kg)	Route	Interval (h)	Duration (days)
Fenbendazole	50	PO	24	5
Ivermectin (1% injectable)	0.2	SC, PO	Once[a]	—

[a]Repeat in 2 weeks.

 # THERAPEUTICS

- Infection is usually self-limiting in both cats and dogs.
- Ova are no longer detectable in the urine sediment of infected dogs after 10–12 weeks if dogs are isolated from reinfection.
- Consider anthelmintic therapy if clinical signs are present.
- Monitor success of therapy by clinical signs and examining urine sediment for ova.

Drugs of Choice

- Fenbendazole—not approved but is effective
- Ivermectin—1% injectable; has been suggested also but is not approved (Table 108-1)

Precautions/Interactions

- If using ivermectin, check for presence of circulating *Dirofilaria* microfilaria before administration to avoid complications.

 # COMMENTS

- Prevalence of infection in kennels can be reduced by replacing soil surfaces with sand, gravel, or cement.

Abbreviations

CBC, complete blood count; PPP, prepatent period.

Suggested Reading

Brown SA, Prestwood KA. Parasites of the urinary tract. In: Kirk RW, ed. *Current Veterinary Therapy IX*. Philadelphia: WB Saunders, 1986:1153–1155.

Whipworms (Trichuriasis)

DEFINITION/OVERVIEW

- A nematode parasite of dogs and cats; adult worms live in the cecum and may cause large bowel diarrhea and pseudohypoadrenocorticism in dogs
- Asymptomatic in cats

ETIOLOGY/PATHOPHYSIOLOGY

- *Trichuris vulpi*—dogs
- *Trichuris campanula* and *Trichuris serrata*—cats
- *T. vulpis*—widely distributed throughout North America
- *T. campanula* and *T. serrata*—occur sporadically in North America, Caribbean Islands, and Australia
- Adult *T. vulpis* worms—embed within the large intestinal and cecal mucosa, causing inflammation
- Cecal mucosal damage—can be severe enough to result in severe bloody mucoid diarrhea and electrolyte abnormalities similar to Addison's disease
- Female worms—lay large numbers (about 2000 per day) of bioperculated eggs, which are passed in feces
- Eggs—extremely resistant to environmental conditions (can remain viable for years)
- Eggs—susceptible to desiccation, extreme temperatures, and ultraviolet radiation
- Infection—dogs ingesting eggs containing mature L1 larvae
- Larvae hatch in the small intestine—migrate to large intestine, molt, and become adults
- *T. vulpis* PPP = 11 weeks.
- *T. campanula* PPP = 9 weeks

SIGNALMENT/HISTORY

- No sex, breed, or age predilection
- Pseudohypoadrenocorticism syndrome due to trichuriasis—middle-aged to older dogs

- Housing—dogs in outside runs, housed on dirt floors, under constant exposure to high build-up of fecal material, and seldom cleaned are predisposed to infection

 CLINICAL FEATURES

Dogs

- Many infections—asymptomatic
- Large-bowel diarrhea—hematochezia; mucus; straining; increased frequency
- Vomiting—secondary to large-bowel inflammation
- Weakness—from dehydration
- Metabolic acidosis
- Electrolyte abnormalities—hyponatremia, hyperkalemia may be present
- Pseudohypoadrenocorticism syndrome—severe diarrhea caused by the parasite results in isotonic GI fluid loss
  - When GI fluid loss replaced by water intake—hyponatremia develops
  - Diarrhea—also leads to dehydration and bicarbonate loss, resulting in metabolic acidosis
  - Metabolic acidosis—causes the translocation of potassium from the intracellular to extracellular fluid, resulting in hyperkalemia
  - If hyponatremia and hyperkalemia severe enough—Na:K ratio falls below 27, resembling Addison's disease

Cats

- Asymptomatic—of little clinical importance

 DIFFERENTIAL DIAGNOSIS

Dogs

- Other causes of large-bowel diarrhea, including idiopathic chronic IBD, immune-mediated eosinophilic colitis, histiocytic colitis, parasites (giardiasis, trichomoniasis, amebiasis, balantidiasis, leishmaniasis), fungal (histoplasmosis, prototheca), bacterial, irritable bowel syndrome, ileocolic and cecocolic intussusception, and neoplasia
- Other causes of reduced Na:K ratio, including hypoadrenocorticism (Addison's disease), renal failure, chylothorax, other GI tract disorders (salmonellosis, perforated duodenal ulcer), pregnancy with diarrhea, and peritoneal effusions

 DIAGNOSTICS

- CBC and serum biochemical profile—No abnormalities if diarrhea is not severe.
- If diarrhea is severe (resulting in pseudohypoadrenocorticism)—hyponatremia, hyperkalemia with a reduced Na:K ratio (<27), normal ACTH response test

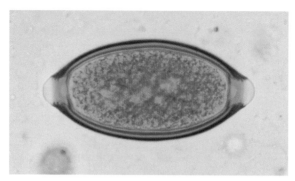

■ **Figure 109-1** *T. vulpis* egg in dog feces. Note the prominent bipolar plugs, brown color, single cell (zygote) within the egg shell membrane, and size, ~90 × 45 m.

- Fecal flotation; trichurid eggs (Fig. 109-1)
- Endoscopy—may view adult parasites in the colonic mucosa (should a clinician be unfortunate enough to miss a diagnosis by fecal flotation or by treatment trial)

THERAPEUTICS

- A dog with severe diarrhea, dehydration, metabolic acidosis, and a reduced Na:K ratio—IV isotonic fluid support (initially isotonic saline)
- Perform ACTH response test—to rule out Addison's disease
- Dogs with trichuriasis-induced pseudohypoadrenocorticism—will not be harmed by treatment with physiologic mineralcorticoid or glucocorticoid supplementation

Drugs of Choice

- Fenbendazole (Panacur Granules 22.2%; Intervet)
- Praziquantel/pyrantel/febantel (Drontal Plus; Bayer)
- Diethylcarbamazine/oxibendazole (Filaribits Plus; Pfizer)
- Milbemycin (Interceptor; Novartis) (Table 109-1)
- Emodepside combined with praziquantel (Profender Tablets; Bayer)—not marketed for use in dogs in the United States, but has been shown to be effective against *T. vulpis* in dogs with no side effects

Precautions/Interactions

- Fenbendazole—can be used in pregnant animals, but praziquantel/pyrantel/febantel should not be
- Diethylcarbamazine/oxibendazole—has been associated with hepatic injury (sometimes fatal) in dogs and should not be used when there is evidence of concurrent hepatic injury

TABLE 109-1 Drug Therapy for Whipworms (Trichuriasis) in Dogs				
Drug	**Dose (mg/kg)**	**Route**	**Interval (h)**	**Duration (days)**
Fenbendazole (Panacur)	50	PO	24	3[a]
Praziquantel/pyrantel/febantel (Drontal Plus)	[b]	PO	24	3[a]
Diethylcarbamazine/oxibendazole (Filaribits Plus)	[c]	PO	Daily[d]	—
Milbemycin (Interceptor)	0.5	PO	Monthly[e]	—

[a]Retreat in 3–4 weeks time.
[b]Praziquantel (5–12), pyrantel (5–12), and febantel (25–65).
[c]Diethylcarbamazine (6.6), and oxibendazole (5).
[d]Given as daily heartworm preventive.
[e]Given as monthly heartworm preventive.

COMMENTS

- Dogs living in chronically infected environment—initially treat with fenbendazole; then place the dog on monthly milbemycin
- Cats—have been successfully treated with fenbendazole

Abbreviations

ACTH, adrenocorticotropic hormone; CBC, complete blood count; GI, gastrointestinal; IBD, inflammatory bowel disease; PPP, prepatent period.

Suggested Reading

Bowman DD, ed. *Georgi's Parasitology for Veterinarians*, 8th ed. Philadelphia: WB Saunders, 2003: 228–229.

DiBartola SP, Johnson SE, Davenport DJ, et al. Clinicopathologic findings resembling hypoadrenocorticism in dogs with primary gastrointestinal disease. *J Am Vet Med Assoc* 1985;187:60–63.

Schimmel A, Altreuther G, Schroeder I, et al. Efficacy of emodepside plus praziquantel tablets (Profender tablets for dogs) against mature and immature adult *Trichuris vulpis* infections in dogs. *Parasitol Res* 2009;105:17–22.

Appendices

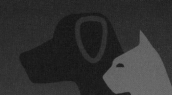

APPENDIX A: VACCINATION SCHEDULE

NOTE: Tailor vaccination schedule for each individual animal based on the following:

1. Age of presentation for the animal's first vaccination
2. Risk of exposure to diseases
3. Risk of developing disease if exposed
4. Likelihood of the owner complying with instructions for revaccination (booster yearly versus every 3 years)
5. Risk of complications developing as a consequence of vaccination (adjuvanted versus nonadjuvanted recombinant vaccines)
6. Modified live vaccine not recommended for pregnant or immunocompromised animals

Feline

	Age of Initial Vaccination[a]		
Vaccine Antigen	**6–12 Weeks**	**12 Weeks**	**Booster Interval**
FVRCP[b]	Every 3 weeks until 12 weeks	1 dose	1 year later, then every 3 years
FeLV[c]	2 doses 3 to 4 weeks apart 9 weeks	2 doses 3 to 4 weeks	1 year later, then annually
Rabies[d]		1 dose	1 year later, then annually or every 3 years[d]

[a] Vaccination of kittens 4–6 weeks of age may be indicated in high-risk environments (catteries, shelters); FVRC recommended in kittens >2 weeks (IN) or >4 weeks (MLV parenteral) if enzootic viral respiratory infections are present.

[b] FVRC: MLV and inactivated for SC administration, and MLV and IN products are available; IN provides more rapid (protection within 48 hours) protection than parenteral dosing but has a high incidence of mild contagious respiratory illness. P: MLV and inactivated for SC administration available; maternal antibody may last to 12 weeks; give last vaccine in initial series at or after 12 weeks of age; if MLV vaccine is used, only one vaccine needed if given after 12 weeks of age until first year booster; booster at 1 year of age, then every 3 years; use inactivated vaccine in the pregnant or immunocompromised.

[c] Recommended for cats at risk (cats that are outdoor, indoor/outdoor, stray/feral, open multicat households, FeLV-positive households, households of unknown FeLV status). All (except Merial's Purevax recombinant leukemia vaccine) products contain inactivated noninfectious viral antigens with an adjuvant, and are given SC distally on the hind limb due to possibility of producing a vaccine-induced sarcoma; Purevax is adjuvant-free in a canarypox vector (reducing risk of tumor formation) and administered in a small volume (0.25 ml) using a transdermal (Vetjet) vaccination system; pretest before considering vaccination (if positive on an ELISA, retest in 4–8 weeks; if negative, start vaccine series).

[d] Inactivated adjuvanted products and one nonadjuvanted recombinant product (Merial) available; adjuvanted products require booster every 3 years; nonadjuvanted recombinant product requires yearly booster (follow manufactures and local law specifications).

ELISA, enzyme-linked immunosorbent assay; FeLV, feline leukemia virus; FVRCP, feline viral rhinotracheitis/calici virus; IN, intranasal; MLV, modified live virus; P, panleukopenia; SC, subcutaneous.

Canine

	Age of Initial Vaccination[a]		
Vaccine Antigen	6 to 12 Weeks	12 to 18 Weeks	Booster Interval
M/DA2Pi[b]	Every 3 weeks until 12 weeks	2 doses 3 to 4 weeks apart	1 year later, then every 3 years[c]
P[d]	2 doses, 3 to 4 weeks apart until 18 weeks	3 doses 3 to 4 weeks apart	1 year later, then every 3 years[e]
Rabies[f]		1 dose	1 year later, then annually or triennially

[a] Vaccination of puppies 4–6 weeks of age may be indicated in high-risk environments (shelters).
[b] M: can be given up to 12 weeks of age, but should be reserved for 6-week-old pups as first vaccine, 3 weeks later by D. D: MLV vaccines and one recombinant in a canary virus vector available; risk of postvaccinal disease for MLV but not for recombinant vaccine; yearly boosters required with recombinant product and every 3 years with MLV. A2: use A-2 MLV vaccines to avoid blue eye (anterior uveitis) seen with A-1 products. Pi: MLV and inactivated for SC administration, and MLV and IN products are available; IN provides more rapid (protection within 48 hours) protection than parenteral dosing but has a high incidence of mild contagious respiratory illness.
[c] Can check titers and booster if titer to D,1:32, Pi,1:16, A2,1:16.
[d] P: killed, MLV, and potentiated MLV vaccines available; use MLV or potentiated in most pups (killed in pregnant animals, immunosuppressed pups, or pups under 5 weeks of age); can begin MLV at 6 weeks, booster every 3 weeks until 16–18 weeks of age; dogs vaccinated with MLV will excrete virus in feces for up to 2 weeks postvaccination.
[e] Can check titer and booster if titer to P <1:80.
[f] Inactivated adjuvanted products available for IM and/or SC administration; require booster 1 year after the first dose at 12 weeks, then annually or triennially (follow manufacturer's and local law specifications).

A, adenovirus type 1 (hepatitis) or type 2 (respiratory); D, distemper; IM, intramuscular; IN, intranasal; M, measles; MLV, modified live virus; P, parvovirus; Pi, parainfluenzap; SC, subcutaneous.

APPENDIX B: PRODUCTS FOR TREATMENT OF CANINE INTESTINAL PARASITES

APPENDIX B: Products for Treatment of Canine Intestinal Parasites

Example Trade Name®	Active Ingredient(s) and Dosage	Toxocara canis	Toxascaris leonina	Ancylostoma caninum	Ancylostoma braziliense	Uncinaria stenocephala	Trichuris vulpis	Taenia pisiformis	Dipylidium caninum	Echinococcus granulosus	Echinococcus multilocularis
Pipfuge	Piperazine (55 mg/kg PO)	+	+								
Nemex	Pyrantel pamoate (5 mg/kg >2.25 kg; 10 mg/kg <2.25 kg PO)	+	+	+		+					
Panacur	Fenbendazole (50 mg/kg PO 3 days)	+	+	+		+	+	+			
Cestex	Epsiprantel (5.5 mg/kg PO)							+	+		
Droncit	Praziquantel (5–7.5 mg/kg PO, SQ, IM)							+	+	+	+
Virbantel	Pyrantel (5 mg) Praziquantel (5 mg/kg PO)	+	+	+	+	+		+	+		
Drontal Plus	Praziquantel (5–12 mg)/pyrantel (5–12 mg)/febantel (25–62 mg/kg PO)	+	+	+		+	+	+	+	+	+

APPENDIX C: PARASITICIDES FOR CATS

APPENDIX C: Parasiticides for Cats

Example Trade Name®	Active Ingredient(s) and Dosage	Age at First Administration (weeks)	Toxocara cati	Toxascaris leonina	Ancylostoma tubaeformis	Dirofilaria immitis (prevention)	Taenia taeinaeformis	Dipylidium caninum	Fleas	Ticks	Otodectes cynotis
Pipa-tabs	Piperazine (55 mg/kg PO)	No age restriction	+	+							
Cestex	Epsiprantel (1.25 mg/kg PO)	7					+	+			
Droncit Feline	Praziquantel (2–10 mg/kg PO, IM SC)	6					+	+			
Drontal	Praziquantel (5 mg)/pyrantel (20 mg/kg PO)	4 >1.5 lb	+	+	+		+	+			
Profender	Emodepside (3 mg) Praziquantel (12 mg/kg topical)	8	+	+	+		+	+			
Program Flavor tabs suspension	Lufenuron (30 mg/kg) monthly	6							+		
Program 6 month Injectable	Lufenuron (10 mg/kg SC) every 6 months	6							+		
Frontline	Fipronil Monthly topical	8							+		
Frontline-plus	Fipronil (S)-methoprene monthly topcial	8							+	+	

(continued)

APPENDIX C: Parasiticides for Cats (Continued)

Example Trade Name®	Active Ingredient(s) and Dosage	Age at First Administration (weeks)	Toxocara cati	Toxascaris leonina	Ancylostoma tubaeformis	Dirofilaria immitis (prevention)	Taenia taeinaeformis	Dipylidium caninum	Fleas	Ticks	Otodectes cynotis
Capstar	Nitenpyram (1 mg/kg PO) daily as needed	4 >2 lb							+		
Heartgard	Ivermectin (0.024 mg/kg) PO monthly	6		+	+	+					
Interceptor	Milbemycin oxime (2 mg/kg) PO monthly	8	+		+	+					
Revolution	Selamectin (6 mg/kg) topical monthly	8	+		+	+			+		+
Advantage Multi	Moxidectin (1 mg) imidoclopride (10 mg/kg) topical monthly	9	+	+	+	+			+		+
Promeris	Metaflumizone topical monthly	8							+		
Acarexx	0.5 ml of 0.01% ivermectin topical per ear	4									+
Milbemite	Milbemycin single dose tube/day topical per ear.	4									+

APPENDIX D: CANINE HEARTWORM PREVENTATIVES

APPENDIX D: Canine Heartworm Preventatives

Example Trade Name®	Active Ingredient(s) and Dosage	Application	Earliest Administration as per Label	Toxocara canis	Toxascaris leonina	Ancylostoma caninum	Ancylostoma braziliense	Uncinaria stenocephala	Trichuris vulpis
Heartgard	Ivermectin (0.006 mg/kg)	Oral/monthly	6 weeks						
Heartgard Plus	Ivermectin + pyrantel for (0.006 + 5 mg/kg, respectively)	Oral/monthly	6 weeks	T	T	T	T	T	
Iverhart Max	Ivermectin + pyrantel + praziquantel (0.006 + 5 + 5 mg/kg, respectively)	PO monthly	8 weeks	T	T	T	T	T	
Interceptor	Milbemycin (0.5 mg/kg)	Oral/monthly >2 lb	4 weeks	T	T	C			T
Revolution†	Selamectin (6 mg/kg)	Topical/monthly	6 weeks	T	T				
Sentinel†	Milbemycin + Lufenuron (0.5 mg + 10 mg/kg, respectively)	Oral/monthly >2 lb	4 weeks	T	T	C			T
Advantage Multi†	Moxidectin + lufenuron (2.2 + 10 mg/kg, respectively)	monthly topical	7 weeks	T	T	T	T		

T, treatment or removal—removes >90% of worms from dogs at the time of dosing.
C, control—removes >90% of existing worms from dogs after two to several treatments.
†, also effective against fleas.

APPENDIX E: CANINE PRODUCTS WITH EFFICACIES AGAINST ARTHROPODS

APPENDIX E: Canine Products with Efficacies Against Arthropods

Example Trade Name®	Active Ingredient(s) and Dosage	FDA or EPA Registered	Application	Age at First Administration	Adult Fleas	Flea Eggs or Larvae	Ticks	Sarcoptes	Otodectes	Mosquitoes
Sentinel	Milbemycin/lufenuron (0.5 mg + 10 mg/kg, respectively)	FDA	Oral/daily	>2 lb	+					
Program	Lufenuron (10 mg/kg)	FDA	Oral/monthly	6 weeks		+				
Revolution	Selamectin (6 mg/kg)	FDA	Oral/monthly	6 weeks	+	+	+	+	+	
Vectra 3D	Dinotefuran/ pyriproxyfen/ permethrin	EPA	Topical/monthly	7 weeks	+	+	+			
Capstar	Nitempyram (1 mg/kg)	FDA	Oral/daily as needed	4 weeks and >2 lb	+	+				
Comfortis	Spinosad (30 mg/kg)	FDA	Oral/monthly	14 weeks	+					
Frontline topical	Fipronil	EPA	Topical/monthly	10 weeks	+	+				
Frontline spray	Fipronil	EPA	Topical/monthly	8 weeks	+	+				
Frontline Plus	Fipronil and (S)-methoprene	EPA	Topical/monthly	8 weeks	+	+	+			
Promeris	Amitraz/ metaflumizone	EPA	Topical/monthly	8 weeks	+	+	+			
Advantage	Imidacloprid	EPA	Topical/monthly	7 weeks	+	+				
K9 Advantix	Imidacloprid/ permethrin	EPA	Topical/monthly	7 weeks	+		+			+
Advantage Multi	Moxidectin/ imidacloprid	FDA	Topical/monthly	7 weeks	+					
Acarexx	Ivermectin	FDA	Topical to ear	4 weeks					+	
MilbeMite Otic Solution	Milbemycin oxime	FDA	Topical to ear	4 weeks					+	

EPA, Environmental Protection Agency; FDA, Food and Drug Administration.

APPENDIX F: DRUG FORMULARY

APPENDIX F: Drug Formulary

Drug Name (Trade or Other Names)	Pharmacology and Indications	Adverse Effects and Precautions	Dosing Information and Comments	Formulations	Dosage
Acemannan	Immunostimulant. A polysaccharide acetylated mannan extract from aloe. Proposed to stimulate T-cell activity in animals. It has been used to treat tumors in dogs and cats. It may stimulate tumor necrosis factor (TNF) and other cytokine release.	No reported side effects	After reconstitution, shake well to dissolve. Use within 4 hr after preparation. Beneficial effect is controversial. There has been a lack of demonstrated effect on lymphocyte blastogenic response in cats.	10-mg vials reconstituted to 1 mg/ml	Intraperitoneal (1 mg/kg) and intralesional injection (2 mg) every week for 6 treatments
Albendazole (Valbazen)	Benzimidazole antiparasitic drug. Inhibits glucose uptake in parasites.	At approved doses, there is a wide margin of safety. Adverse effects can include anorexia, lethargy, and bone marrow toxicity. At high doses, has been associated with bone marrow toxicity (*J Am Vet Med Assoc* 1998;213:44–46). Adverse effects are possible when administered for longer than 5 days.	Used primarily as antihelmintic, but also has demonstrated efficacy for giardiasis	113.6 mg/ml suspension and 300 mg/ml paste	25–50 mg/kg q12h PO × 3 days For giardia, use 25 mg/kg q12h × 2 days
Allopurinol (Lopurin, Zyloprim)	Decreases production of uric acid by inhibiting enzymes responsible for uric acid.	May cause skin reactions (hypersensitivity).	Used in humans primarily for treating gout. In animals, used to decrease formation of uric acid uroliths and treatment of leishmaniasis.	100, 300 mg tablets	10 mg/kg q8h, then reduce to 10 mg/kg q24h, PO. For leishmaniasis, use 10 mg/kg q12h PO for at least 4 months.

(Continued)

APPENDIX F: Drug Formulary (continued)

Drug Name (Trade or Other Names)	Pharmacology and Indications	Adverse Effects and Precautions	Dosing Information and Comments	Formulations	Dosage
Amikacin (Amiglyde-V [veterinary] and Amikin [human])	Aminoglycoside antibacterial drug (inhibits protein synthesis). Mechanism is similar to that of other aminoglycosides (see Gentamicin sulfate), but may be more active than gentamicin.	May cause nephrotoxicosis with high doses or prolonged therapy. May also cause ototoxicity and vestibulotoxicity. (See Gentamicin sulfate.)	Once-daily doses are designed to maximize peak minimum inhibitory concentration (MIC) ratio. Consider therapeutic drug monitoring for chronic therapy. (See also Gentamicin sulfate.)	50, 250 mg/ml injection	Dog and cat: 6.5 mg/kg q8h IV, IM, SC. Dog: 15–30 mg/kg q24h IV, IM, SC. Cat: 10–14 mg/kg q24h IV, IM, SC.
Amitraz (Mitaban)	Antiparasitic drug for ectoparasites. Used for treatment of mites, including Demodex. Inhibits monoamine oxidase in mites.	Causes sedation in dogs (α_2-agonist), which may be reversed by yohimbine or atipamezole. When high doses are used, other side effects reported include pruritus, polyuria and polydipsia (PU/PD), bradycardia, hypothermia, hyperglycemia, and (rarely) seizures.	Manufacturer's dose should be used initially. But, for refractory cases, this dose has been exceeded to produce increased efficacy. Doses that have been used include: 0.025, 0.05, and 0.1% concentration applied 2× week and 0.125% solution applied to half of body every day for 4 weeks to 5 months.	10.6 ml concentrated dip (19.9%)	10.6 ml per 7.5 L water (0.025% solution). Apply 3 to 6 topical treatments q14d. For refractory cases, this dose has been exceeded to produce increased efficacy. Doses that have been used include: 0.025, 0.05, and 0.1% concentration applied 2× week and 0.125% solution applied to half of body every day for 4 weeks to 5 months.
Amoxicillin (Amoxi-Tabs, Biomox, and other brands. [Omnipen, Principen, Totacillin are human forms])	β-Lactam antibiotic. Inhibits bacterial cell wall synthesis. Generally broad-spectrum activity. Used for a variety of infections in all species.	Usually well tolerated. Allergic reactions are possible. Diarrhea is common with oral doses.	Dose recommendations vary depending on the susceptibility of bacteria and location of infection. Generally, more frequent or higher doses needed for gram-negative infections.	50, 100, 150, 200, 400 mg tablets. 250 and 500 mg capsules (human forms)	6.6–20 mg/kg q8–12h PO.

Amoxicillin trihydrate (Amoxi-Tabs, Amoxi-Drops, Amoxil, and others)	β-Lactam antibiotic. Inhibits bacterial cell wall synthesis. Generally broad-spectrum activity, but resistance is common.	Use cautiously in animals allergic to penicillin-like drugs.	Dose requirements vary depending on susceptibility of bacteria	50, 100, 200, 400 mg tablets, 50 mg/ml oral suspension	6–20 mg/kg, q8–12h, PO
Amoxicillin + clavulanate potassium (Clavamox)	β-Lactam antibiotic + β-Lactamase inhibitor (clavulanate/clavuanic acid).	Same as for amoxicillin	Same as for amoxicillin	62.5, 125, 250, 375 mg tablets and 62.5 mg/ml suspension	Dog: 12.5–25 mg/kg, q12h, PO. Cat: 62.5 mg/cat, q12h, PO. Consider administering these doses q8h for gram-negative infections.
Amphotericin B (Fungizone)	Antifungal drug. Fungicidal for systemic fungi, by damaging fungal membranes.	Produces a dose-related nephrotoxicosis. Also produces fever, phlebitis, and tremors.	Administer IV via slow infusion diluted in fluids, and monitor renal function closely. When preparing IV solution, do not mix with electrolyte solutions (use D5W, for example); administer NaCl fluid loading before therapy. (One study administered this drug subcutaneously: *Aust Vet J* 1996;73:124)	50 mg injectable vial	0.5, mg/kg, IV (slow infusion) q48h to a cumulative dose of 4–8 mg/kg.

(Continued)

APPENDIX F: Drug Formulary (continued)

Drug Name (Trade or Other Names)	Pharmacology and Indications	Adverse Effects and Precautions	Dosing Information and Comments	Formulations	Dosage
Amphotericin B, liposomal formulation (ABLC, Abelcet)	Same indications as for conventional amphotericin B. Liposomal formulations may be used at higher doses, and safety margin is increased. Expense is much higher than for conventional formulations.	Renal toxicity is the most dose-limiting effect.	Higher doses can be used compared to conventional formulation of amphotericin B. Dilute in 5% dextrose in water to 1 mg/ml and administer IV over 1–2 hr.	100 mg/20 ml in lipid formulation	Dog: 2–3 mg/kg, IV, 3×/week for 9–12 treatments to a cumulative dose of 24–27 mg/kg. Cat: 1 mg/kg IV 3×/week for 12 treatments.
Ampicillin (Omnipen, Principen, others [human forms])	β-Lactam antibiotic. Inhibits bacterial cell wall synthesis.	Use cautiously in animals allergic to penicillin-like drugs.	Dose requirements vary depending on susceptibility of bacteria. Absorbed approximately 50% less, compared with amoxicillin, when administered orally. Generally, more frequent or higher doses needed for gram-negative infections.	250, 500 mg capsules; 125, 250, 500 mg vials of ampicillin sodium. Ampicillin trihydrate: 10 and 25 g vials for injection.	Ampicillin sodium: 10–20 mg/kg, q6–8h, IV, IM, SC or 20–40 mg/kg, q8h, PO. Ampicillin trihydrate: Dog: 10–50 mg/kg, q12–24h, IM, SC. Cat: 10–20 mg/kg q12–24h IM, SC. Dogs and cats: doses as high as 100 mg/kg have been used for some resistant infections, such as those caused by enterococci.
Ampicillin + sulbactam (Unasyn)	Ampicillin plus a β-lactamase inhibitor (sulbactam). Sulbactam has similar activity as clavulanate.	Same as for ampicillin.	Same as for amoxicillin + clavulanate.	2:1 combination for injection. 1.5 and 3 g vials.	10–20 mg/kg IV, IM q8h.
Ampicillin trihydrate (Polyflex)	β-Lactam antibiotic. Inhibits bacterial cell wall synthesis.	Use cautiously in animals allergic to penicillin-like drugs.	Absorption is slow and may not be sufficient for acute serious infection.	10, 25 mg vials for injection	Dog: 10–50 mg/kg q12–24h IM, SC. Cat: 10–20 mg/kg q12–24h IM, SC.

Drug	Description	How supplied	Dosage
Amprolium (Amprol, Corid)	Antiprotozoal drug. Antagonizes thiamine in parasites. Used for treatment of coccidiosis, especially in puppies.	Toxicity observed only at high doses (CNS signs due to thiamine deficiency). Eye irritation —flush with water.	Usually administered as feed additive to livestock. For dogs, 30 ml 9.6% amprolium added to 3.8 L of drinking water for control of coccidiosis.	9.6% (9.6 g/100 ml) oral solution; 20% soluble powder.	1.25 g of 20% amprolium powder to daily feed, or 30 ml of 9.6% amprolium solution to 3.8 L of drinking water for 7 days.
Azithromycin (Zithromax)	Azalide antibiotic. Similar mechanism of action as macrolides (erythromycin), which is to inhibit bacteria protein synthesis via inhibition of ribosome. Spectrum is primarily gram-positive.	Has not been in common use in veterinary medicine to establish adverse effects. Vomiting is likely with high doses. Diarrhea may occur in some patients.	Azithromycin may be better tolerated than erythromycin. Primary difference from other antibiotics is the high intracellular concentrations achieved.	250 mg capsules, 250 and 600 mg tablets, 100 or 200 mg/5 ml oral suspension, and 500 mg vials for injection.	Dog: 10 mg/kg PO once every 5 days or 3.3 mg/kg q24h for 3 days. Cat: 5 mg/kg PO q48h.
AZT (Azidothymidine)	See Zidovudine.				
Bactrim (sulfamethoxazole + trimethoprim) (See Trimethoprim-sulfonamide combinations.)					
Benznidazole (Ragonil)	Antiprotozoal drug with activity against Trypanosoma cruzi. Thought to inhibit protein and RNA synthesis in the parasite.	Vomiting is the main side effect. May cause hepatic and renal toxicity; monitor organ function while treating.	Available in United States only from the CDC. Best efficacy in acute cases; little effect on outcome of chronic disease.	100 mg tablet	5–10 mg/kg q24h PO for 2 months.

(Continued)

APPENDIX F: Drug Formulary (continued)

Drug Name (Trade or Other Names)	Pharmacology and Indications	Adverse Effects and Precautions	Dosing Information and Comments	Formulations	Dosage
Cefaclor (Ceclor)	Cephalosporin antibiotic. Action is similar to that of other b-lactam antibiotics, inhibiting synthesis of bacterial cell wall, leading to cell death. Cephalosporins are divided into 1st, 2nd, or 3rd generation, depending on spectrum of activity. Consult package insert or specific reference for spectrum of activity of individual cephalosporin. Cefaclor is a 2nd-generation cephalosporin.	All cephalosporins are generally safe; however, sensitivity can occur in individuals (allergy). Rare bleeding disorders have been known to occur with some cephalosporins.	Used primarily when resistance has been demonstrated to 1st-generation cephalosporins.	250, 500 capsules and 25 mg/ml oral suspension.	15 mg/kg q8h PO.
Cefadroxil (Cefa-Tabs, Cefa-Drops)	See Cefaclor. Cefadroxil is a 1st-generation cephalosporin antibiotic.	See Cefaclor. Cefadroxil has been known to cause vomiting after oral administration in dogs.	Spectrum of cefadroxil is similar to that of other 1st-generation cephalosporins. For susceptibility test, use cephalothin as test drug.	50 mg/ml oral suspension; 50, 100, 200, 1000 mg tablet.	Dog: 22 mg/kg q12h, up to 30 mg/kg q12h PO. Cat: 22 mg/kg q24h PO.
Cefazolin sodium (Ancef, Kefzol, and generic)	See Cefadroxil. Cefazolin is a 1st-generation cephalosporin antibiotic.	Adverse effects uncommon.	Commonly used 1st-generation cephalosporin as injectable drug for prophylaxis for surgery, as well as for acute therapy for serious infections.	50 and 100 mg/50 ml for injection	20–35 mg/kg q8h IV, IM. For perisurgical use: 22 mg/kg q2h during surgery.

			Dose regimen based on pharmacokinetics in dogs.	500 mg, 1 g, 2 g vials for injection.	Dog: 40 mg q6h IM or IV
Cefepine (Maxipine)	4th generation cephalosporin antbiotic. Broader spectrum than other cephalosporins.	Similar adverse effects to other cephalosporins	Dose regimen based on pharmacokinetics in dogs.	500 mg, 1 g, 2 g vials for injection.	Dog: 40 mg q6h IM or IV
Cefixime (Suprax)	See Cefaclor. Cefixime is an oral 3rd-generation cephalosporin antibiotic	See Cefaclor.	Although not approved for veterinary use, pharmacokinetic studies in dogs have provided recommended dosages.	20 mg/ml oral suspension and 200 and 400 mg tablets	10 mg/kg q12h PO. For cystitis: 5 mg/kg q12–24h PO.
Cefotaxime sodium (Claforan)	See Cefaclor. Cefotaxime is a 3rd-generation cephalosporin. Cefotaxime is used when resistance to other antibiotics is encountered or when infection is in CNS.	See Cefaclor.	3rd-generation cephalosporin used when resistance encountered to 1st- and 2nd-generation cephalosporins.	500 mg; 1, 2, and 10 g vials for injection.	Dog: 50 mg/kg IV, IM, SC q12h. Cat: 20–80 mg/kg q6h IV, IM.
Cefotetan disodium (Cefotan)	See Cefaclor. Cefotetan is a 2nd-generation cephalosporin antibiotic.	See Cefaclor.	2nd-generation cephalosporin similar to cefoxitin, but may have longer half-life in dogs.	1, 2, and 10 g vials for injection.	30 mg/kg q8h IV, SC.
Cefovecin (Convenia)	Injectable 3rd generation cephalosporin antibiotic for use in dogs and cats. Very long half-life compared to other cephalosporins.	Adverse effects may include transient GI problems.	Dose intervals: Usually 14 days in dogs and cats, or a single injection.	80 mg/ml vial for injection.	8 mg/kg SC usually as a single injection, or repeated in 14 days.

(Continued)

APPENDIX F: Drug Formulary (*continued*)

Drug Name (Trade or Other Names)	Pharmacology and Indications	Adverse Effects and Precautions	Dosing Information and Comments	Formulations	Dosage
Cefoxitin sodium (Mefoxin)	See Cefaclor. Cefoxitin is a 2nd-generation cephalosporin. May have increased activity against anaerobic bacteria.	See Cefaclor.	2nd-generation cephalosporin, which is often used when activity against anaerobic bacteria is desired.	1, 2, and 10 g vials for injection	30 mg/kg q6–8h IV
Cefpodoxime proxetil (Vantin)	Oral 3rd-generation cephalosporin. Activity includes gram-negative bacilli resistant to 1st-generation cephalosporins. Activity also includes staphylococcus.	No adverse effects reported for animals, but be aware of possibility of reactions seen with other oral cephalosporins (e.g., vomiting, diarrhea, allergy).	Use for infections (e.g., UTI) resistant to other oral drugs.	100, 200 mg tablets; 10 or 20 mg/ml oral suspension.	Systemic infections: 10 mg/kg q8h PO. Urinary tract infections: 10 mg/kg q12h PO.
Ceftazidime (Fortaz, Ceptaz, Tazicef)	3rd-generation cephalosporin. Ceftazidime has more activity than other cephalosporins against Pseudomonas aeruginosa.	See Cefaclor.	3rd-generation cephalosporin. May be reconstituted with 1% lidocaine for IM injection.	Vials (0.5, 1, 2, 6 g) reconstituted to 280 mg/ml.	Dog and cat: 30 mg/kg q6h IV, IM. Dog: 30 mg/kg q4–6h SC.
Ceftiofur (Naxcel [ceftiofur sodium]; Excenel [ceftiofur HCl]).	See Cefaclor. Ceftiofur is a unique cephalosporin that does not fit into a distinct class; however, its spectrum resembles that of many of the 3rd-generation cephalosporins.	See Cefaclor. Ceftiofur is primarily used only for urinary tract infections.	Available as powder for reconstitution before injection. After reconstitution, stable for 7 days when refrigerated or 12 hr at room temperature, or frozen for 8 weeks. Excenel is not approved for use in dogs.	50 mg/ml injection.	2.2–4.4 mg/kg SC q24h (for urinary tract infections).

Drug	Description	Susceptibility	Other Information	How Supplied	Dosage
Cephalexin (Keflex and generic forms)	See Cefaclor. Cephalexin is a 1st-generation cephalosporin.	See Cefaclor. For cephalexin, use cephalothin to test susceptibility.	Although not approved for veterinary use, trials in dogs with pyoderma show similar efficacy.	250, 500 mg capsules; 250, 500 mg tablets; 100 mg/ml or 125, 250 mg/ 5 ml oral suspension.	10–30 mg/kg q6–12h PO; for pyoderma, 22–35 mg/kg q12h PO.
Cephalothin sodium (Keflin)	See Cefaclor.		1st-generation cephalosporin. Used as test drug for susceptibility tests of other 1st-generation cephalosporins.	1 and 2 g vials for injection	10–30 mg/kg q4–8h IV, IM
Cephapirin (Cefadyl)	See Cefaclor. Cephapirin is a 1st-generation cephalosporin.			500 mg, 1, 2, 4 g vials for injection.	10–30 mg/kg q4–8h IV, IM.
Cephradine (Velosef)	See Cefaclor. Cephradine is a 1st-generation cephalosporin.			250, 500 mg capsules, and 250, 500 mg, 1 and 2 g vials for injection.	10–25 mg/kg q6–8h PO.
Chloramphenicol and chloramphenicol palmitate (Chloromycetin, generic forms)	Antibacterial drug. Mechanism of action is via inhibition of protein synthesis via binding to ribosome. Broad spectrum of activity. Florfenicol acts via similar mechanism and has been substituted in some animals. (See Florfenicol.)	Bone marrow suppression is possible with high doses or prolonged treatment (especially in cats). Avoid use in pregnant or neonatal animals. Drug interactions with other drugs (e.g., barbiturates) possible because chloramphenicol will inhibit hepatic microsomal enzymes.	Chloramphenicol use based on susceptibility data. Chloramphenicol palmitate requires active enzymes and should not be administered to fasted (or anorectic) animals. Note: Some forms of chloramphenicol are no longer available in the United States.	30 mg/ml oral suspension (palmitate), 250 mg capsules, and 100, 250, and 500 mg tablets	Dog: 50 mg/kg q8h PO. Cat: 12.5–20 mg/kg q12h PO.

(Continued)

APPENDIX F: Drug Formulary (continued)

Drug Name (Trade or Other Names)	Pharmacology and Indications	Adverse Effects and Precautions	Dosing Information and Comments	Formulations	Dosage
Chloramphenicol sodium succinate (Chloromycetin, generic)	Injection form of choramphenicol. Converted by liver to parent drug.	Same as for chloramphenicol.	Injectable solution converted to chloramphenicol by hepatic metabolism.	100 mg/ml injection.	Dog: 40–50 mg/kg q6–8h IV, IM.
Chlortetracycline (generic)	Tetracycline antibacterial drug. Inhibits bacterial protein synthesis by interfering with peptide elongation by ribosome. Bacteriostatic agent with broad spectrum of activity.	Avoid use in young animals; may bind to bone and developing teeth. High doses have caused renal injury.	Broad-spectrum antibiotic. Used for routine infections and intracellular pathogens.	Powdered feed additive.	Cat: 12.5–20 mg/cat q12h IV, IM. 25 mg/kg q6–8h PO.
Cimetidine (Tagamet)	Histamine-2 antagonist. Blocks histamine stimulation of gastric parietal cells to decrease gastric acid secretion. Used to treat ulcers and gastritis.	Adverse effects usually seen only with decreased renal clearance. Drug interactions: may increase concentration of other drugs used concurrently (theophylline) because of inhibition of hepatic P450 enzymes.	Precise doses needed to treat gastric ulcers have not been established.	100, 200, 300, 400, and 800 mg tablets. 80 mg/ml oral suspension. 6 mg/ml injectable solution.	10 mg/kg q6-8h, IV, IM, PO.
Ciprofloxacin (Cipro)	Fluoroquinolone antibacterial. Acts to inhibit DNA gyrase and inhibit cell DNA and RNA synthesis. Bactericidal. Broad antimicrobial activity.	Avoid use in dogs 4 weeks to 7 months of age. High concentrations may cause CNS toxicity, especially in animals with renal failure. Causes occasional vomiting. IV solution should be given slowly (over 30 min).	Doses are based on plasma concentrations needed to achieve sufficient plasma concentration above MIC. Efficacy studies have not been performed in dogs or cats. Ciprofloxacin is not absorbed orally as well as enrofloxacin.	250, 500, 750 mg tablets; 2 mg/ml injection or 10 mg/ml injection.	Dogs: 20-25 mg/kg PO q24h, or 10-15 mg/kg IV q24h. Cats: 20 mg/kg PO q24h, or 10 mg/kg IV q24h.

Clarithromycin (Biaxin)	Macrolide antibiotic with bacteriostatic activity. Spectrum includes primarily gram-positive bacteria. Resistance is expected for most gram-negative bacteria. Efficacy is not established for animals. Most common use in humans is for treatment of Helicobacter gastritis, and respiratory infections.	Well tolerated in animals. Most common side side effects are vomiting, nausea, and diarrhea.	Doses are not established for animals because of lack of clinical trials. Dose recommendations are extrapolated from human or empirical use.	250, 500 mg tablets; 25 and 50 mg/ml oral suspension.	7.5 mg/kg q12h PO.
Clavamox	See Amoxicillin/ clavulanate potassium.				
Clindamycin (Antirobe [veterinary], Cleocin [human])	Antibacterial drug of the lincosamide class (similar in action to macrolides). Inhibits bacterial protein synthesis via inhibition of bacterial ribosome. Primarily bacteriostatic, with spectrum of activity primarily against gram-positive bacteria and anaerobes.	Generally well tolerated in dogs and cats. Oral liquid product may be unpalatable to cats. Lincomycin and clindamycin may alter bacterial population in intestine and cause diarrhea; for this reason, do not administer to rodents or rabbits.	Most doses are based on manufacturer's drug approval data and efficacy trials. See dosing column for specific infections.	Oral liquid 25 mg/ml; 25, 75, and 150 mg capsules; and 150 mg/ml injection (Cleocin).	Dog: 11–33 mg/kg PO; for periodontal and soft tissue infection, 5.5–33 mg/kg q12h PO. Cat: 11–33 mg/kg q24h PO; for skin and anaerobic infections, 11 mg/kg q12h PO; for toxoplasmosis, 12.5–25 mg/kg PO q12h.

(Continued)

APPENDIX F: Drug Formulary *(continued)*

Drug Name (Trade or Other Names)	Pharmacology and Indications	Adverse Effects and Precautions	Dosing Information and Comments	Formulations	Dosage
Clofazimine (Lamprene)	Antimicrobial agent used to treat feline leprosy. Slow bactericidal effect on Mycobacterium leprae.	Adverse effects have not been reported in cats. In humans, the most serious adverse effects are GI.	Doses based on empiricism or extrapolation of human studies.	50 and 100 mg capsules.	Cat: 1 mg/kg up to a maximum of 4 mg/kg/day PO.
Clotrimazole (Lotrimin)	Azole antifungal agent for topical (dermal candidasis) or infusion use (nasal for aspergillosis, urinary bladder for candidasis). Inhibits ergosterol formation in fungal cell wall.	Propylene glycol or isopropyl alcohol carrier in infusion solution can cause irritation of mucous membranes and esophagitis if swallowed. May prolong barbiturate anesthesia.	Topical solutions contain propylene glycol and isopropyl alcohol carrier. Various creams and lotion also. All products available from most pharmacies.	1% topical solution in 10 ml and 30 ml, creams, lotion, and vaginal tablets.	Nasal infusion (aspergillosis): 60 ml (2 × 30 ml bottles of 1% solution) usually sufficient to infuse into each nasal cavity (120 ml total) of a large-breed dog; maintain infusion over 60 min while animal is under general anesthesia. Drain out drug completely once completed. Topical: apply q12h for 3–4 weeks. 20–40 mg/kg q8h PO
Cloxacillin sodium (Cloxapen, Orbenin, Tegopen)	Beta-lactam antibiotic. Inhibits bacterial cell wall synthesis. Spectrum is limited to gram-positive bacteria, especially staphylococci.	Use cautiously in animals allergic to penicillin-like drugs.	Doses based on empiricism or extrapolation from human studies. No clinical efficacy studies available for dogs or cats. Oral absorption is poor; if possible, administer on empty stomach.	250, 500 mg capsules, 25 mg/mL oral solution	

Drug	Description / Action	Cautions / Notes	Additional notes	Formulation	Dose
Dapsone (generic)	Antimicrobial drug used primarily for treatment of mycobacterium infection. May have some immunosuppressive properties or inhibit function of inflammatory cells. Used primarily for dermatologic diseases in dogs and cats.	Hepatitis and blood dyscrasias may occur. Toxic dermatologic reactions have been seen in humans. Drug interactions: Do not administer with trimethoprim (may increase blood concentrations).	Doses are derived from extrapolation of human doses or empiricism. No well-controlled clinical studies have been performed in veterinary medicine.	25 and 100 mg tablets.	1.1 mg/kg q8–12h PO.
Decoquinate (Deccox)	Coccidiostat with activity against Hepatozoon spp. Disrupts electron transport in mitochondrial cytochrome system.	Should not be given to pregnant animals.	Efficacy against Hepatozoon spp. unknown.	0.8% medicated powder, 6% medicated feed.	Long-term treatment of Hepatozoon infection: 10–20 mg/kg q12h PO for 33 months (1/4 oz of the 6% feed additive preparation will medicate 20–40 kg body weight of dog).
Dichlorvos (Task)	Antiparasitic drug, used primarily to treat hookworms, roundworms, and whipworms. Kills parasites by anticholinesterase action.	Do not use in heartworm-positive patients. Overdoses can cause organophosphate intoxication. (treat with 2-PAM, atropine).	Doses based on manufacturer's recommendations.unknown.	10, 25 mg tablets.	Dog: 26.4–33 mg/kg PO. Cat: 11 mg/kg PO.

(Continued)

APPENDIX F: Drug Formulary (continued)

Drug Name (Trade or Other Names)	Pharmacology and Indications	Adverse Effects and Precautions	Dosing Information and Comments	Formulations	Dosage
Dicloxacillin sodium (Dynapen)	Beta-Lactam antibiotic. Inhibits bacterial cell wall synthesis. Spectrum is limited to gram-positive bacteria, especially staphylococci.	Use cautiously in animals allergic to penicillin-like drugs.	No clinical efficacy studies available for dogs or cats. In dogs, oral absorption is very low and may not be suitable for therapy (J Vet Pharmacol Ther 21:414–417, 1998). Administer, if possible, on empty stomach.	125, 250, 500 mg capsules, 12.5 mg/ml oral suspension.	11–55 mg/kg q8h PO.
Diethylcarbamazine (DEC) (Caricide, Filaribits)	Heartworm preventive but no longer used commonly. For action, see Piperazine.	Safe in all species. Reactions can occur in animals with positive microfilaria.	Doses based on manufacturer's recommendations. Specific protocols for heartworm administration may be based on region of country.	50, 60, 180, 200, 400 mg chewable tablets but many preparations have been removed from market.	Heartworm prophylaxis: 6.6 mg/kg q24h PO.
Difloxacin hydrochloride (Dicural)	Fluoroquinolone antibacterial drug. Acts via inhibition of DNA gyrase in bacteria to inhibit DNA and RNA synthesis. Bactericidal, with broad spectrum of activity. Used for variety of infections, including skin infections, wound infections, and pneumonia.	Adverse effects include seizures in epileptic animals, arthropathy in young animals, vomiting at high doses. Drug interactions: May increase concentrations of theophylline if used concurrently. Coadministration with di- and trivalent cations (e.g., sucralfate) may decrease absorption. Ocular safety not established in cats.	Dose range can be used to adjust dose, depending on severity of infection and susceptibility of bacteria. Bacteria with low MIC can be treated with low dose; susceptible bacteria with higher MIC should be treated with higher dose. Difloxacin is primarily eliminated in feces rather than urine (urine is 5% of clearance). Sarafloxacin is an active desmethyl metabolite.	11.4, 45.4, and 136 mg tablets.	Dog: 5–10 mg/kg q24h PO (see dosing information guidelines).

Doramectin (Dectomax)	Macrocyclic antiparasitic agent (similar to ivermectin) active against Spirocerca spp. Neurotoxic to parasites by potentiating effects of inhibitory neurotransmitter GABA.	Not approved for use in dogs. Cattle or swine injectable product effective in treating spirocercosis if used early in disease. Can administer PO or SC in dogs.	1% (10 mg/ml) injectable solution.	Regimen 1: 0.2 mg/kg SC every 14 days for 3 treatments—resolves clinical signs and nodules in most dogs. If not fully resolved, use 0.5 mg/kg q24h PO for 6 wk. Regimen 2: 0.4 mg/kg SC every 14 days for 6 treatments and then monthly until all esophageal granulomas are gone (2 years in some cases).
Doxycycline (Vibramycin and generic forms)	Tetracycline antibiotic. Mechanism of action of tetracyclines is to bind to 30S ribosomal subunit and inhibit protein synthesis. Usually bacteriostatic. Broad spectrum of activity, including bacteria, some protozoa, Rickettsia, and Ehrlichia. Also used as adjunctive treatment for heartworm disease in dogs.	Severe adverse reactions not reported with doxycycline. Tetracyclines in general may cause renal tubular necrosis at high doses. Tetracyclines can affect bone and teeth formation in young animals. Drug interactions: Tetracyclines bind to calcium-containing compounds, which decreases oral absorption.	Many pharmacokinetic and experimental studies have been conducted in small animals, but no clinical studies. Ordinarily considered the drug of choice for Rickettsia and Ehrlichia infections in dogs. Doxycycline IV infusion is stable for only 12 hr at room temperature and 72 hr if refrigerated.	10 mg/ml oral suspension; 100 mg tablets; 100 mg injection vial.	3–5 mg/kg q12h PO IV or 10 mg/kg q24h PO. For Rickettsia or Ehrlichia in dogs: 5 mg/kg q12h. Heartworm treatment: 10 mg/kg PO q24h, intermittently at 4 – 6 week intervals, usually with a macrocyclic lactone.

(Continued)

APPENDIX F: Drug Formulary (continued)

Drug Name (Trade or Other Names)	Pharmacology and Indications	Adverse Effects and Precautions	Dosing Information and Comments	Formulations	Dosage
Enilconazole (Imaverol, Clinafarm EC)	Azole antifungal agent for topical use only. Like other azoles, inhibits membrane synthesis (ergosterol) in fungus. Highly effective for dermatophytes.	Administered topically. Adverse effects have not been reported.	Imaverol is available only in Canada as 10% emulsion. In the United States, Clinafarm EC is available for use in poultry units as 13.8% solution. Dilute solution to at least 50:1, and apply topically every 3–4 days for 2–3 wk. Enilconazole also has been instilled as 1:1 dilution into nasal sinus for nasal aspergillosis.	10% or 13.8% emulsion.	Nasal aspergillosis: 10 mg/kg q12h instilled into nasal sinus for 14 days (10% solution diluted 50/50 with water). Dermatophytes: dilute 10% solution to 0.2%, and wash lesion with solution 4 times at 3- to 4-day intervals.
Enrofloxacin (Baytril)	Fluoroquinolone antibacterial drug. Acts via inhibition of DNA gyrase in bacteria to inhibit DNA and RNA synthesis. Bactericidal. Broad spectrum of activity.	Adverse effects include seizures in epileptic animals, arthropathy in dogs aged 4–28 wk, vomiting in dogs and cats at high doses. Blindness in cats has been reported. Drug interactions: May increase concentrations of theophylline if used concurrently. Coadministration with di- and trivalent cations (e.g., sucralfate) may decrease absorption.	In dogs, low dose of 5 mg/kg/day is used for sensitive organisms with MIC of 0.12 mcg/ml or less, or urinary tract infection; dose of 5–10 mg/kg/day is used for organisms with MIC of 0.12–0.5 mcg/ml; dose of 10–20 mg/kg/day is used for organisms with MIC of 0.5–1.0 mcg/ml. Solution is not approved for IV use but has been administered via this route safely if given slowly.	68, 22.7, and 5.7 mg tablets. Taste Tabs are 22.7 and 68 mg. 22.7 mg/ml injection.	Dog: 5–20 mg/kg/ q24h PO, IV, IM (see dosing information guidelines). Cat: 5 mg/kg q24h PO, IM Do not administer to cats at doses higher than 5 mg/kg and do not administer to cats IV.

Epsiprantel (Cestex)	Antehelmintic with activity against cat and dog tapeworms, including Dipylidium caninum, Taenia taeniaformis, T, pisiformis, and T. hydatigena.	No known contraindications. Very safe drug. Do not use in kittens or pups under age 7 wk.	A single oral dose is effective. Fasting is not necessary or recommended. Treatment of D. caninum should be coupled with an effective flea control program.	12.5, 25, 50, 100 mg film-coated tablets.	Dogs: 5.5 mg/kg PO once, repeat as necessary. Cats: 2.75 mg/kg PO once, repeat as necessary. Convenient dosing chart available.
Ertapenum (Invanz)	Carbapenum antibiotic of the beta-lactam group. Like meropenum and imipenus, it is highly active against a broadspecbtrum of bacteria, including those resistant to other drugs. Ertapenum is not as active against Pseudomonas as imipenum or meropenum.	Well tolerated in animals. CNS toxicity maybe possible with high doses. Allergy to beta-lactam antibiotics is possible.	Dosing information is extrapoloated from human medicine or limited empirical use in veterinary medicine. As with other carbapenums, use only when organisms are resistant to other drugs.	1 g vials for injection.	30 mg/kg q8h, IV or SC.
Erythromycin (many brands and generic)	Macrolide antibiotic. Inhibits bacteria by binding to 50S ribosome and inhibiting protein synthesis. Spectrum of activity limited primarily to gram-positive aerobic bacteria. Used for skin and respiratory infections.	Most common side effect is vomiting (probably caused by cholinergic-like effect or motilin-induced motility). May cause diarrhea in some animals. Do not administer PO to rodents or rabbits.	There are several forms of erythromycin, including the ethylsuccinate and estolate esters, and stearate salt for oral administration. There are no convincing data to suggest that one form is absorbed better than another, and one dose is included for all. Only erythromycin gluceptate and lactate are to be administered IV. Motilin-like effect on GI motility occurs at low dose.	250 mg capsules or tablets.	10–20 mg/kg q8–12h PO; GI motility effects at 0.5–1.0 mg/kg q8–12h PO.

(Continued)

APPENDIX F: Drug Formulary (continued)

Drug Name (Trade or Other Names)	Pharmacology and Indications	Adverse Effects and Precautions	Dosing Information and Comments	Formulations	Dosage
Famotidine (Pepsid)	Histamine H$_2$-receptor antagonist. (See Cimetidine for details.)	See Cimetidine.	See Cimetidine. Clinical studies for famotidine have not been performed; therefore optimal dose for ulcer prevention and healing is not known.	10 mg tablet; 10 mg/ml injection.	0.1–0.2 mg/kg q12h PO, IV, SC, IM.
Febantel-praziquantel-pyrantel (Drontal Plus)	Broad-spectrum anthelmintic for dogs, with activity against tapeworms, hookworms, roundworms, and whipworms (label use) and Giardia spp. (off-label use). Febantel blocks parasites energy metabolism. See praziquantel and pyrantel for mechanism of action.	Febantel – metabolized to fenbendazole and oxfendazole by liver. Acute toxic dose in dogs is 10 g/kg. See praziquantel and pyrantel for adverse effects. Do not use in pregnant dogs, in dogs, 1 kg, or puppies, 3 wk of age.	Product formulated to deliver 25–30 mg of febantel, 5–7 mg of praziquantel, and 5–7 mg of pyrantel pomoate per kg.	Tablets for small dogs contain: 22.7 mg praziquantel, 22.7 mg pyrantel, and 113.4 mg febantel. Tablets for medium and large dogs contain: 68 mg praziquantel, 68 mg pyrantel, and 340.2 mg febantel.	Single oral dose for on label use. Giardiasis: 1 tablet q24h PO for 3 consecutive days.
Fenbendazole (Panacur, Safe-Guard)	Benzimidazole antiparasite drugs. (See Albendazole). Effective for treatment of Giardia (Am J Vet Res 59:61–63, 1998).	Good safety margin, but vomiting and diarrhea have been reported. No known contraindication.	Dose recommendations based on clinical studies by manufacturer. Granules may be mixed with food. In studies for treatment of Giardia, it was safer than other treatments.	Panacur granules 22.2% (222 mg/ g); 100 mg/ ml oral suspension.	50 mg/kg/day 3 3 days PO

Drug	Mechanism	Adverse effects	Comments	Dose form	Dosage
Florfenicol	Chloramphenicol derivative with same mechanism of action as chloramphenicol (inhibition of protein synthesis) and broad antibacterial spectrum. Infrequently used in small animals.	Because of limited use in small animals, there are few reports of adverse effects. Chloramphenicol linked to bone marrow depression (possible for florfenicol) and aplastic anemia (not seen with florfenicol).	Dose form is only approved for use in cattle; not evaluated in small animals. Doses listed are derived from pharmacokinetic studies.	300 mg/kg injectable solution.	Dog: 20 mg/kg q6h IM or PO. Cat: 22 mg/kg q8h IM or PO.
Fluconazole (Diflucan)	Azole antifungal drug. Similar mechanism as other azole antifungal agents. Inhibits ergosterol synthesis in fungal cell membrane. Fungistatic. Efficacious against dermatophytes and variety of systemic fungi.	Adverse effects have not been reported from fluconazole administration. Compared to ketoconazole, it has less effect on endocrine function. However, increased liver enzyme plasma concentrations and hepatopathy are possible. Compared with other oral azole antifungals, fluconazole is absorbed more predictably and completely, even on an empty stomach.	Doses for fluconazole are primarily based on studies performed in cats for treatment of cryptococcosis. Efficacy for other infections has not been reported. The primary difference between fluconazole and other azoles is that fluconazole attains higher concentrations in the CNS.	50, 100, 150, or 200 mg tablets; 10 or 40 mg/ml oral suspension; 2 mg/ml IV injection.	Dog: 10–12 mg/kg q24h, PO. Cat: 50 mg/cat q12h–24h.
Flucytosine (Ancobon)	Antifungal drug. Used in combination with other antifungal drugs for treatment of cryptococcosis. Action is to penetrate fungal cells. Converted to fluorouracil, which acts as antimetabolite.	Adverse effects have not been reported in animals.	Flucytosine is used primarily to treat cryptococcosis in animals. Efficacy is based on flucytosine's ability to attain high concentrations in CSF. Flucytosine may be synergistic with amphotericin B.	250 mg capsule; 75 mg/ml oral suspension.	25–50 mg/kg q6–8h PO (up to a maxiumum dose of 100 mg/kg q12h PO).

(Continued)

APPENDIX F: Drug Formulary (continued)

Drug Name (Trade or Other Names)	Pharmacology and Indications	Adverse Effects and Precautions	Dosing Information and Comments	Formulations	Dosage
Furazolidone (Furoxone)	Oral antiprotozoal drug with activity against Giardia. May have some activity against bacteria in intestine. Not used for systemic therapy	Adverse effects not reported in animals. In humans, mild anemia, hypersensitivity, and disturbance of intestinal flora have been reported.	Clinical studies have not been reported for animals. Doses and recommendations are based on extrapolation from humans. Other drugs, such as fenbendazole, may be preferred for Giardia.	100 mg tablets.	4 mg/kg q12h for 7–10 days PO
Gentamicin sulfate (Gentocin)	Aminoglycoside antibiotic. Action is to inhibit bacteria protein synthesis via binding to 30S ribosome. Bactericidal. Broad spectrum of activity except streptococci and anaerobic bacteria	Nephrotoxicity is the most dose-limiting toxicity. Ensure that patients have adequate fluid and electrolyte balance during therapy. Ototoxicity and vestibulotoxicity also are possible. Drug interactions: When used with anesthetic agents, neuromuscular blockade is possible. Do not mix in vial or syringe with other antibiotics.	Dosing regimens are based on sensitivity of organisms. Some studies have suggested that once-daily therapy (combining multiple doses into a single daily dose) is as efficacious as multiple treatments. Activity against some bacteria (e.g., Pseudomonas) is enhanced when combined with a b-lactam antibiotic. Nephrotoxicity is increased with persistently high trough concentrations persistently high trough concentrations.	50 and 100 mg/ ml solution for injection	Dog: 2–4 mg/kg q8h or 9–14 mg/kg q24h IV, Im, SC. Cat: 3 mg/kg q8h or 5–8 mg/kg q24h IV, IM, SC.

| Griseofulvin (microsize) (Fulvicin U/F, Fulvicin P/G, Gris-PEG) | Antifungal drug. Incorporates into skin layers and inhibits mitosis of fungi. Antifungal activity is limited to dermatophytes. | Adverse effects in animals include teratogenicity in cats; anemia and leukopenia in cats; anorexia, depression, vomiting, and diarrhea. Do not administer to pregnant cats. | A wide range of doses has been reported. Doses listed here represent the current consensus. Griseofulvin should be administered with food to enhance absorption. Ultramicro size dose is absorbed to a greater extent and doses should be less than microsize. | 125, 250, 500 mg tablets; 25 mg/ml oral suspension; 125 mg/ml oral syrup. 100, 125, 165, 250, 330 mg tablets, or ultramicro sizes. | 50 mg/kg q24h PO (up to a maximum dose of 110–132 mg/kg/day in divided treatments) Ultramicro size does: 30 mg/kg/day in divided treatments. |
| Imidocarb dipropionate (Imazol) | Injectable parasiticide with activity against Babesia (on label use), ehrlichiosis, and cytauxzoonosis (off-label use). Interferes with nucleic acid metabolism. | Pain/ulceration at injection site; periorbital edema, hypersalivation, lacrimation, shivering, diarrhea, vomiting, depression, or mental agitation (signs similar to organophosphate toxicity because it has anticholinesterase activity); posttreatment vomiting (consistent side effect). Preadminister atropine. Rarely, renal tubular necrosis develops. High doses (10 mg/kg) toxic with cardiac effects and hepatic necrosis. | Reduce doses if renal or hepatic insufficiency present. Avoid use with preexisting pulmonary impairment. Not for IV use. May be synergistic with diminazene (which is not available in the United States). | 12% (120 mg/ml) solution, in multidose 10 ml vial for SC or IM injection. | Babesiosis: 5–6.6 mg/kg IM or SC once, repeat in 14 days. Cytauxzoonosis (cats): 2 mg/kg IM once, repeat in 3–7 days. Ehrlichiosis (dogs and cats): 5 mg/kg IM once, repeat in 14 days. |

(Continued)

APPENDIX F: Drug Formulary (continued)

Drug Name (Trade or Other Names)	Pharmacology and Indications	Adverse Effects and Precautions	Dosing Information and Comments	Formulations	Dosage
Imipenem (Primaxin)	β-Lactam antibiotic with broad-spectrum activity. Action is similar to other β-lactam (see Amoxicillin). Imipenem is the ost active of all β-lactams. Used primarily for serious, multiple-resistant infections.	Allergic reactions may occur with β-lactam antibiotics. With rapid infusion or in patients with renal insufficiency, neurotoxicity may occur (seizures). Vomiting and nausea are possible. IM or SC injections may cause pain in dogs.	Doses and efficacy studies have not been determined in animals. Recommendations are based on studies performed in humans and extrapolation from humans. Reserve the use of this drug for only resistant, refractory infections. Observe manufacturer's instructions carefully for proper administration. For IV administration, add to IV fluids. For IM administration, add 2 ml lidocaine (1%); suspension is stable for only 1 hr.	250 or 500 mg vials for injection.	Dog: 5 mg/kg IV, IM, or SC q4h. Cat: Dose not established, but often used at same dose as in dogs.
Interferon (interferon-α, HuIFN-α) (Roferon)	Human interferon. Used to stimulate the immune system in patients.	Adverse effects have not been reported in animals.	Doses and indications for animals have primarily been based on extrapolation of human recommendations or limited experimental studies. (J Am Vet Med Assoc 199:1477, 1991.) To prepare, add 3 million U to 1 L sterile saline and divide into aliquots and freeze. Thaw as needed for 30 U/ml solution.	3 million U/vial.	Cat: 15–30 U per cat SC or IM q24h for 7 days and repeated every other week.

Drug	Description	Formulation	Dosage
Itraconazole (Sporanox)	Azole (triazole) antifungal drug. See Ketoconazole for mechanism of action. Active against dermatophytes and systemic fungi, such as Blastomyces, Histoplasma, and Coccidioides.	Itraconazole is better tolerated than ketoconazole. However, vomiting and hepatotoxicosis are possible, especially at high doses. In one study, hepatotoxicosis was more likely at high doses. 10%–15% of dogs will develop high liver enzyme levels. High doses in cats caused vomiting and anorexia.	Doses are based on studies in animals in which itraconazole has been used to treat blastomycosis in dogs. In cats, lower doses have been effective for dermatophytes (see dosage section). Other uses or doses are based on empiricism or extrapolation from the literature on humans.	100 mg capsules and 10 mg/ml oral liquid	Dog: 2.5 mg/kg q12h or 5 mg/kg q24h PO. Malassezia dermatitis: 5 mg/kg q24h PO for 2 days, repeated each week for 3 weeks. Cat: 5 mg/kg q12h PO. Dermatophyte infection in cats: 1.5–3.0 mg/kg (up to 5 mg/kg) q24h PO for 15 days.
Ivermectin (Heartgard, Ivomec, Eqvalan liquid)	Antiparasitic drug and heartworm prevention. Neurotoxic to parasites by potentiating glutamate gated chloride channels.	Toxicity may occur at high doses and in breeds in which ivermectin crosses blood–brain barrier. Sensitive breeds include collies, Australian shepherds, shelties, and Old English sheepdogs. Toxicity is neurotoxic, and signs include depression, ataxia, difficulty with vision, coma, and death. Ivermectin appears to be safe for pregnant animals. Do not administer to animals under 6 wk of age. Animals with high microfilaremia may show adverse reactions to high doses.	Doses vary, depending on use. Heartworm prevention is lowest dose, other parasites require higher doses. Heartgard is only form approved for small animals; for other indications, large animal injectable products are often administered PO, IM, or SC to small animals.	1% (10 mg/ml) injectable solution; 10 mg/ml oral solution; 18.7 mg/ml oral paste; 68, 136, and 272 mcg tablets.	Heartworm preventive: 6 mcg/kg every 30 days PO in dogs and 24 mcg/kg every 30 days PO in cats. Microfilaricide: 50 mcg/kg PO 2 wks after adulticide therapy. Ectoparasite therapy (dogs and cats): 200–300 mcg/kg IM, SC, PO. Endoparasites (dogs and cats): 200–400 mcg/kg weekly SC, PO. Cats: heartworm prevention; 25 mcg/kg PO every 30 days

(Continued)

APPENDIX F: Drug Formulary (*continued*)

Drug Name (Trade or Other Names)	Pharmacology and Indications	Adverse Effects and Precautions	Dosing Information and Comments	Formulations	Dosage
Kanamycin (Kantrim)	Aminoglycoside antibiotic. (See Gentamicin, Amikacin for details.)	Shares same properties with other aminoglycosides (see Amikacin, Gentamicin).	See Gentamicin.	200, 500 mg/ml injection.	10 mg/kg q12h or 20 mg/kg q24h IV IM, SC.
Ketoconazole (Nizoral)	Azole (imidazole) antifungal drug. Similar mechanism of action as other azole antifungal agents. Inhibits ergosterol synthesis in fungal cell membrane. Fungistatic. Efficacious against dermatophytes and variety of systemic fungi, such as Histoplasma, Blastomyces, and Coccidioides.	Adverse effects in animals include dose-related vomiting, diarrhea, and hepatic injury. Enzyme elevations are common. Do not administer to pregnant animals. Ketoconazole causes endocrine abnormalities, especially, inhibition of cortisol synthesis. Drug interactions: Ketoconazole will inhibit metabolism of other drugs (anticonvulsants, cyclosporine, cisapride).	Oral absorption depends on acidity in stomach. Do not administer with antisecretory drugs or antacids. Because of endocrine effects, ketoconazole has been used for short-term treatment of hyperadrenocorticism.	200 mg tablets; 100 mg/ml oral suspension (available only in Canada).	Dog: 10–15 mg/kg q8–12h PO. Malassezia canis infection: 5 mg/kg q24h PO. For hyperadrenocorticism: Start with 5 mg/kg q12h for 7 days, then 12–15 mg/kg q12h PO. Cat: 5–10 mg/kg q8–12h PO.
Levamisole (Levasole, Tramisol, Ergamisol)	Antiparasitic drug of the imidazothiazole class. Mechanism of action is neuromuscular toxicity to parasites. Levamisole has been used for endoparasites in dogs and as a microfilaricide. In humans, levamisole is used as immunostimulant to aid in treatment of colorectal carcinoma and malignant melanoma.	May produce cholinergic toxicity. May cause vomiting in some dogs.	In heartworm-positive dogs, it may sterilize female adult heartworms. Levamisole has also been used as an immunostimulant; however, clinical reports of its efficacy are not available.	0.184 g bolus; 11.7 g per 13-g packet; 50 mg tablet (Ergamisol).	Dog: Hookworms: 5–8 mg/kg once PO (up to 10 mg/kg PO for 2 days). Microfilaricide: 10 mg/kg q24h PO for 6–10 days. Immunostimulant: 0.5–2 mg/kg 3 times/week PO. Cat: Endoparasites: 4.4 mg/kg once PO. Lungworms: 20–40 mg/kg q48h for 5 treatments PO. 15–25 mg/kg q12h PO. 10 mg/kg q8-12h, PO or IV

Linezolid (Zyvox)	Oxazolidinone antibiotic. Gram positive spectrum that includes drug resistant strains of Enterococcus and Staphylococcus. High expense limits routine use.	Adverse reactions include diarrhea and nausea. Rarely, anemia and leucopenia in people. Use cautiously with monoamine oxidase inhibitors and serotonergic drugs.	Use in animals is reserved only for drug resistant infections (eg methicillin-resistant Staphylococcus spp.) for which other drugs are ineffective.	400 and 600 mg tablets. 20 mg/ml oral suspension. 2 mg/ml injectable solution.	For pyoderma, doses as low as 10 mg/kg q12h have been used.
Lincomycin (Lincocin)	Lincosamide antibiotic, similar in mechanism to clindamycin and erythromycin. Spectrum includes primarily gram-positive bacteria. Used for pyoderma and other soft tissue infections.	Adverse effects uncommon. Lincomycin has caused vomiting and diarrhea in animals. Do not administer orally to rodents and rabbits.	Actions of lincomycin and clindamycin are similar enough that clindamycin can be substituted for lincomycin.	100, 200, 500 mg tablets.	Dog: 10 mg/kg PO every 30 days. Antifungal: 80 mg/kg. Cat: 30 mg/kg PO every 30 days.
Lufenuron (Program)	Antiparasitic. Used for controlling fleas in animals. Inhibits development in hatching fleas. May be used for dermatophytes in dogs and cats, although efficacy has been questioned by some experts.	Adverse effects have not been reported. Appears to be relatively safe during pregnancy and in young animals	Lufenuron may control flea development with administration once every 30 days in animals.	45, 90, 135, 204.9, 409.8 mg tablets; 135 and 270 mg suspension per unit pack.	Cat injection: 10 mg/kg SC every 6 months. Antifungal: 100 mg/kg. In endemic areas (e.g., catteries) treat cats once a month.

(Continued)

APPENDIX F: Drug Formulary (continued)

Drug Name (Trade or Other Names)	Pharmacology and Indications	Adverse Effects and Precautions	Dosing Information and Comments	Formulations	Dosage
Lufenuron + milbemycin oxime (Sentinel tablets and Flavor Tabs)	Combination of two antiparasitic drugs. (See Lufenuron or Milbemycin oxime.) Used to protect against fleas, heartworms, roundworms, hookworms, and whipworms.	See Lufenuron or Milbemycin oxime.	See Lufenuron or Milbemycin oxime.	Milbemycin oxime/ lufenuron ratio is as follows: 2.3/46 mg tablets; 5.75/115, 11.5/230, and 23/460 mg Flavor Tabs.	Dog: Administer 1 tablet every 30 days. Each tablet formulated for size of dog. Cat: This product is not registered for cats.
Marbofloxacin (Zeniquin)	Fluoroquinolone antimicrobial. Same mechanism as enrofloxacin and ciprofloxacin. Spectrum includes staphylococci, gram-negative bacilli, and some Pseudomonas.	Same precautions as enrofloxacin. May cause some nausea and vomiting at high doses. Avoid use in young animals. Safe for cats (ocular safety) at recommended dose.	Same dosing guidelines as for other fluoroquinolones. Higher doses are needed for organisms with higher MIC values. Safety data not available for cats. Doses published for European use may be lower than those U.S. approved for dogs.	25, 50, 100, and 200 mg tablets	2.75–5.55 mg/kg q24h PO
Meglumine antimonite (Glucantime)	Antiprotozoal pentavalent antimonial agent that interferes with energy metabolism in Leishmania spp.	Pain and swelling at injection site if given IM; SC preferred. Contraindications include renal and hepatic insufficiency, cardiac arrhythmias, and leukopenia.	May not always be available in the United States—contact CDC. Resistance to drug may develop during treatment. Use with allopurinol.	5 ml vials (300 mg/ml) for injection.	Multiple dosing regimens for leishmaniasis. 100 mg/ kg q24h SC for 10 to 30 days. 200 mg/kg q48h SC or IV for 20–40 days. More effective if combined with oral allopurinol.

Drug	Description	Adverse effects / Notes		Formulation	Dose
Melarsomine (Immiticide)	Organic arsenical compound used for heartworm therapy. Heartworm adulticide. Arsenicals alter glucose uptake and metabolism in heartworms.	Adverse effects: pulmonary thromboembolism (7–20 days after therapy), anorexia (13% incidence), injection site reaction (myositis) (32% incidence), lethargy or depression (15% incidence). Causes elevation of hepatic enzymes. High doses (3×) can cause pulmonary inflammation and death. If high doses are administered, dimercaprol (3 mg/kg IM) may be used as antidote.	Dose regimens are based on severity of heartworm disease. Consult current reference to determine class of disease (class I–IV). Class I and II are least severe. Class IV is most severe, and should not be treated with adulticide before surgery. Avoid human exposure. (Wash hands after handling or wear gloves.) Do not freeze solutions after they are prepared.	25 mg/ml injection. After reconstitution, retains potency for 24 hr.	Dog: Administer via deep IM injection. Class I and II dogs: 2.5 mg/kg q24h for 2 consecutive days. Class III dogs: 2.5 mg/kg once, then in 1 month, two additional doses 24 hr apart.
Meropenem (Merrem IV)	Broad-spectrum carbapenem antibiotic; indicated primarily for resistant infections caused by bacteria resistant to other drugs. Bactericidal. More active than imipenem and ertapenem.	Risks similar to those of other b-lactam antibiotics. Meropenem does not cause seizures as frequently as imipenem. SC injections may cause slight hair loss at injection site.	Dosage guidelines have been extrapolated from pharmacokinetic studies in animals and not tested for efficacy in animals. Meropenem is more soluble than imipenem and can be injected via bolus rather than administered in fluid solutions.	500 mg/20 ml or 1 g/30 ml vial for injection.	8 mg/kg q12h SC up to 12 mg/kg q8h SC (for Pseudomonas infection); IV dose, 12 mg/kg q8h.

(Continued)

596   BLACKWELL'S FIVE-MINUTE VETERINARY CONSULT CLINICAL COMPANION

APPENDIX F: Drug Formulary (continued)

Drug Name (Trade or Other Names)	Pharmacology and Indications	Adverse Effects and Precautions	Dosing Information and Comments	Formulations	Dosage
Metronidazole (Flagyl and generic)	Antibacterial and antiprotozoal drug. Disrupts DNA in organism via reaction with intracellular metabolite. Action is specific for anaerobic bacteria and some protozoa such as Giardia.	Most severe adverse effect is caused by toxicity to CNS. High doses have caused lethargy, CNS depression, ataxia, vomiting, and weakness. Metronidazole may be mutagenic. Fetal abnormalities have not been demonstrated in animals with recommended doses, but use cautiously during pregnancy.	Metronidazole is one of the most commonly used drugs for anaerobic infections and giardia. CNS toxicity is dose-related. Maximum dose that should be administered is 50–65 mg/kg/day in any species. Although tablets have been broken or crushed for oral administration to cats, they find these unpalatable.	250, 500 mg tablet; 50 mg/ml suspension; 5 mg/ml injection.	Dog: Anaerobes: 15 mg/kg q12h or 12 mg/kg q8h PO. Giardia spp.: 12–15 mg/kg q12h for 8 days PO. Cat: Anaerobes: 10–25 mg/kg q24h PO. Giardia spp.: 17 mg/kg (1–3 tablet per cat) q24h for 8 days.
Miconazole (Conifite, Candistat, Daktarin, Monistat)	Imidazole fungistatic agent, inhibits ergosterol biosynthesis and damages fungal cell wall with activity against Candida albacans (inhibits transformation of blastospores into invasive mycelial form).	Topical: may cause skin irritation (blistering, redness, irritation).	Available from human pharmacies as a cream, lotion, powder, spray liquid, and spray powder to be applied to the skin. Many preparations.	Topical creams: Monistat-derm 2%; Daktarin cream 2% (20 g); 2% Candistat (15 g)	Apply locally q12–24h for 3 wk.

Milbemycin oxime (Interceptor, Interceptor Flavor Tabs, and SafeHeart)	Antiparasitic drug of the macrocyclic lactone group with mechanism of action similar to ivermectin. Used as heartworm preventive, miticide, and microfilaricide. Used to control hookworm, roundworm, and whipworm infections. At high doses, it has been used to treat Demodex infection in dogs.	In susceptible dogs (collie breeds), milbemycin may cross the blood–brain barrier and produce CNS toxicosis (depression, lethargy, coma). At doses used for heartworm prevention, this effect is less likely.	Doses vary, depending on parasite treated. Consult dose column. Treatment of Demodex requires high dose administered daily (J Am Vet Med Assoc 207:1581, 1995). (See also Lufenuron 1 milbemycin oxime.)	2.3, 5.75, 11.5, and 23 mg tablet.	Dog: Microfilaricide: 0.5 mg/kg; Demodex: 2 mg/kg q24h PO for 60–120 days. Heartworm prevention and control of endoparasites: 0.5 mg/kg every 30 days PO. Cat: Heartworm and endoparasite control: 2 mg/kg every 30 days PO.
Minocycline (Minocin)	Tetracycline antibiotic. Similar to doxycycline in pharmacokinetics. (See Doxycycline.)	Adverse effects have not been reported for minocycline. Oral absorption is not affected by calcium products as with other tetracyclines.	Clinical use has not been reported, but properties are similar to those of doxycycline.	50, 100 mg tablets; 10 mg/ml oral suspension.	5–12.5 mg/kg q12h PO.
Moxidectin (canine form: ProHeart; equine oral gel: Quest; cattle pour-on: Cydectin)	Antiparasitic drug. Neurotoxic to parasites by potentiating glutamate gated chloride ion channels in parasites. Used for endo- and ectoparasites, as well as heartworm prevention.	Toxicity may occur at high doses and in species in which ivermectin crosses blood–brain barrier (collie breeds). Toxicity is neurotoxic, and signs include depression, ataxia, difficulty with vision, coma, and death.	Similar use as ivermectin. Extreme caution is recommended if equine formulation is considered for use in small animals. Toxic overdoses are likely because the equine formulation is highly concentrated.	30, 68, 136 mcg tablets for dogs; 20 mg/ml equine oral gel; and 5 mg/ml cattle pour-on.	Dog: Heartworm prevention: 3 mcg/kg q30d PO. Endoparasites: 25–300 mcg/kg Demodex: 500 mcg/kg/day for 21–22 wk. Long acting ProHeart-6: 0.17 mg/kg SC every 6 months

(Continued)

APPENDIX F: Drug Formulary (continued)

Drug Name (Trade or Other Names)	Pharmacology and Indications	Adverse Effects and Precautions	Dosing Information and Comments	Formulations	Dosage
Moxifloxacin (Avelox)	Fluoroquinolone antibiotic similar to other fluoroquinolones, except with greater activity against gram-positive and anaerobic bacteria.	Similar to those of other fluoroquinolones. Because of the increased spectrum of action on anaerobic bacteria, greater GI disturbance is possible from oral dose.	Doses and recommendations based primarily on limited clinical experience and extrapolation from human studies.	400 mg tablet.	10 mg/kg q24h PO.
Nandrolone decanoate (Deca-Durabolin)	Anabolic steroid. Derivative of testosterone. Anabolic agents are designed to maximize anabolic effects while minimizing androgenic action (see Methyltestosterone). Anabolic agents have been used for reversing catabolic conditions, increasing weight gain, increasing muscling in animals, and stimulating erythropoiesis.	Adverse effects from anabolic steroids can be attributed to the pharmacologic action of these steroids. Increased masculine effects are common. Increased incidence of some tumors has been reported in people. 17a-Methylated oral anabolic steroids (oxymetholone, stanozolol, and oxandrolone) are associated with hepatic toxicity.	Results of clinical studies in animals have not been reported. Use in animals (and doses) is based on experience in humans or anecdotal experience in animals.	50, 100, 200 mg/ml injection	Dog: 1–1.5 mg/kg/wk IM. Cat: 1 mg/kg/wk IM.
Neomycin (Biosol)	Aminoglycoside antibiotic. For mechanism, and other effects, see Gentamicin, Amikacin. Neomycin differs from other aminoglycosides because it is only administered topically or orally. Systemic absorption is minimal from oral absorption.	Although oral absorption is so small that systemic adverse effects are unlikely, some oral absorption has been demonstrated in young animals (calves). Alterations in intestinal bacterial flora from therapy may cause diarrhea.	Neomycin is primarily used for oral treatment of diarrhea. Efficacy for this indication (especially for nonspecific diarrhea) is questionable. Used also for treatment of hepatic encephalopathy.	500 mg bolus; 200 mg/ml oral liquid.	10–20 mg/kg q6–12h PO.

Nifurtimox (Lampit)	Antiprotozoal drug with activity against *Trypanosoma cruzi*. Experimental drug. Exact mechanism unknown.	Side effects are common and usually limit treatment to 3–4 wk; side effects include anorexia, vomiting, weight loss, CNS signs, polyneuritis, pulmonary infiltrates, and skin eruptions.	Available in United States only from the CDC. If side effects become too severe, stop treatment. May be given with glucocorticoids to treat acute myocarditis.	30 mg, 100 mg tablets.	2–7 mg/kg q6h PO for 3 to 5 months or until side effects become too severe.
Nitazoxanide (Alinia)	Antiprotozoal drug with activity against Cryptosporidium. Activity believed to be due to interference with the enzyme-dependent electron transfer reaction essential for energy metabolism.	Often causes vomiting in cats. Use with caution in hepatic or renal insufficiency. May also cause abdominal pain, diarrhea, and anorexia.	Has only been used in a few experimentally infected cats with mixed but promising results (Am J Vet Res 62:1690–1607, 2001).	100 mg/5 ml oral solution.	25 mg/kg q24h PO for 1–4 wk.
Nitenpyram (Capstar)	Antiparasitic drug that rapidly kills adult fleas.	No adverse reactions are reported. Safe in dogs and cats at 10 X the dose. Transient pruritis observed shortly after administration co-inciding with rapid flea death.	Do not use in dogs and cats under 1 kg in body weight, or less than 4 weeks of age.	11.4 and 57 mg tablets.	1 mg/kg PO daily as needed to kill fleas.
Nitrofurantoin (Macrodantin, Furalan, Furatoin, Furadantin, and generic)	Antibacterial drug. Urinary antiseptic. Action is via reactive metabolites that damage DNA. Therapeutic concentrations are reached only in the urine. Not to be used for systemic infections. May be active against some bacteria that are resistant to other antimicrobials.	Adverse effects include nausea, vomiting, and diarrhea. Turns urine color rust-yellow brown. Do not administer during pregnancy.	Two dosing forms exist. Microcrystalline is rapidly and completely absorbed. Macrocrystalline (Macrodantin) is more slowly absorbed and causes less GI irritation. Urine should be at acidic pH for maximum effect. Administer with food to increase absorption.	Macrodantin and generic: 25, 50, 100 mg capsules; Furalan, Furatoin, and generic: 50, 100 mg tablets; Furadantin: 5 mg/ml oral suspension.	10 mg/kg/day divided into 4 daily treatments for 10 – 14 days, then 1 mg/kg at night PO.

(Continued)

APPENDIX F: Drug Formulary (continued)

Drug Name (Trade or Other Names)	Pharmacology and Indications	Adverse Effects and Precautions	Dosing Information and Comments	Formulations	Dosage
Norfloxacin (Noroxin)	Fluoroquinolone antibacterial drug. Same action as ciprofloxacin, except spectrum of activity is not as broad as with enrofloxacin or ciprofloxacin.	Adverse effects have not been reported in animals. Some effects are expected to be similar to enrofloxacin and other veterinary fluoroquinolones.	Use in animals (and doses) is based on pharmacokinetic studies in experimental animals, experience in humans, or anecdotal experience in animals.	400 mg tablets.	22 mg/kg q12h PO.
Nystatin (Nilstat, many others)	Fungistatic and fungicidal agent topically used to treat candidiasis. Binds to sterols in the fungal cell membrane; prevents membrane's inability to function as a selective barrier, allowing loss of essential intracellular constituents.	May cause mild skin irritation. If swallowed, can cause GI tract upsets with vomiting, diarrhea.	Can use oral products (Nystatin Oral Suspension) to swab out mouth ulcers caused by candidiasis (e.g., dogs post parvovirus infections).	Multiple topical cream preparations in 15, 30, and 540 g sizes (100,000 U/g); oral suspension (100,000 U/g).	Apply topically q6–12h for 2 wk.
Orbifloxacin (Orbax)	Fluoroquinolone antimicrobial. Same mechanism as enrofloxacin and ciprofloxacin. Spectrum includes staphylococci, gram-negative bacilli, and some Pseudomonas spp.	Same precautions as enrofloxacin. May cause some nausea and vomiting at high doses. Avoid use in young animals. Blindness in cats has not been reported with doses ≤15 mg/kg/day.	Dose range is wide to account for susceptibility of bacteria. Most susceptible bacteria should be treated with low dose. More resistant bacteria, such as Pseudomonas, should be treated with high dose.	5.7, 22.7, and 68 mg tablets. Oral suspension: 30 mg/mg.	2.5–7.5 mg/kg q24h PO. Cats: 7.5 mg/kg q24h PO oral suspension.
Ormetoprim + sulfadimethoxine	Trimethoprim-like drug used in combination with sulfadimethoxine. (See Primor.)				

Oxacillin (Prostaphlin and generic)	β-lactam antibiotic. Inhibits bacterial cell wall synthesis. Spectrum is limited to gram-positive bacteria, especially staphylococci.	Use cautiously in animals allergic to penicillin-like drugs.	Doses based on empiricism or extrapolation from human studies. No clinical efficacy studies available for dogs or cats. Administer on empty stomach, if possible.	250, 500 mg capsules; 50 mg/ml oral solution.	22–40 mg/kg q8h PO.
Oxfendazole (Synanthic)	Benzimidazole anthelmintic for use in cattle and horses. Exclusively used in dogs to treat canine tracheal worm (Oslerus [Filaroides] osleri).	Good safety margin, but vomiting and diarrhea have been reported.	Available in the United States as a cattle deworming suspension (Synanthic). Oral LD$_{50}$ is 1.6 g/kg for dogs.	9.06 % (90.6 mg/ml) oral suspension.	10 mg/kg q24h PO for 28 days. Couple with physical removal of nodules from the trachea and bifurcation using endoscopy.
Oxymetholone (Anadrol)	Anabolic steroid derived from testosterone. Used to stimulate androgenic activity, increase weight gain and stimulate erythropoiesis.	Produces androgenic side effects. Liver damage is possible.	Use is based primarily on anecdotal experience.	50 mg tablets.	1–5 mg/kg q24h PO.
Oxytetracycline (Terramycin)	Tetracycine antibiotic. (See Tetracycline). Same mechanism and spectrum as tetracycline. Oxytetracycline may be absorbed to higher extent.	Generally safe. Use cautiously in young animals.	Oral dose forms are from large-animal use. Use of injectable long-acting forms has not been studied in small animals. For most indications, doxycycline or minicycline can be substituted.	250 mg tablets; 100, 200 mg/ml injection.	7.5–10 mg/kg IV q12h; 20 mg/kg q12h PO.

(Continued)

APPENDIX F: Drug Formulary (continued)

Drug Name (Trade or Other Names)	Pharmacology and Indications	Adverse Effects and Precautions	Dosing Information and Comments	Formulations	Dosage
Paromomycin (Humatin)	Aminoglycoside antibiotic with no absorption from the GI tract unless damaged. Activity against GI tract bacteria and Cryptosporidium spp.	Good safety margin in animals with intact GI tract. If absorbed (very young and patients showing blood in stool)—nephrotoxicity.	Careful assessment of patient is needed to determine if drug is likely to be absorbed from GI tract. Monitor for nephrotoxicity by examining urine for cast.	250 mg capsules.	125–165 mg/kg q12h PO for 5 days.
Penicillin G potassium; Penicillin G sodium (many brands)	β-Lactam antibiotic. Action is similar to that of other penicillins (see Amoxicillin). Spectrum of penicillin G is limited to gram-positive bacteria and anaerobes.	Injections may induce allergic reactions.	Penicillin G does not have good activity against most small animal pathogens.	5–20 million U vials.	20,000–40,000 U/kg q6–8h IV or IM.
Penicillin G procaine (generic)	Procaine penicillin is absorbed slowly, producing concentrations for 12–24 hr after injection.	IM and SC injections can produce injection-site reactions.	Avoid SC injection with procaine penicillin G.	300,000 U/mL suspension.	20,000–40,000 U/kg q12–24h IM.
Pentamidine isethionate (Lomidine, Pentam)	An aromatic diamidine; interferes with synthesis of DNA, RNA, proteins, and phospholipids, with activity against Pneumocystis spp.	After systemic administration: hypotension, systemic anaphylaxis, nausea, vomiting, diarrhea, hypoglycemia, myelosuppression, renal failure, hypocalcemia, hypokalemia.	Pretreat with antihistamines to avoid allergic reactions. IM use can cause pain at injection site. Use sterile water or 5% dextrose for reconstitution because other solutions cause precipitation.	Lomidine: 20 ml vials (40 mg/ml) for injection. Pentam: 300 mg vials of powder (reconstitute with sterile water or 5% dextrose).	Pneumocystis infection: 4 mg/kg IM q24h for 2 weeks.

Drug	Description	Precautions	Comment	Formulation	Dosage
Piperacillin (Pipracil)	β-Lactam antibiotic of the acylureidopenicillin class. Similar to other penicillins, except with high activity against Pseudomonas aeruginosa. Also good activity against streptococci.	Same precautions as for other injectable penicillins (e.g., ampicillin).	Reconstituted solution should be used within 24 hr (or 7 days if refrigerated). Piperacillin is combined with tazobactam (β-lactamase inhibitor) in Zosyn.	2, 3, 4, 40 g vials for injection.	40 mg/kg IV or IM q6h.
Piperazine (many)	Antiparasitic compound. Produces neuromuscular blockade in parasite through inhibition of neurotransmitter, which causes paralysis of worms. Used primarily for treatment of helminth (ascarid) infections.	Remarkably safe in all species.	Used to treat all species for roundworms.	860 mg powder; 140 mg capsules; 170, 340, and 800 mg/ml oral solution.	44–66 mg/kg PO, administered once.
Polymyxin B sulfate.	Broad spectrum antibiotic; distrupts bacterial cell membranes.	Renal injury possible. IM injection is painful.	Primarily used topically, but systemic use may be indicated for resistant infections.	500,000 U/vial for injection. 10,000 U = 1 mg.	Dogs and cats: 15,000 – 25,000 U/kg IV q12h. Monitor renal function.
Potassium iodide (SSKI, Pima Syrup, many other generic).	Antifungal (exact mechanism unknown) with activity against Sporothrix spp.	Relatively safe in dogs. Cats may develop signs of iodism—vomiting, anorexia, muscle twitching, cardiomyopathy. Contraindicated in hyperthyroidism, iodine hypersensitivity, renal failure, and pregnancy.	Concurrent use with potassium-containing medications may cause hyperkalemia. Can formulate own super saturated solution of KI by dissolving 1 g/ml in water.	Oral solutions: SSKI, many other generic (1 g/ml in 300 ml bottles). Pima Syrup (325 mg/5 ml).	Dogs: 40 mg/kg q8h PO for at least 30 days, usually 60 days. Cats: 20 mg/kg q12h PO for at least 30 days, usually 60 days.

(Continued)

APPENDIX F: Drug Formulary *(continued)*

Drug Name (Trade or Other Names)	Pharmacology and Indications	Adverse Effects and Precautions	Dosing Information and Comments	Formulations	Dosage
Praziquantel (Droncit)	Antiparasitic drug. Action on parasites related to neuromuscular toxicity and paralysis via altered permeability to calcium. Used primarily to treat infection caused by tapeworms.	Vomiting occurs at high doses. Anorexia and transient diarrhea have been reported. Safe in pregnant animals.	Dose recommendations based on label dose supplied by manufacturer.	23, 34 mg tablet; 56.8 mg/ml injection	Dog: Oral dose—6.8 kg: 7.5 mg/kg PO, once; .6.8 kg: 5 mg/kg PO, once. Injection—≤2.3 kg: 7.5 mg/kg IM or SC, once; 2.7–4.5 kg: 6.3 mg/kg IM or SC, once; ≤5 kg: 5 mg/kg IM or SC, once. Cat: Oral dose—1.8 kg: 6.3 mg/kg PO, once; 1.8 kg: 5 mg/kg PO, once. Paragonimus infection: 25 mg/kg q8h PO for 2–3 days. Injection: 5 mg/kg IM or SC.
Primaquine phosphate	Antiprotozoal agent that binds DNA and alters mitrocondria with activity against Babesia spp.	Methemoglobinemia, hemolysis, myelosuppression. Contraindicated when concurrent hemolysis or bone marrow suppression, or when other myelosuppressive drugs are used.	Check CBC once weekly while treating (monitor for myelosuppression). Give with food to avoid GI side effects.	26.3 mg (15 mg active base) tablets.	Babesia infection: 0.3 mg/kg q24h PO for 14 days.

Drug	Mechanism	Adverse effects	Notes	Formulation	Dose
Primor (ormetoprim + sulfadimethoxine) (Primor)	Antibacterial drug. Ormetoprim inhibits bacterial dihydrofolate reductase, sulfonamide competes with p-aminobenzoic acid (PABA) for synthesis of nucleic acids. Bactericidal/bacteriostatic. Broad antibacterial spectrum and active against some coccidia.	Several adverse effects have been reported from sulfonamides. No adverse effects reported from ormetoprim.	Doses listed are based on manufacturer's recommendations. Controlled trials have demonstrated efficacy for treatment of pyoderma on once-daily schedule.	Combination tablet (ormetoprim + sulfadimethoxine). 120, 240, 600, and 1200 mg tablets in 1:5 ratio.	Dogs: 55 mg/kg, PO, on first day, then 27.5 mg/kg q24h PO. Daily doses can be divided BID.
Pyrantel pamoate (Nemex, Strongid)	Antiparasitic drug. Acts to block ganglionic neurotransmission via cholinergic action.	No adverse effects reported.	Dose recommendations based on manufacturer's recommendations.	180 mg/ml paste; 50 mg/ml suspension. Also combined with praziquantel.	Dog: 5 mg/kg once PO and repeat in 7–10 days. Cat: 20 mg/kg once PO.
Pyrimethamine (Daraprim)	Antibacterial, antiprotozoal drug. Blocks dihydrofolate reductase enzyme, which inhibits synthesis of reduced folate and nucleic acids. Activity of pyrimethamine is more specific against protozoa than bacteria.	When administered with trimethoprim-sulfonamide combinations, anemia has been observed. Folic or folinic acid has been supplemented to prevent anemia, but benefit of this treatment is unclear.	Used either alone or in combination with sulfonamides.	25 mg tablets.	Dog: 1 mg/kg q24h PO for 14–21 days (5 days for Neosporum caninum). Cat: 0.5–1 mg/kg q24h PO for 14–28 days.

(Continued)

APPENDIX F: Drug Formulary (*continued*)

Drug Name (Trade or Other Names)	Pharmacology and Indications	Adverse Effects and Precautions	Dosing Information and Comments	Formulations	Dosage
Ranitidine (Zantac)	Histamine H_2-antagonist. See Cimetidine for details. Same as cimetidine except 4–10× more potent and longer acting.	See Cimetidine. Ranitidine may have fewer effects on endocrine function and drug interactions, compared to cimetidine.	See Cimetidine. Pharmacokinetic information in dogs suggests that ranitidine may be administered less often than cimetidine to achieve continuous suppression of stomach acid secretion. Ranitidine may stimulate stomach emptying and colon motility via anticholinesterase action.	75, 150, 300 mg tablets; 150, 300 mg capsules; 25 mg/ml injection.	Dog: 2 mg/kg q8h IV, PO. Cat: 2.5 mg/kg q12h IV; 3.5 mg/kg q12h PO.
Rifampin (Rifadin)	Antibacterial. Action is to inhibit bacterial RNA synthesis. Spectrum of action includes staphylococci and mycobacteria. Other susceptible bacteria include streptococci. Used in humans primarily for treatment of tuberculosis.In dogs, used to treat Staphylococcus including methiciline resistant strains.	Adverse effects not reported in animals, but in humans, hypersensitivity and flulike symptoms are reported. Drug interactions: Multiple drug interactions are possible. Induces cytochrome P-450 enzymes. Drugs affected include Transient barbiturates, chloramphenicol, and corticosteroids.	Results of clinical studies in animals have not been reported. Use in animals (and doses) is based on experience in humans or anecdotal experience in animals. Rifampin is highly lipid soluble and has been used to treat intracellular infections. Administer on an empty stomach.	150, 300 mg capsules; injection solution: 600 mg Rifadin IV.	5 mg/kg q12h PO, or 10 mg/kg q24h PO.

Drug				
Ronidazole	Antiprotozoan drug. Mechanism of action similar to other nitromidazoles (metronidazole). Used to treat enteric tritrichomoniasis in cats.	Neurotoxicity at high doses.	Do no exceed 60 mg/kg/day in cat to avoid neurotoxicity. Doses based on experimental studies.	No commercial formulations but compounding pharmacies will formulate compounds for cats.	30 mg/kg q12h PO for 2 weeks. Once daily treatment may also be effective.
Selamectin (Revolution)	Topical parasiticide and heartworm prevention.	Transient localized alopecia with or without inflammation at or near the site of application was observed in approximately 1% of 691 treated cats. Other signs observed rarely included GI signs, anorexia, lethargy, salivation, tachypnea, and muscle tremors.	Recommended for use in dogs 6 wk of age or older and in cats 8 wk of age or older.	Available in six separate dose strengths.	The recommended minimum dose is 6 mg/kg topically; see insert.
Sodium stibogluconate (Pentostam)	Antiprotozoal pentavalent antimonial agent that interferes with energy metabolism in Leishmania spp.	Muscle pain at injection site, pancreatitis, myocardial injury, hemolytic anemia, leukopenia, vomiting, diarrhea, cardiac arrhythmias, renal dysfunction, shock, sudden death, thrombophlebitis (if given IV), elevated ALT.	May not always be available in the United States—contact CDC. Resistance to drug may develop during treatment. Use with allopurinol.	100 ml multidose vials (100 mg/ml).	30–50 mg/kg q24h SC or IV for 30 days. More effective if combined with oral allopurinol.

(Continued)

APPENDIX F: Drug Formulary (*continued*)

Drug Name (Trade or Other Names)	Pharmacology and Indications	Adverse Effects and Precautions	Dosing Information and Comments	Formulations	Dosage
Spinosub (Comfortis).	Oral antiparasitic drug used for flea control. Kills fleas rapidly after administration.	Occasional vomiting after administration.	Administer with food.	140, 270, 560, 810, and 1620 mg tablets.	Dog: 30 mg/kg PO once per month. No dose established for cats.
Sulfadiazine (generic, combined with trimethoprim in Tribrissen)	Sulfonamides compete with PABA for enzyme that synthesizes dihydrofolic acid in bacteria. Synergistic with trimethoprim. Broad spectrum of activity, including some protozoa. Bacteriostatic.	Adverse effects associated with sulfonamides include allergic reactions, type II and III hypersensitivity, hypothyroidism (with prolonged therapy), keratoconjunctivitis sicca, and skin reactions.	Usually, sulfonamides are combined with trimethoprim or ormetoprim in 5:1 ratio. There is no clinical evidence that one sulfonamide is more or less toxic or efficacious than another.	500 mg tablets.	100 mg/kg PO (loading dose), followed by 50 mg/kg q12h PO.
Sulfadimethoxine (Albon, Bactrovet, and generic)	See Sulfadiazine.	See Sulfadiazine.	See Sulfadiazine. Sulfadimethoxine is combined with ormetoprim in Primor.	125, 250, 500 mg tablets; 400 mg/ml injection; 50 mg/ml suspension.	55 mg/kg PO (loading dose), followed by 27.5 mg/kg q12h PO.
Sulfamethazine (many brands [e.g., Sulmet])	See Sulfadiazine.	See Sulfadiazine.	See Sulfadiazine.	30 g bolus.	100 mg/kg PO (loading dose), followed by 50 mg/kg q12h PO.

(*Continued*)

Drug	Description/Mechanism	Adverse Effects	Comments	Supplied	Dosage
Sulfamethoxazole (Gantanol)	See Sulfadiazine.		See Sulfadiazine.	500 mg tablets.	100 mg/kg IV, PO (loading dose), followed by 50 mg/kg q12h IV, PO.
Sulfisoxazole (Gantrisin)	See Sulfadiazine. Sulfisoxizole is primarily used only for treating urinary tract infections.		See Sulfadiazine.	500 mg tablets; 500 mg/5 ml syrup.	50 mg/kg q8h PO (urinary tract infections).
Terbinafine (Lamisil)	Fungicidal agent that interferes with ergosterol biosynthesis by inhibiting squalene epoxidase in the fungal cell membrane.	High margin of safety. May cause GI tract disturbances (vomiting, diarrhea). Hepatic failure, pancytopenia, toxic epidermal necrolysis reported in humans.	Used for the systemic treatment of pythiosis and cryptococcosis.	125, 250 mg tablets. 1% topical solution and cream.	Dogs: 30–40 mg/kg PO with food for 3 weeks. Cats: 30–40 mg/kg q24h PO for at least 2 weeks.
Tetracycline (Panmycin)	Tetracycline antibiotic. Mechanism of action of tetracyclines is to bind to 30S ribosomal subunit and inhibit protein synthesis. Usually bacteriostatic. Broad spectrum of activity, including bacteria, some protozoa, Rickettsia spp., and Ehrlichia spp.	Tetracyclines can affect bone and teeth formation in young animals. Tetracyclines have been implicated in drug fever in cats. Hepatotoxicity may occur at high doses in susceptible individuals. Drug interactions: Tetracyclines bind to calcium-containing compounds, which decreases oral absorption.	Pharmacokinetic and experimental studies have been conducted in small animals, but no clinical studies. Do not use outdated solutions. Doxycycline can be substituted in most cases.	250, 500 mg capsules; 100 mg/ml suspension.	15–20 mg/kg q8h PO; or 4.4–11 mg/kg q8h IV, IM.
Tetramizole hydrochloride (Nilverm)	A broad-spectrum imidazothiazole anthelmintic. Mechanism of action is neuromuscular toxicity to parasites. In humans, used as an immunostimulant to aid in the treatment of colorectal carcinoma.	Similar side effects of levamisole (potentiates cholinergic toxicity). May cause vomiting.	Rarely used in small animals. Still recommended for treatment of Ollulanus infections in cats. Available in Australia and New Zealand as a cattle and sheep drench (Nilverm).	Nilverm Oral drench: 32 g/L.	5 mg/kg PO once administer as a 2.5% (25 mg/ml) solution.

(Continued)

APPENDIX F: Drug Formulary (continued)

Drug Name (Trade or Other Names)	Pharmacology and Indications	Adverse Effects and Precautions	Dosing Information and Comments	Formulations	Dosage
Thenium diosylate (Canopar)	Antiparasitic drug used to treat hookworms.	Tablet is bitter if coating is broken. May cause vomiting.	Doses are based on manufacturer recommendations.	500 mg tablets.	Dogs > 4.5 kg: 500 mg PO once; repeat in 2–3 weeks. Dogs between 2.5 and 4.5 kg: 250 mg PO, q12h for 1 day, repeated in 2–3 weeks.
Thiabendazole (Omnizole, Equizole)	Benzimidazole anthelmintic. (See Fenbendazole, Albendazole.)	Adverse effects uncommon. Can cause graying of hair at high doses.	Ordinarily administered to horses and cattle. Experience in small animals is limited.	2 or 4 g per oz (30 ml) suspension or liquid.	Dog: 50 mg/kg q24h for 3 days, repeat in 1 month. Respiratory parasites: 30–70 mg/kg q12h PO Cat: Strongloides spp.: 125 mg/kg q24h for 3 days.
Ticarcillin (Ticar, Ticillin)	Beta-Lactam antibiotic. Action similar to ampicillin/amoxicillin. Spectrum similar to that of carbenicillin. Ticarcillin is primarily used for gram-negative infections, especially those caused by Pseudomonas spp.	Adverse effects are uncommon. However, allergic reactions are possible. High doses can produce seizures and decreased platelet function. Drug interactions: Do not combine in same syringe or in vial with aminoglycosides.	Ticarcillin is synergistic and often combined with aminoglycosides (e.g., amikacin, gentamicin). 1% lidocaine may be used for reconstitution to decrease pain from IM injection.	6 g/50 ml vial; vials containing 1, 3, 6, 20, and 30 g.	33–50 mg/kg q4–6h IV, IM.
Ticarcillin + clavulanate (Timentin)	Same as ticarcillin, except clavulanic acid has been added to inhibit bacterial b-lactamase and increase spectrum. Clavulanate does not increase activity against Pseudomonas spp., however.	Same as for ticarcillin.	Same as for ticarcillin.	3 g per vial for injection.	Dose according to rate for ticarcillin.

Drug	Description	Adverse effects	Dosing notes	Formulations	Dosage
Tinidazole (Tindamax)	Antiprotozoal drug similar to metronidazole but considered to be 2nd generation. Used to treat tritrichomoniasis and giardiasis.	Like metronidazole, high doses can cause neurotoxicity	Dosing in dogs and cats is mainly based on anecdotal information or extrapolated from human medicine.	250 and 500 mg tablets.	Dog: 15 mg/kg PO q12h. Cat: 15 mg/kg PO q24h.
Tobramycin (Nebcin)	Aminoglycoside antibacterial drug. Similar mechanism of action and spectrum as amikacin and gentamicin.	Adverse effects similar to those of amikacin, gentamicin.	Dosing requirements vary depending on bacterial susceptibility. See dose schedules for gentamicin and amikacin.	40 mg/ml injection.	Dog 9–14 mg/kg q24h IV, IM, SC. Cat 5–8 mg/kg q24h, IV, IM, SC.
Trimethoprim + sulfadiazine (Tribrissen, Tucoprim, and others)	Combines the antibacterial drug action of trimethoprim and a sulfonamide. Together, the combination is synergistic, with a broad spectrum of activity.	Adverse effects primarily caused by sulfonamide component. (See Sulfadiazine.)	Dosage recommendations vary. There is evidence that 30 mg/kg/day is efficacious for pyoderma; for other infections, 30 mg/kg twice daily has been recommended.	30, 120, 240, 480, 960 mg tablet (all formulations have ratio of 5:1 sulfa:trimethoprim).	15 mg/kg q12h PO or 30 mg/kg q12–24h PO. Toxoplasma: 30 mg/kg q12h PO.
Trimethoprim + sulfamethoxazole (Bactrim, Septra, and generic forms)	Combines the antibacterial drug action of trimethoprim and a sulfonamide. Together, the combination is synergistic, with a broad spectrum of activity.	Adverse effects primarily caused by sulfonamide component. (See Sulfadiazine.)	Dosage recommendations vary. There is evidence that 30 mg/kg/day is efficacious for pyoderma; for other infections, 30 mg/kg twice daily has been recommended.	480, 960 mg tablet; 240 mg/5 ml oral suspension (all formulations have ratio of 5:1 sulfa:trimethoprim).	15 mg/kg q12h PO or 30 mg/kg q12–24h PO.
Tylosin (Tylocine, Tylan, Tylosin tartrate)	Macrolide antibiotic. (See Erythromycin for mechanisms of action and spectrum of activity.)	May cause diarrhea in some animals. Do not administer orally to rodents or rabbits.	Tylosin is rarely used in small animals. Powdered formulation (tylosin tartrate) has been administered on food for control of signs of colitis in dogs. Tablets are approved in Canada for treatment of colitis.	Available as soluble powder 2.2 tylosin per tsp (tablets for dogs in Canada)	Dog and cat: 7–15 mg/kg q12–24h PO. Dog (for colitis): 10–20 mg/kg q8h with food; if there is a response, increase the interval to q12–24h

(Continued)

APPENDIX F: Drug Formulary (continued)

Drug Name (Trade or Other Names)	Pharmacology and Indications	Adverse Effects and Precautions	Dosing Information and Comments	Formulations	Dosage
Vancomycin (Vancocin, Vancoled)	Antibacterial drug. Mechanism of action is to inhibit cell wall and cause bacterial cell lysis (via mechanism different from that of b-lactams). Spectrum includes staphylococci, streptococci, and enterococci (but not gram-negative bacteria). Used primarily for treatment of resistant staphylococci and enterococci including methiciline-resistant strains.	Adverse effects have not been reported in animals. Administer IV; causes severe pain and tissue injury if administered IM or SC. Do not administer IM or SC. Do not administer rapidly; use slow infusion, if possible (e.g., over 30 min). Adverse effects in humans include renal injury (more common with older products that contained impurities) and histamine release.	Vancomycin use is not common in animals, but is valuable for treatment of enterococci or staphylococci that are resistant to other antibiotics. Doses are derived from pharmacokinetic studies in dogs. Monitoring of trough plasma concentrations is recommended to ensure proper dose. Maintain trough concentration above 5 mcg/ml. Infusion solution can be prepared in 0.9% saline or 5% dextrose, but not alkalinizing solutions.	Vials for injection (0.5 to 10 g).	Dog: 15 mg/kg q6–8h IV infusion. Cat: 12–15 mg/kg q8h IV Infusion.
Voriconazole (Vfend)	Azole (triazole) antifungal agent. Action is similar to other antifungal azole drugs which inhibit ergosterol synthesis. Active against systemic fungi, dermatophytes, and aspergillosis.	Well tolerated by dogs but is associated with neurotoxicity in cats. May cause drug interations by inhibiting cytochrome P450 enzymes.	Clinical use is based on limited clinical experience, anecdotal use, and extrapolation from human medicine.	50 and 200 mg tablets. 10 mg/ml injectable solution.	Dogs: 4.5 mg/kg q12h PO. Cats: Safe dose has NOT been established.

Abbreviations: ALT, alanine aminotransferase; CDC, Centers for Disease Control and Prevention; CNS, central nervous system; CSF, cerebrospinal fluid; DNA, deoxyribonucleic acid; GABA, g-aminobutyric acid; GI, gastrointestinal; IM, intramuscular; IV, intravenous; MIC, minimum inhibitory concentration; PO, per os (oral), PU/PD, polyuria/polydipsia; q, every, as in q8h 5 every 8 hours; SC, subcutaneous; U, units.

Disclaimer for Dose Tables: Doses listed are for dogs *and* cats, unless otherwise listed. Many of the doses listed are extra-label or are human drugs not approved for animals administered in an extra-label manner. Doses listed are based on best available information at the time of table editing. The author cannot ensure efficacy or absolute safety of drugs used according to recommendations in this table. Adverse effects may be possible from drugs listed in this table of which authors were not aware at the time of table preparation. Veterinarians using this table are encouraged to consult current literature, product labels and inserts, and the manufacturer's disclosure information for additional information on adverse effects, interactions, and efficacy that were not identified at the time these tables were prepared.

Index

cyclophosphamide
  feline foamy virus infection, 221
  feline infectious peritonitis, 240
cyproheptadine, FIV, 232
Cytauxzoon felis, 177, 178*f*
cytauxzoonosis
  clinical features, 177–178
  defined, 177
  diagnostics, 178–179, 178*f*, 179*f*
  differential diagnosis, 178
  etiology, pathophysiology, 177
  signalment, history, 177
  therapeutics, 179–180, 180*f*
  vs. babesiosis, 35
  vs. hemotropic mycoplasmosis, 290
  vs. plague, 402
cythioate
  Chagas disease, 128
  fleas, 261

dapsone
  mycobacterial infections, 365–367
  Rhinosporidium infection, 442
decoquinate, hepatozoonosis, 299
Demodex spp, 181, 182*f*
demodicosis
  clinical features, 183–185, 183*f*, 184*f*
  defined, 181
  diagnostics, 185
  differential diagnosis, 185
  etiology, pathophysiology, 181–182, 182*f*
  signalment, history, 182–183
  therapeutics, 185–188
  vs. dermatophytosis, 195–196
  vs. sporotrichosis, 485
Dermacentor andersoni, 517, 520. *see also* ticks, tick control
Dermacentor variabilis, 177, 517, 520, 522. *see also* ticks, tick control
dermatophilosis
  clinical features, 189–190
  defined, 189
  diagnostics, 190–191
  differential diagnosis, 190
  etiology, pathophysiology, 189
  prognosis, 191–192
  signalment, history, 189
  therapeutics, 191
Dermatophilus congolensis, 189
dermatophytosis: keratinophilic mycosis
  client education, 199
  clinical signs, 194, 195*f*
  defined, 193
  diagnostics, 196–197
  differential diagnosis, 194–195
  etiology, pathophysiology, 193
  signalment, 193–194, 194*f*

  therapeutics, 197–199
dewormer, hookworms, 312–313
diarrhea
  amebiasis, 4–5
  astrovirus infection, 29–30
  balantidiasis, 40–41
  clostridial enterotoxicosis, 139–140
  coccidiosis, 152
  cryptosporidiosis, 168
  giardiasis, 264
  Helicobacter infection, 283–284
  histoplasmosis, 303
  reovirus infection, 433–434
  rotavirus infection, 450–451
  roundworm, 456
  salmonellosis, 463
  salmon poisoning, 469
  strongyloides, 501–502
  whipworms, 557
diazepam, FIV, 232
dichlorophene, roundworms, 458–459
dichlorvos
  hookworms, 312–313
  roundworms, 458–460
diclazuril, coccidiosis, 154–155
diethylcarbamazine
  heartworm disease, dogs, 281
  roundworms, 458–459
  whipworms, 558–559
dihydrostreptomycin, mycobacterial infections, 365–367
diminazene acetate, cytauxzoonosis, 179–180
Diminazine aceturate, babesiosis, 37–38
dinotefuran, flea control, 260, 509
Dioctyophyma renale, 325, 327*f. see also* kidney worm
Dipetalonema reconditum, 537
Dipylidium caninum, 260, 505–506, 507*f. see also* fleas, flea control
Dirofilaria immitis, 270, 275, 277*f. see also* heartworm disease, cats; heartworm disease, dogs
  urinary capillariasis complications, 555
  vs. Angiostrongylus infection, 12
  vs. blastomycosis, 53
  vs. canine lungworm, 102, 107
  vs. canine tracheal worm, 118
  vs. histoplasmosis, 303
  vs. infectious canine tracheobronchitis, 321
  vs. lung fluke infection, 349
  vs. pneumocystosis, 406
  vs. respiratory capillariasis, 437
  vs. *Trichinella,* 537
diskospondylitis
  vs. aspergillosis, systemic, 24
  vs. brucellosis, 69–70, 70*f*
  vs. hepatozoonosis, 296
disseminated nocardiosis, 391. *see also* nocardiosis